Primary Care

America's Health in a New Era

Molla S. Donaldson, Karl D. Yordy, Kathleen N. Lohr, and
Neal A. Vanselow, *Editors*

Committee on the Future of Primary Care

Division of Health Care Services

INSTITUTE OF MEDICINE

NATIONAL ACADEMY PRESS
Washington, D.C. 1996

NATIONAL ACADEMY PRESS • 2101 Constitution Avenue, NW • Washington, DC 20418

NOTICE: The project that is the subject of this report was approved by the Governing Board of the National Research Council, whose members are drawn from the councils of the National Academy of Sciences, the National Academy of Engineering, and the Institute of Medicine. The members of the committee responsible for this report were chosen for their special competencies and with regard for appropriate balance.

This report has been reviewed by a group other than the authors according to procedures approved by a Report Review Committee consisting of members of the National Academy of Sciences, the National Academy of Engineering, and the Institute of Medicine.

The Institute of Medicine was chartered in 1970 by the National Academy of Sciences to enlist distinguished members of the appropriate professions in the examination of policy matters pertaining to the health of the public. In this, the Institute acts under both the Academy's 1863 congressional charter responsibility to be an adviser to the federal government and its own initiative in identifying issues of medical care, research, and education. Dr. Kenneth I. Shine is president of the Institute of Medicine.

See the Acknowledgments for a complete listing of the organizations that provided support for this study.

The stand-alone Summary is available in limited quantities from the Institute of Medicine, Division of Health Care Services, 2101 Constitution Avenue, NW, Washington, DC 20418. It is available on-line at **http://www.nap.edu/nap/online**.

The complete volume of *Primary Care: America's Health in a New Era* is available for sale from the National Academy Press, 2101 Constitution Avenue, NW, Lock Box 285, Washington, DC 20055. Call 1-800-624-6242 or 202-334-3313 (in the Washington metropolitan area).

Library of Congress Cataloging-in-Publication Data

Institute of Medicine (U.S.). Division of Health Care Services
    Committee on the Future of Primary Care.
      Primary care : America's health in a new era / Molla S. Donaldson
    . . . [et al.], editors ; Committee on the Future of Primary Care
    Services, Division of Health Care Services, Institute of Medicine.
      p. cm
      Includes bibliographical references and index.
      ISBN 0-309-05399-4
      1. Primary health care—United States. I. Donaldson, Molla S.
    II. Title.
      [DNLM: 1. Primary Health Care—United States. W 84.6 I587p 1996]
    RA427.9.I56   1996
    362.1′0973—dc20
    DNLM/DLC   96-25823
for Library of Congress   CIP

The serpent has been a symbol of long life, healing, and knowledge among almost all cultures and religions since the beginning of recorded history. The image adopted as a logotype by the Institute of Medicine is based on a relief carving from ancient Greece, now held by the Staatlichemuseen in Berlin.

COMMITTEE ON THE FUTURE OF PRIMARY CARE

NEAL A. VANSELOW, *Chair*,* Professor of Medicine and Adjunct Professor, Department of Health Systems Management, School of Public Health and Tropical Medicine, Tulane University Medical Center, New Orleans, Louisiana

JOEL J. ALPERT,* Professor of Pediatrics and Public Health (Health Law), Department of Pediatrics, Boston University School of Medicine, Boston, Massachusetts

CHERYL Y. BOYKINS, Director, National Black Women's Health Project, Atlanta, Georgia

cAROLYN V. BROWN, Private practice, Burlington, Vermont

KEN CAMERON, Chairman of the Board, Group Health Cooperative of Puget Sound, Seattle, Washington

PETE T. DUARTE, Chief Executive Officer, Thomason Hospital, El Paso, Texas

PETER ELLSWORTH, President and CEO, Sharp HealthCare, San Diego, California

RAYMOND S. GARRISON, JR., Associate Professor and Chairman, Department of Dentistry, Bowman Gray School of Medicine, Winston-Salem, North Carolina

LARRY A. GREEN,* Professor and Woodward-Chisholm Chairman of Family Medicine, University of Colorado Health Sciences Center, Denver

PAUL F. GRINER,* Vice President and Director, Center for the Assessment and Management of Change in Academic Medicine, Association of American Medical Colleges, Washington, D.C.

JEAN JOHNSON, Associate Dean, Health Sciences Programs, The George Washington University Medical Center, Washington, D.C.

P. EUGENE JONES, Associate Professor and Director, Physician Assistant Program, Department of Health Care Sciences, University of Texas Southwestern Medical Center at Dallas

HENK LAMBERTS,* Professor of Family Medicine, Academic Medical Centre, University of Amsterdam, The Netherlands

PAUL W. NANNIS, Commissioner of Health, City of Milwaukee Health Department, Milwaukee, Wisconsin

R. HEATHER PALMER, Director, Center for Quality of Care Research and Education, Harvard School of Public Health, Boston, Massachusetts

BARBARA ROSS-LEE, Dean, College of Osteopathic Medicine, Ohio University, Athens

---

*Institute of Medicine member.

iii

SHEILA A. RYAN,* Dean, School of Nursing, Director, Medical Center Nursing, University of Rochester, Rochester, New York

RICHARD M. SCHEFFLER, Professor, Health Economics and Public Policy, School of Public Health, University of California at Berkeley

WILLIAM L. WINTERS, JR., Clinical Professor of Medicine, Baylor College of Medicine, Houston, Texas

Study Staff

KATHLEEN N. LOHR, Director, Division of Health Care Services

KARL D. YORDY, Study Co-Director

MOLLA S. DONALDSON, Study Co-Director

LISA M. CHIMENTO, Program Officer (until July 1994)

ROBIN L. RIVKIND, Research Associate (until September 1995)

DIANE PRESCOTT, Research Assistant (as of September 1995)

HELEN C. ROGERS, Project Assistant (until January 1995)

ANITA M. ZIMBRICK, Project Assistant (as of January 1995)

H. DONALD TILLER, Administrative Assistant

Preface

After decades of relative neglect in a health care system that placed most of its emphasis on specialization, high technology, and acute care medicine, the value of primary care is again being recognized as part of the wave of reform that is sweeping the U.S. health care industry. There are numerous indications of the increasingly important role being played by primary care. Health care reform proposals developed by both the federal government and several state governments have included measures to strengthen the delivery of primary care. More important in view of current trends has been the emphasis that market forces have placed on a vigorous primary care system. A further indication of the current level of interest has been the number and variety of public and private sponsors of this Institute of Medicine (IOM) study of the future of primary care.

The current IOM study can be divided into two phases. During the first phase the study committee, which included members with diverse backgrounds and interests, agreed upon a number of underlying principles related to primary care and also reviewed and updated the definition of primary care that had been developed by the IOM in 1978. The underlying principles are listed in Chapter 1 of this report. Of particular importance is the committee's consensus that primary care represents the logical foundation for the U.S. health care system of the future.

The revised definition of primary care was published in a September 1994 preliminary report and is also contained in Chapter 2 of this final report. It takes into consideration the numerous changes in health care that have occurred in the nearly two decades since the original IOM definition was published. It would be impossible to overemphasize the importance the committee attached to the new definition. Committee members continually referred to it when formulating recommendations on issues such as who is a primary care clinician, what should be the content of education and training programs in primary care, and what items should be included in the research agenda for primary care.

The second phase, which occupied the final 18 months of the study, involved visits to urban and rural primary care delivery sites, a public hearing, the preparation and review of several commissioned papers, and two workshops. It included an examination of topics such as the nature and content of primary care and the value of primary care to both individual patients and to the health care system as a whole. Also considered were the delivery of primary care, the needs of the primary care workforce, education and training in primary care, and primary care research requirements. Finally, the committee recognized that additional steps will be needed to implement the 31 recommendations contained in this report and therefore developed the implementation strategy outlined in Chapter 9.

The committee wishes to acknowledge the superb support it received from the IOM staff. Study Co-directors Karl Yordy and Molla Donaldson, and Kathleen Lohr, Director of the IOM Division of Health Care Services, all played major roles in gathering data, helping to define the issues, and writing the report. The committee was impressed with both their knowledge and their professionalism. Other IOM personnel who provided valuable assistance were Lisa Chimento, Robin Rivkind, Diane Prescott, Helen Rogers, Anita Zimbrick, and Don Tiller.

Although it is impossible to predict what the U.S. health care system will look like when the current pace of rapid change ends and a period of relative stability is reached, the committee is confident that primary care will remain an essential component of efforts to improve the quality of care, increase access to health care, and control health care costs. It hopes that this report will both convey the value, complexity, and richness of primary care and catalyze concrete steps to strengthen this crucial part of the delivery system.

Neal A. Vanselow, M.D.
Chair

Acknowledgments

The Committee on the Future of Primary Care is appreciative of the assistance it and the study staff received from many individuals and organizations during its site visits. All were gracious in offering their time and insights regarding the direction of primary care. The committee also made much use of the written statements and testimony given at a public hearing held by the committee in December 1994. These testimonies provided thoughtful reactions to the committee's interim report and information about current and planned primary care activities.

The committee benefited from thoughtful presentations by several experts invited to its meetings. At its first meeting, in March 1994, the committee heard from John M. Eisenberg, M.D., Chairman and Physician-in-Chief of the Department of Medicine at Georgetown University and Chairman of the Physician Payment Review Commission. Guest speakers at its second meeting, in May 1994, were Susan Schooley, M.D., Chair, Department of Family Practice, Henry Ford Health System; Patricia Simmons, M.D., Associate Professor, Department of Pediatrics and Adolescent Medicine, and Member, Board of Governors, Mayo Clinic and Foundation; and Jack M. Colwill, M.D., Professor and Chairman, Department of Family and Community Medicine, University of Missouri–Columbia, and Member, Council on Graduate Medical Education (COGME).

At its July 1994 meeting the committee heard a presentation by Dana Gelb Safran, Sc.D., Senior Policy Analyst, Division of Health Improvement, The Health Institute, New England Medical Center. She and the committee engaged in a lively discussion about a background paper she wrote for the committee on defining primary care. Material in that paper was derived in part from a consensus conference convened in May 1994 by Dr. Safran and Dr. Alvin Tarlov of The Health Institute.

Fitzhugh Mullan, M.D., Director, Bureau of the Health Professions, Health Resources and Services Administration (U.S. Public Health Service) gave a presentation on the changing primary care workforce at its June 1995 workshop on roles in primary care. Drs. Kerr White and Barbara Starfield were extraordinarily helpful to the committee in responding to requests for information and generous with ideas about primary care based on their long experience in this field. Joyce Fitzpatrick, while the Distinguished Nurse-Scholar-in-Residence at the IOM, provided very helpful material to the committee on interdisciplinary education and practice.

The committee would like particularly to acknowledge the help of several organizations and individuals who provided data and conducted analyses for the committee: Carolyn Clancy, M.D., Agency for Health Care Policy and Research (USPHS); Paul A. Nutting, M.D., Ambulatory Sentinel Practice Network; Robert Larsen, M.D., FHP International, Inc.; Pauline Nefcy and Sarmad Pirzada of the Group Health Cooperative of Puget Sound; William Rush, Ph.D., and Leif I. Solberg, M.D., the Group Health Foundation; David Nerenz, Ph.D., the Henry Ford Health System; Merwyn R. Greenlick, Ph.D., and Nancy Clarke, the Kaiser Permanente Center for Health Research; Les Zendle, M.D., the Southern California Permanente Medical Group; Kathy Martin of Sharp HealthCare; Marcia J. Wilson of Sharp Rees-Stealy Medical Center, Inc.; and Peter Franks, M.D., University of Rochester/Highland Park Hospital.

Major funding for this study was received from the following: Department of Veterans Affairs, The Josiah Macy, Jr., Foundation, The Pew Charitable Trusts, The Robert Wood Johnson Foundation, and the U.S. Public Health Service, the Agency for Health Care Policy and Research and the Health Resources and Services Administration (HRSA). HRSA provided additional funding for a workshop on the scientific basis of primary care held in January 1995. The committee and staff are appreciative of the help provided by the contract officers whose organizations sponsored the study.

Additional funding for special study activities was received from Blue Cross of California, the Irvine Health Foundation, and the Pew Health Professions Commission for support of a constructive and informative workshop on roles in primary care that was held in Irvine, California, in June 1995. Funding for the committee's very useful and illuminating site visits was provided by the W.K. Kellogg Foundation.

Additional funding was received from a large set of organizations. Many of these organizations also provided helpful materials and data in response to our numerous questions. These sponsors are the Ambulatory Pediatric Association, American Academy of Family Physicians, American Academy of Pediatrics, American Academy of Physician Assistants, American Association of Colleges of Nursing, American Association of Colleges of Osteopathic Medicine, American Association of Dental Schools, American College of Osteopathic Family Physicians, American College of Physicians, American Geriatrics Society, American Medical Informatics Association, American Nurses Association, American Optometric Association, American Osteopathic Association, American Physical Therapy Association, and the Society of General Internal Medicine.

Finally, the committee would like to express its gratitude to the IOM staff who facilitated the work of the committee. We are grateful for the secretarial and logistical support provided by Helen Rogers and Anita Zimbrick, to H. Donald Tiller, Administrative Assistant to the Division, and for the assistance during the report review and preparation stage of Claudia Carl and Michael Edington of the IOM's Reports and Information Office; the steady help of Nina Spruill, Financial Associate for the Division of Health Care Services, is also greatly appreciated.

Contents

SUMMARY   1
  Definition of Primary Care, 2
  Value of Primary Care, 3
  The Nature of Primary Care, 3
  The Delivery of Primary Care, 4
  The Primary Care Workforce, 4
  Education and Training for Primary Care, 5
  Research and Evaluation in Primary Care, 6
  A Strategy for Implementation, 6

1 INTRODUCTION   13
  The Institute of Medicine Study, 15
  Underlying Assumptions, 18
  Historic Roots and the Contemporary Context for Primary Care, 19
  Organization of the Report, 25
  References, 25

2 DEFINING PRIMARY CARE   27
  Early Definitions, 28
  The First IOM Definition, 29
  Distinguishing Public and Personal Health Services, 29
  The 1984 Report on Community-Oriented Primary Care, 30
  Changes in Health Care Delivery Today, 31
  The New Definition and an Explanation of Terms, 31
  Achieving the Goals of Primary Care as Defined, 50
  References, 50

3 THE VALUE OF PRIMARY CARE   52
   The Value of Primary Care for Individuals, 53
   Primary Care and Costs, Access, and Quality, 62
   The Limits of Primary Care in Improving Population Health, 71
   Summary, 72
   References, 72

4 THE NATURE OF PRIMARY CARE   76
   Content of Primary Care, 77
   Characteristics of Primary Care, 80
   Summary, 88
   Appendix: Data on the Majority of Personal Health Care Needs, 89
   References, 102

5 THE DELIVERY OF PRIMARY CARE   104
   Current Pathways for Primary Care, 105
   Moving Toward Delivery of Primary Care as Defined, 112
   Summary, 144
   References, 145

6 THE PRIMARY CARE WORKFORCE   148
   Workforce Trends and Supply Projections: Physicians, 149
   Workforce Trends and Supply Projections: Nurse Practitioners, 158
   Workforce Trends and Supply Projections: Physician Assistants, 162
   Other First-Contact Providers, 165
   Comment on Workforce Estimation, 165
   Conclusions and Recommendations about the Supply of
      Primary Care Clinicians, 167
   Summary, 175
   References, 175

7 EDUCATION AND TRAINING FOR PRIMARY CARE   179
   Appropriate Training in Primary Care, 180
   The Education of Physicians, 180
   Other Content Issues in Training for Primary Care, 187
   Financial Support for Graduate Training in Primary Care, 196
   Interdisciplinary Education of Primary Care Clinicians, 203
   Integrated Delivery Systems and Primary Care Training, 206
   Continuing Medical Education, 207
   Physician Retraining, 208
   Summary, 211
   References, 212

8   RESEARCH AND EVALUATION IN PRIMARY CARE   216
    Support for the Infrastructure for Primary Care Research, 218
    Priority Areas for Primary Care Research, 234
    Summary, 244
    References, 244

9   IMPLEMENTATION STRATEGY   247
    Guiding Perspectives, 247
    A Primary Care Consortium, 250
    Implementation of Specific Recommendations, 252
    Final Comment on Implementation, 261

APPENDIXES   263

A   Site Visits   265
B   Public Hearing   268
C   Workshops   274
D   Mental Health Care in the Primary Care Setting   285
    Frank deGruy III, M.D.
E   Life in the Kaleidoscope: The Impact of Managed Care
    on the U.S. Health Care Workforce and a New Model
    for the Delivery of Primary Care   312
    Richard M. Scheffler, Ph.D.
F   Integrating Our Primary Care and Public Health Systems:
    A Formula for Improving Community and Population Health   341
    William E. Welton, M.H.A., Theodore A. Kantner, M.D.,
    and Sheila Moriber Katz, M.D., M.B.A.
G   Committee Biographies   374

INDEX   387

Primary Care

Summary

Primary care is the provision of integrated, accessible health care services by clinicians who are accountable for addressing a large majority of personal health care needs, developing a sustained partnership with patients, and practicing in the context of family and community. To bring this vision of the future of primary care closer to reality, the Institute of Medicine (IOM) appointed an expert committee to carry out a two-year study intended to address the opportunities for and challenges of reorienting health care in the United States. The above definition (published in the committee's interim report in 1994) guided its deliberations and its consideration of the conclusions and recommendations offered in the main part of this report (see Box S-1). Specifically, the report

• gives a clear definition of the function of primary care that can guide public and private actions to improve health care;

• encourages certain organizational arrangements for health care, built on a foundation of strong primary care, that will facilitate the coordination of the full array of services that are essential for maintaining and improving the health status of patients;

• argues for development and dissemination of improved information systems and quality assurance programs for primary care;

• advocates development and sustained support of means to make primary care available to all Americans, regardless of economic status, geographic location, or language and cultural differences;

1

- suggests financing mechanisms that encourage good primary care rather than episodic interventions late in the disease process;
- encourages support for training of a primary care workforce, sufficient in numbers to meet the needs for primary care, equipped with the skills and competencies that match the function as the committee has defined it, and prepared to work in the context of a team that includes primary care physicians, nurse practitioners, physician assistants, community health workers, and other health professionals;
- favors enhancement of the knowledge base for primary care based on clinical and health services research; and
- speaks to the development of primary care as a continually improving system in an era of rapid change through program evaluations, dissemination of innovations, and continued education of the clinician and patient.

The chapters of this report constitute a road map for reaching the committee's goals, as reflected in five assumptions. First, primary care is the logical foundation of an effective health care system because primary care can address the large majority of the health problems present in the population. Second, primary care is essential to achieving the objectives that together constitute value in health care—quality of care (including achievement of desired health outcomes), patient satisfaction, and efficient use of resources. Third, personal interactions that include trust and partnership between patients and clinicians are central to primary care. Fourth, primary care is an important instrument for achieving stronger emphasis on (a) health promotion and disease prevention and (b) care of the chronically ill, especially among the elderly with multiple problems. Fifth, the trend toward integrated health care systems in a managed care environment will continue and will provide both opportunities and challenges for primary care.

DEFINITION OF PRIMARY CARE

The committee's definition of primary care (see Chapter 2), which the committee formally recommends be adopted (see Box S-1), is presented in terms of the *function* of primary care, not solely in terms of who provides it. The definition calls attention to several attributes that provide the structure within which the broad themes of this report are addressed. The critical elements include

- integrated and accessible health care services;
- services provided by primary care clinicians—generally considered to be physicians, nurse practitioners, and physician assistants—but involving a broader array of individuals in a primary care team;
- accountability of clinicians and systems for quality of care, patient satisfaction, efficient use of resources, and ethical behavior;

- the majority of personal health care needs, which include physical, mental, emotional, and social concerns;
  - a sustained partnership between patients and clinicians; and
  - primary care in the context of family and community.

VALUE OF PRIMARY CARE

The committee's case for primary care (see Chapter 3) is made in two ways. The first concerns the value of primary care for individuals. The committee uses fictional scenarios to illustrate the terms in the definition and argues that primary care (a) provides a place to which patients can bring a wide range of health problems; (b) guides patients through the health system; (c) facilitates ongoing relationships between patients and clinicians within which patients participate in decision making about their health and health care; (d) opens opportunities for disease prevention and health promotion as well as early detection of disease; and (e) builds bridges between personal health care and patients' families and communities.

The second way to approach the question of the value of primary care is by recourse to empirical evidence. The committee amasses considerable evidence that primary care improves the quality and efficiency of care and expands access to appropriate services; it also forms an important bridge between personal health care and public health, to the advantage of both.

THE NATURE OF PRIMARY CARE

The complexity of primary care is reflected in six core attributes explored in Chapter 4 of the report:

1. Excellent primary care is grounded in both the biomedical and the social sciences.
2. Clinical decision making in primary care differs from that in specialty care.
3. Primary care has at its core a sustained personal relationship between patient and clinician.
4. Primary care does not consider mental health separately from physical health.
5. Important opportunities to promote health and prevent disease are intrinsic to primary care practice.
6. Primary care is information intensive.

In the committee's view, no health care system can be complete without primary care. In the United States, the time is right for primary care to undergo more systematic and creative development and to expand as the foundation of health care delivery. It is amenable to improvement through methods of science, implementation of key supporting elements of the health care infrastructure, and use of relevant management and organizational principles. Much of the remainder of the report explores these points in more detail.

THE DELIVERY OF PRIMARY CARE

The features of the U.S. health care scene that will influence the extent to which primary care evolves in this country are myriad: the spread of managed care, the expansion of integrated health care delivery systems, the consolidation of health plans and systems, growth in for-profit ownership of health plans and integrated delivery systems, the diversity among and within health care markets, the special challenges of primary care in rural areas and for the urban poor, the need for primary care to coordinate with other types of services, current and evolving roles for health care professionals, and the role of academic health centers in primary care delivery.

Key aspects of these trends and themes are explored in Chapter 5. Based on its analysis of these topics, the committee arrived at a series of recommendations concerning actions it believes would be necessary to overcome the barriers, or exploit the advantages, that these above factors pose for full implementation of the committee's vision of primary care. In all, the committee advances 11 separate recommendations in Chapter 5 (see Box S-1). The first group concerns the financing of primary care services, and the committee makes a strong statement about the availability of the services of a primary care clinician and the need for health care coverage for all Americans. Another recommendation concerns the organization of primary care and emphasizes the importance of the primary care team. With respect to underserved populations, the committee returned to its earlier themes to underscore the importance of primary care for populations who have special health care needs or who are traditionally underserved. Another major thesis of this chapter is the need for primary care to develop strong relationships with three other types of health activities—public health, mental health, and long-term care—and the committee offers three specific recommendations intended to reinforce the coordination and collaboration of efforts in these areas. Another recommendation calls for specific steps to develop tools and approaches for monitoring and improving the quality of primary care and to make performance information available to a wide audience. The final recommendation concerning the delivery of primary care calls on academic health centers to make primary care a core element of their mission and to provide leadership in education, research, and service delivery related to primary care.

THE PRIMARY CARE WORKFORCE

The committee concludes in Chapter 6 that the nation probably has a slight shortage, overall, in supply of the principal types of primary care clinicians—physicians, nurse practitioners, and physician assistants—but it underscores the great difficulties of developing reliable and valid estimates of supply of and, especially, requirements for clinicians or clinicians' services. The committee states four recommendations concerning important directions for the production and use of primary care clinicians (see Box S-1). These involve: (1) continuing the current level of effort to increase the supply of primary care clinicians but ensuring that primary care training programs and delivery systems focus their efforts on improving the competency of primary care clinicians and on increasing access for populations not now receiving adequate primary care; (2) encouraging state and federal agencies to monitor carefully the supply of and requirements for primary care clinicians; (3) exploring ways in which managed care and integrated health care systems might be used to alleviate the geographic maldistribution of primary care clinicians; and (4) examining how state practice acts for nurse practitioners and physician assistants might be amended to eliminate outmoded restrictions on practices that currently impede efficient and effective functioning of primary care teams and access to needed health care.

EDUCATION AND TRAINING FOR PRIMARY CARE

If primary care is to move in the directions advocated by this committee, then many aspects of health professions education and training will need to be restructured. Chapter 7 explores the changes likely to be required in undergraduate and graduate training, argues that clinical training ought to involve multidisciplinary team practice, and examines issues of retraining physicians for primary care. The committee used the broad scope of primary care to suggest that all trainees should be equipped to practice competently in the following areas: periodic assessment of asymptomatic persons; screening and early disease detection; evaluation and management of acute illness; assessment and either management or referral of patients with more complex problems that call for the diagnostic and therapeutic tools of medical specialists and other professionals; ongoing management of patients with established chronic diseases; coordination of care among specialists; and provision of acute hospital and long-term care.

To reach this goal, the committee puts forward several recommendations (see Box S-1). With respect to undergraduate medical education, the committee is concerned about students gaining experience in primary care settings; with respect to graduate training, the committee explores issues of residency programs in family practice, internal medicine, and pediatrics. More broadly, the committee examines questions of advanced training for all primary care clinicians and calls attention to the need to develop a set of common core competencies for all primary care clinicians. In addition, the committee highlights its concerns about two special areas of emphasis—communication skills and cultural sensitivity. A major concern for the committee is financial support for primary care training, and consistent with earlier recommendations about universal coverage for health care, the committee calls for an all-payer system to support health professions education and training, with some of this support reserved for primary care and directed to training in nonhospital sites such as offices, clinics, and extended care facilities. Other elements of education and training include developing more innovative and interdisciplinary training programs and creating mechanisms by which physicians can be formally retrained for primary care.

RESEARCH AND EVALUATION IN PRIMARY CARE

Despite the committee's clear vision for the future of primary care and the consensus it reached on many steps toward bringing that vision to fruition, the committee still acknowledges that primary care represents a largely uncharted frontier awaiting discovery and exploration. Expanded research in this area is timely because of the accelerating movement toward a variety of managed care and integrated delivery systems, most of which will rely on primary care models and clinicians. To the degree that this is so, improved primary care that can bring about a better balance between patients' and populations' needs and the health care services they receive is critical.

As noted in Chapter 8, the science base for primary care is modest, and the infrastructure underlying the knowledge base is skeletal at best. Thus, the committee proposes four recommendations intended to strengthen the underpinnings of a primary care research enterprise (see Box S-1). These relate to (1) federal support for primary care research, including the designation of a lead agency in this effort; (2) development of a national database on primary care, ideally through some form of ongoing survey mechanism; (3) support of research through practice-based primary care research networks; and (4) development of standards for data collection, including attention to data element definition and improved coding.

The committee also identified a number of subjects that it believes warrant high priority in any primary care research agenda. Prominent among these is the committee's fifth recommendation in Chapter 8 concerning specialist provision of primary care. Other subjects involve major elements of the committee's conceptualization of primary care, such as the large majority of personal health care needs, the sustained partnership between clinicians and patients, accountability, and practicing in a family and community context.

A STRATEGY FOR IMPLEMENTATION

The recommendations described so far are regarded by the committee as essential steps toward strengthening primary care as the firm foundation for health care in this country, but only effective implementation will permit the nation to realize their benefits. To provide focus for the implementation effort,

Chapter 9 of the report discusses specific means for implementation and identifies the many parties whose commitment will be necessary. This plan for implementation is guided by several perspectives that, in the view of the committee, are essential for success: the need for a coordinated strategy, a long-term perspective, and involvement of a large set of change agents and interested parties.

Coordinated implementation by many participants over time is unlikely to take place unless an entity exists whose purposes are to build appropriate coalitions, stimulate action, and monitor and facilitate implementation. To this end, the committee recommends the formation of a public-private, nonprofit primary care consortium (see Box S-1). Its broad functions would be (among other things) to

- coordinate efforts to promote and enhance primary care;
- conduct research and development projects, provide technical assistance, and disseminate information on issues such as primary care infrastructure, innovative models of primary care, and methods to monitor primary care performance; and
- organize national meetings through which interested parties can report on progress in implementing the primary care agenda.

The committee's view of this entity as a public-private partnership was arrived at advisedly. Government at all levels has a deep interest in seeing the primary care vision of this committee succeed, but many aspects of the strategy proposed in this report require action and commitment by many entities in the private sector.

With the apparent demise of comprehensive national health care reform, the climate for moving ahead on a reform agenda affecting primary care might seem to be unfavorable. Yet, the pace of change in the health care systems of communities around the country remains very rapid. In those changes and the restructuring being proposed for Medicare and Medicaid, opportunities exist to make the American health care system more effective and efficient. Important parts of the agenda proposed in this report require federal action, but for many elements the key decisionmakers are to be found in the states and cities of this country, in health care plans, in educational institutions, in professions, and in private foundations. Many of these parties are already committed to a renewed emphasis on primary care. In this situation, opportunities for coalition building for implementation should be present, and that is one reason the committee has recommended establishment of a primary care consortium.

This is a time when creative effort and collaboration can influence the forces driving health care change in the directions defined by this committee. It will not be a time for weak hearts or quick fixes—but the promise of improving health care for Americans should be motivation enough to stay the course set out in this report.

BOX S-1 **Committee Recommendations**

Chapter 2

2.1 *To Adopt the Committee's Definition*
This committee has defined primary care as the provision of integrated, accessible health care services by clinicians who are accountable for addressing a large majority of personal health care needs, developing a sustained partnership with patients, and practicing in the context of family and community. The committee recommends the adoption of this definition by all parties involved in the delivery and financing of primary care and by institutions responsible for the education and training of primary care clinicians.

Chapter 5

5.1 *Availability of Primary Care for All Americans*
The committee recommends development of primary care delivery systems that will make the services of a primary care clinician available to all Americans.

5.2 *Health Care Coverage for All Americans*
To assure that the benefits of primary care are more uniformly available, the committee recommends that the federal government and the states develop strategies to provide health care coverage for all Americans.

5.3 *Payment Methods Favorable to Primary Care*
The committee recommends that payment methods favorable to the support of primary care be more widely adopted.

5.4 *Payment for Primary Care Services*
The committee recommends that when fee-for-service is used to reimburse clinicians for patient care, payments for primary care be upgraded to reflect better the value of these services.

5.5 *Practice by Interdisciplinary Teams*
The committee believes that the quality, efficiency, and responsiveness of primary care are enhanced by the use of interdisciplinary teams and recommends the adoption of the team concept of primary care wherever feasible.

5.6 *The Underserved and Those with Special Needs*
The committee recommends that public or private programs designed to cover underserved populations and those with special needs include the provision of primary care services as defined in this report. It further recommends that the agencies or organizations funding these programs carefully monitor them to ensure that such primary care is provided.

BOX S-1 **Continued**

5.7 *Primary Care and Public Health*

The committee recommends that health care plans and public health agencies develop specific written agreements regarding their respective roles and relationships in (a) maintaining and improving the health of the communities they serve and (b) ensuring coordination of preventive services and health promotion activities related to primary care.

5.8 *Primary Care and Mental Health Services*

The committee recommends the reduction of financial and organizational disincentives for the expanded role of primary care in the provision of mental health services. It further recommends the development and evaluation of collaborative care models that integrate primary care and mental health services more effectively. These models should involve both primary care clinicians and mental health professionals.

5.9 *Primary Care and Long-Term Care*

To improve the continuity and effectiveness of services for those requiring long-term care, the committee recommends that third-party payers (including Medicare and Medicaid), health care organizations, and health professionals promote the integration of primary care and long-term care by coordinating or pooling financing and removing regulatory or other barriers to such coordination.

5.10 *Quality of Primary Care*

The committee recommends the development and adoption of uniform methods and measures to monitor the performance of health care systems and individual clinicians in delivering primary care as defined in this report. Performance measures should include cost, quality, access, and patient and clinician satisfaction. The results should be made available to public and private purchasers of care, provider organizations, clinicians, and the general public.

5.11 *Primary Care in Academic Health Centers*

The committee recommends that academic health centers explicitly accept primary care as one of their core missions and provide leadership in the development of primary care teaching, research, and service delivery programs.

Chapter 6

6.1 *Programs Regarding the Primary Care Workforce*

The committee recommends (a) that the current level of effort to increase the supply of primary care clinicians be continued and (b) that these primary care training programs and delivery systems focus their efforts on improving the competency of primary care clinicians and on increasing access for populations not now receiving adequate primary care.

BOX S-1 Continued

6.2 *Monitoring the Primary Care Workforce*
The committee recommends that state and federal agencies carefully monitor the supply of and requirements for primary care clinicians.

6.3 *Addressing Issues of Geographic Maldistribution*
The committee recommends that federal and state governments and private foundations fund research projects to explore ways in which managed care and integrated health care systems can be used to alleviate the geographic maldistribution of primary care clinicians.

6.4 *State Practice Acts for Nurse Practitioners and Physician Assistants*
The committee recommends that state governments review current restrictions on the scope of practice of primary care nurse practitioners and physician assistants and eliminate or modify those restrictions that impede collaborative practice and reduce access to quality primary care.

Chapter 7

7.1 *Training in Primary Care Sites*
All medical schools should require their undergraduate medical students to experience training in settings that deliver primary care as defined by this committee.

7.2 *Common Core Competencies*
The committee recommends that common core competencies for primary care clinicians, regardless of their disciplinary base, be defined by a coalition of appropriate educational and professional organizations and accrediting bodies.

7.3 *Emphasis on Common Core Competencies by Accrediting and Certifying Bodies*
The committee recommends that organizations that accredit primary care training programs and certify individual trainees support curricular reforms that teach the common core competencies and essential elements of primary care.

7.4 *Special Areas of Emphasis in Primary Care Training*
The committee recommends that the curricula of all primary care education and training programs emphasize communication skills and cultural sensitivity.

7.5 *All-Payer Support for Primary Care Training*
The committee recommends the development of an all-payer system to support health professions education and training. A portion of this pool of funds should be reserved for education and training in primary care.

BOX S-1 **Continued**

7.6 *Support for Graduate Medical Education in Primary Care Sites*
The committee recommends that a portion of the funds for graduate medical education be reallocated to provide explicit support for the direct and overhead costs of primary care training in nonhospital sites such as health maintenance organizations, community clinics, physician offices, and extended care facilities.

7.7 *Interdisciplinary Training*
The committee recommends that (a) the training of primary care clinicians include experience with the delivery of health care by interdisciplinary teams; and (b) academic health centers work with health maintenance organizations, group practices, community health centers, and other health care delivery organizations using interdisciplinary teams to develop clinical rotations for students and residents.

7.8 *Experimentation and Evaluation*
The committee recommends that private foundations, health plans, and government agencies support ongoing experimentation and evaluation of interdisciplinary teaching of collaborative primary care to determine how such teaching might best be done.

7.9 *Retraining*
The committee recommends that (a) curricula of retraining programs in primary care include instruction in the core competencies proposed for development in Recommendations 7.2 and 7.3 and (b) certifying bodies in the primary care disciplines develop mechanisms for testing and certifying clinicians who have undergone retraining for primary care.

Chapter 8

8.1 *Federal Support for Primary Care Research*
The committee recommends that (a) the Department of Health and Human Services identify a lead agency for primary care research and (b) the Congress of the United States appropriate funds for this agency in an amount adequate to build both the infrastructure required to conduct primary care research and fund high-priority research projects.

8.2 *National Database and Primary Care Data Set*
The committee recommends that the Department of Health and Human Services support the development of and provide ongoing support for a national database (based on a sample survey) that reflects the majority of health care needs in the United States and includes a uniform primary care data set based on episodes of care. This national survey should capture data on the entire U.S. population, regardless of insurance status.

BOX S-1 **Continued**

8.3 *Research in Practice-Based Primary Care Research Networks*
The committee recommends that the Department of Health and Human Services provide adequate and stable financial support to practice-based primary care research networks.

8.4 *Data Standards*
The committee recommends that the federal government foster the development of standards for data collection that will ensure the consistency of data elements and definitions of terms, improve coding, permit analysis of episodes of care, and reflect the content of primary care.

8.5 *Study of Specialist Provision of Primary Care*
The committee recommends that the appropriate federal agencies and private foundations commission studies of (a) the extent to which primary care, as defined by the IOM, is delivered by physician specialists and sub-specialists, (b) the impact of such care delivery on primary care workforce requirements, and (c) the effects of these patterns of health care delivery or such care on the costs and quality of and access to health care.

Chapter 9

9.1 *Establishment of a Primary Care Consortium*
The committee recommends the formation of a public-private, nonprofit primary care consortium consisting of professional societies, private foundations, government agencies, health care organizations, and representatives of the public.

1

Introduction

Rapid and profound changes are under way in the organization and financing of health care in the United States. Driven largely by concerns about the rising costs of health care, some of these changes are intended to control the growth of expensive, specialized services and to favor growth in the role of primary care. The desirability of greater emphasis on primary care has long been recognized by the Institute of Medicine (IOM) and other groups and reflected in public policies at the federal and state levels. Efforts to encourage primary care in the past have included federal and state support for training of primary care clinicians, direct support for the organization of primary care services to disadvantaged populations, and development of health maintenance organizations (HMOs) and other financing mechanisms that encourage primary care.

These policies and steps have not, however, been the major force in bringing about renewed emphasis on primary care. In fact, pronouncements, studies, and public policies intended to encourage primary care have seemed remarkably ineffective as the health care system continued its drift of the past 50 years toward ever greater dependency on services provided by medical specialists and the related growth of hospital-based care. Meanwhile, a growing body of evidence suggested that this trend toward expanded use of specialized services has contributed significantly to an unsustainable increase in health care costs, has aggravated problems of access to basic services for some of our population, and has failed to address effectively common health problems that cause disability and death in the population.

Many factors encourage specialization. Among them are growth of medical knowledge based on biomedical research; methods of reimbursement of physicians and hospitals that support the expanded use of medical technologies; and a training system based in specialized care settings. Prior reports by the IOM (1978) and other organizations (e.g., the Physician Payment Review Commission [PPRC] in its annual reports of the 1980s and 1990s; the Council on Graduate Medical Education [COGME] in its periodic reports over the same time period) have documented these trends and demonstrated how, until fairly recently, they overwhelmed the factors that promote primary care.

Today, powerful economic forces in the health care market, especially the actions of large purchasers of group health benefits, are driving a shift away from specialized services and toward primary care. In the absence of comprehensive health care reform, these market forces are likely to remain dominant in reshaping health care. Because cost is the major concern behind these market forces, primary care is seen as desirable because it is less expensive. Although wholeheartedly endorsing the emphasis on primary care, the IOM study committee appointed to produce this report (see below) is concerned about spotlighting primary care as a means to control the use of expensive, specialized services rather than as a better way to meet the health care needs of people.

In the longer run, the American people will accept only a system that meets their needs for good health care, and they will resist changes that are perceived as aimed principally at controlling costs. The committee believes that primary care is the foundation of that health care system—one that is effective and responsive *as well as* efficient in the use of expensive resources. Medical science will continue to improve its ability to diagnose and treat diseases, but primary care can assure that advances in diagnosis and treatment are used in a way that emphasize personal values in our diverse society; that emphasize health promotion, disease prevention, and early intervention; that enhance the ability of the individual to maintain effective functioning in daily life; and that facilitate links among individuals, their families, and their communities.

In this report, the committee sets out its vision of primary care, taking full advantage of the forces that have brought primary care to the fore after decades in eclipse. Its focus is on ensuring that primary care is shaped by concern for meeting people's needs for health care in the best traditions of the health professions. This vision includes continuous innovation and improvement in the performance of the health system. The committee cannot answer all questions that might arise about primary care, but it can and does identify the directions in which to go and the means by which to get there. As laid out in this report, these objectives include:

- a clear definition of the function of primary care that can guide public and private actions to improve health care;
- organizational arrangements for health care that are built on a foundation of strong primary care and that facilitate the coordination of the full array of services essential for maintaining and improving individuals' health status;

- improved information systems and quality assurance programs for primary care;
- ways to make primary care available to all Americans, regardless of economic status, geographic location, language, or cultural background;
- financing mechanisms that encourage quality primary care rather than episodic interventions late in the disease process;
- a primary care workforce sufficient in numbers to meet the needs for primary care, equipped with appropriate skills and competencies, and prepared to work in teams that include primary care physicians, nurse practitioners, physician assistants, community health workers, and other health professionals;
- an enhanced knowledge base for primary care, drawn from clinical and health services research; and
- program evaluation, dissemination of innovations, and continued education of both clinician and patient as means continually to improve the primary care system in an era of rapid change.

As can be seen from these objectives, primary care is not just a label for a set of clinicians. Rather, the committee views primary care as a system of services guided by a common vision. Realizing this vision poses a complex agenda—one that requires a coordinated strategy for implementation, many actors, and both short- and long-term steps. Primary care must include the appropriate organizational and financing arrangements, the necessary infrastructure, the knowledge base, a way of thinking and acting for the clinicians, and the understanding and support of patients and consumers. The committee hopes that this report will serve as a road map for a journey that will continue for many years.

THE INSTITUTE OF MEDICINE STUDY

Funding

The IOM initiated this study with major funding provided by the U.S. Public Health Service (the Health Resources and Services Administration [HRSA] and the Agency for Health Care Policy and Research [AHCPR]), the Department of Veterans Affairs, The Robert Wood Johnson Foundation, The Pew Charitable Trusts, and The Josiah Macy, Jr. Foundation. All these foundations and government agencies as well as the IOM have had a long-standing interest in issues relating to primary care such as workforce, financing, organization and delivery, education and training, and research. As the study proceeded, the committee identified additional activities that would contribute to its deliberations, and additional support for these activities was received from a number of professional organizations and foundations (see list of sponsors in acknowledgments).

The Study Committee and Its Charge

In early 1994, the IOM appointed a study committee that conducted the major part of its work between March 1994 and October 1995. The committee, chaired by Neal A. Vanselow, M.D., consisted of 19 individuals (see roster on pp. iii–iv) with diverse expertise in the administration and governance of hospitals, HMOs, medical centers, and academic health centers; the practice of medicine (including the fields of family practice, general internal medicine, general pediatrics, cardiology, obstetrics-gynecology, and osteopathy); public health; nursing; physician assistant training; dentistry; health economics; long-term care; health services research; epidemiology; and consumer wellness. During its nine meetings and other study activities, the committee addressed the following charge:

> [P]rovide guidance for augmenting and improving primary care as an essential component of an effective and efficient health care system. The study will focus on the health needs of the population and the functions of primary care in meeting those needs, not just on the numbers and roles of health care professionals choosing primary care careers. Attention will be given to the issues of the overall financing and organization of services as well as to the training and deployment of the primary care work force. An interim report providing the initial conclusions of the committee concerning the definition of the primary care function will be issued in September, 1994. The study will draw on the related work of federal agencies, foundations, and other organizations carrying out related studies and program initiatives.

Study Activities

Commissioned Papers

To avail itself of expert and detailed analysis of several issues beyond the time resources of its members, the committee commissioned three major background papers. The first, by Inge Hofmans-Okkes, M.A., Ph.D. and Henk Lamberts, M.D., Ph.D., provides data on the majority of personal health service needs and is summarized as an appendix to Chapter 4. The second, by Frank deGruy III, M.D., examines the relationship between primary care and mental health and appears as Appendix D. The third, by William E. Welton, M.H.A., Theodore A. Kantner, M.D., and Sheila M. Katz, M.D., M.B.A., explores issues of primary care and public health and appears as Appendix F. In addition, a paper commissioned by HRSA and written by committee member Richard M. Scheffler, Ph.D., provides an economic analysis of workforce issues and appears as Appendix E.

Interim Report

In September 1994 the committee released *Defining Primary Care: An In-*

terim Report (IOM, 1994). The definitions of primary care and the terms used in the definition acted as a reference point for the committee during its deliberations. The definition has been disseminated widely, and the committee has received considerable feedback from a variety of individuals, professional groups, and organizations. That work is incorporated in Chapter 2.

Site Visits

When IOM studies with national significance involve activities initiated at the state and community level, the IOM often makes a concerted effort to reach out to those engaged in such activities in those locales. The aims are (a) to learn about the activities and to understand the views of interested parties about issues pertinent to the local efforts and then (b) to apply those lessons, as appropriate, to broad national, professional, and policy-related issues. The IOM takes care, in these circumstances, not to evaluate or draw public judgments about organizational efforts.

During late 1994 and through the summer of 1995, the committee conducted site visits. Three major visits were made to the following areas: Minnesota, southern California, and Texas and New Mexico. Shorter visits were made to rural North Carolina and Boston. (See Appendix A.) The sites were chosen to provide a firsthand view of primary care in these very different settings. Information gathered there confirmed the swift and profound changes that are under way in the financing and organization of health care in this country. Discussions with people engaged in the organization and delivery of primary care and involved in educational programs, as well as patients, reinforced the committee's view that primary care is a very rapidly moving target.

Public Hearing

In December 1994 the full committee held a public hearing to gather information about a broad set of issues, including (a) the scope of primary care; (b) who should deliver primary care; (c) the organization and financing of primary care; (d) education, training, and research in primary care; (e) the committee's definition of primary care; and (f) other issues before the committee. A range of organizations were invited to express their views, describe their experiences, and comment on these matters, as well as to submit articles, descriptive materials, and position statements on primary care. In all, 86 organizations submitted written testimony and 31 organizations presented oral testimony at the public hearing. (See Appendix B.)

Workshops

An invitational workshop held in January 1995 (see Appendix C) provided an opportunity for thoughtful discourse among a knowledgeable and diverse group of experts concerning the scope and directions for research that can best strengthen the base of scientific knowledge for primary care, and it yielded insights that the committee incorporated in its conclusions and recommendations concerning primary care research and the infrastructure necessary to the research enterprise (see Chapter 8). A special issue of the *Journal of Family Practice* (February 1996) comprises papers based on many of the workshop presentations.

A second invitational workshop held in June 1995 (see Appendix C) featured a structured discussion by a diverse group of health professionals about the roles of the various health professions in carrying out the function of primary care. Materials and views from this workshop are reflected throughout this report (and especially in Chapters 3 through 7).

UNDERLYING ASSUMPTIONS

To guide its development of this report, the committee adopted five assumptions. These are, in the committee's judgment, critical for the future of primary care in this nation's health care system, and they are consistent with the evidence and logic presented throughout the report. The principles are:

1. Primary care is the logical foundation of an effective health care system because it can address the large majority of the health problems present in the population.
2. Primary care is essential to achieving the objectives that together constitute value in health care: high quality of care, including achievement of desired health outcomes; patient satisfaction; and efficient use of resources.
3. Personal interactions that include trust and partnership between patients and clinicians are central to primary care.
4. Primary care is an important instrument for achieving stronger emphasis on both ends of the spectrum of care: (a) health promotion and disease prevention and (b) care of the chronically ill, especially among the elderly with multiple problems.
5. The trend toward integrated health care systems in a managed care environment will continue and will provide both opportunities and challenges for primary care.

HISTORIC ROOTS AND THE CONTEMPORARY CONTEXT
FOR PRIMARY CARE

Historic Roots

Before World War II

Before World War II, health care in the United States was based on what would now be described as primary care. The Committee on the Costs of Medical Care, a private group established with support from foundations, carried out the first comprehensive study of health care in this country and, in 1932, stated that "each patient would be primarily under the charge of the family practitioner . . . [and] . . . would look to his physician for guidance and counsel on health matters and ordinarily would receive attention from specialists when referred . . ." (CCMC, 1932, p. 63). Through the 1930s and 1940s general care was increasingly provided by pediatricians and internists (whose specialty boards were established in 1933 and 1936, respectively) in addition to general practitioners. In many locales, the public health nurse also provided important aspects of what we now call primary care.

The 1960s

The term *primary care* began to appear in the literature in the early 1960s. Kerr White and his associates made important contributions to the concept and study of primary care. The important 1961 article "The Ecology of Medical Care," written at a time when the growth of specialized care was well under way, used epidemiological analysis to show that most health care problems were appropriately addressed in the primary care setting (White et al., 1961).

Concerned by the decline of general practitioners as key providers of primary care, several major commissions issued reports in the 1960s[1] that encouraged the establishment of family practice as a new primary care specialty. Nevertheless, the decline in the numbers of general practitioners continued (from 71,366 in 1965 to 42,374 in 1975), and the numbers of physicians trained in the new specialty of family practice did not make up for this decline. Meanwhile, the total number of physicians grew rapidly as medical education expanded, encouraged by federal and state policies and financial support that resulted from a perceived general shortage of physicians; most of this growth went into specialty care (COGME, 1992).

---

[1]Important publications on primary care issues dating back 25 to 30 years or so include the Coggeshall report (1965), the Millis Commission report (1966), and the Willard Committee report (1966).

The training of physician assistants and nurse practitioners also began in this period, with the objective of filling part of the perceived gap in the shortage of physicians. Federal support, such as that authorized in Titles VII and VIII of the Public Health Act, encouraged these training programs.

Public sector financing of health services also emerged in the 1960s. To target the problem of access to health services for the poor, federal programs were launched to assist in the development of community-based comprehensive primary care centers for both the urban and rural poor. More well-known efforts to expand access to care were the Medicare and Medicaid programs for, respectively, the elderly and selected parts of the poor population.

The 1970s

By 1976, a growing belief that primary care physicians were in short supply led to federal support for the training of general internists and general pediatricians in addition to family practitioners. Several major private foundations, particularly the Robert Wood Johnson Foundation, devoted substantial funds to the encouragement of primary care and training for primary care.

The IOM report *A Manpower Policy for Primary Care* made a number of recommendations to shift the emphasis of medical care toward primary care (IOM, 1978). Drawing heavily on the earlier work of Alpert and Charney (1973), the report contained a definition of primary care that became widely used, but the report's policy recommendations were not implemented.

During this period, specialty care grew in most industrialized countries, but the proportion of physicians delivering primary care remained substantially higher in other nations than in the United States (Starfield, 1991, 1992). In 1978, the World Health Organization, in the so-called Alma-Ata declaration, put primary care at the center of its strategy of "health for all by the year 2000."

In the United States, the growth of HMOs was encouraged by the Health Maintenance Organization Act of 1973. Drawing on the experience of capitated group practice models, HMOs emphasized primary care services and lower hospital utilization. Their growth accelerated in the 1970s and 1980s (from 3 million members in 1973 to more than 29 million in 1987) largely through encouragement by business interests looking for a way to control their expenditures for employee health benefits. Much of this growth was in loose models based on networks of physicians and hospitals; the primary care physician filled a "gatekeeper" role as the required path to specialized services.

Despite these many independent efforts, primary care did not prosper in the midst of economic and professional incentives that continued to favor specialty care. Specialized services continued to increase as a proportion of all medical care.

Current Forces

Health Care Reform

When this study began, comprehensive reform of the U.S. health system seemed a likely prospect. A number of the proposals for comprehensive reform, including that of the Clinton administration, contained specific provisions intended to increase the emphasis on primary care. Whatever the specific arrangements, such extensive reform would have addressed the issue of health coverage for the growing numbers of uninsured. It would also have provided a specific framework for changes in health care and clearer patterns of accountability for the results of those changes.

Comprehensive reform initiated by the government did not come to pass, however, and it now seems unlikely for some years. Although some states have moved to develop and implement their own reform plans, the future of these plans is also uncertain in light of both the failure of national comprehensive reform and efforts to constrain spending at all levels of government. Incremental changes in the rules for the health insurance market may still occur at the national and state levels, but how these changes will affect the arrangements for primary care is unclear.

Other Forces

Despite the failure of comprehensive reform efforts, rapid changes in the organization and financing of health care continue, driven primarily by powerful forces in the health care marketplace. These forces are likely to continue and constitute the context in which the future of primary care will be determined. The major forces for change, as seen by the committee, involve the following eight sets of factors:

1. Continuing concerns of payers of group health benefits about the costs and effectiveness of medical care. Group payers include both private sector employers and federal, state, and local governments. All are concerned about what they perceive as unsustainable rates of increases in medical care expenditures. Derivative from cost concerns are questions about the effectiveness and necessity of specific health services.

These considerations have led to various approaches to managing care and capping expenditures, which often emphasize reducing the use of specialized services and hospital care and shifting more clinical responsibility to the primary care clinician. Health care plans and governments have also used their economic power to reduce levels of payment to providers. These actions have the aggregate effect of creating excess capacity in hospitals, reducing the demand for many specialized services, and creating economic pressures to reduce these capacities.

Although the more aggressive actions have been taken by private payers, several states are moving their Medicaid programs into managed care arrangements. The Medicare program has lagged in this movement; overall, only about 9 percent of beneficiaries are enrolled in plans with Medicare risk contracts (HMOs), but the proportion is much higher in some markets where managed care penetration is high. By contrast, Medicare has taken the lead on changes in methods of reimbursement in the fee-for-service sector, including changes in physician reimbursement that were intended to increase the payment for primary care services relative to specialty procedures. Discussions of substantial reductions in Medicare and Medicaid funding are likely to accelerate the move of these public programs into managed care arrangements.

The result of these actions is a strong growth in enrollments in HMOs and other forms of managed care, but the rates of HMO enrollment vary considerably across different areas of the country and there is little penetration of rural markets. In markets in which managed care penetration is high, intense cost-based competition results.

2. Development of integrated delivery systems and consolidation of providers and health plans. To compete effectively for patients and to meet the concerns of health plans, employers, and governments to hold down costs, physicians and institutional providers are increasingly forming integrated delivery systems built on a foundation of primary care. As the committee observed in its site visits to areas where markets have advanced far into this competitive managed care environment, physicians and hospitals are finding it difficult to survive without joining some form of organized arrangement for health care. Plans and delivery systems are also consolidating into larger aggregates that can access capital, market and compete effectively in broader areas, and develop the infrastructure (including data systems and clinical decision systems) needed for improved efficiency and effectiveness of services.

3. Growing influence of the private capital markets. The creation of large plans and integrated systems requires access to substantial capital. The need for capital has the practical effect of introducing a new set of decision makers who focus chiefly on financial viability. For for-profit plans, which are a growing proportion of the health care industry, growth in profitability over time is another major goal and criterion of success to which the health plans must be attentive.

4. Legislative actions affecting primary care in an era of reductions of public budgets. The federal government has encouraged primary care in several ways: subsidies for the training of primary care clinicians, changes in Medicare reimbursements for physicians, and grant support for organized primary care services at the community level. Unprecedented efforts to balance the federal budget make future funding of these federal programs uncertain. Efforts to reduce the growth of Medicare and Medicaid may contribute to the inability of health care institutions and organizations to meet the primary care needs (let alone the full range of health care needs) of the growing numbers of uninsured throughout the country, and these steps to curtail federal programs will complicate, if not undermine, the actions that states and localities might wish to take to support and expand primary care services.

Meanwhile, various states have considered or taken actions intended to increase the proportion of primary care physicians and other clinicians being trained. Laws have also been passed or are being considered that designate certain specialties as part of primary care. State legislative actions have also expanded the scope of practice of nurse practitioners and physician assistants in many states, which has implications for the role of these clinicians in the provision of primary care. These state actions are often linked to concerns about rural health care and access to care by the poor in the inner cities, but the process serves to raise the level of awareness of primary care issues in the legislature.

5. *A surplus of specialist practitioners.* As the health care system shifts toward primary care and the demand for specialized care diminishes, a surplus of physicians and nurses who have been providing specialty services seems likely to emerge. Certainly this is true for physicians (IOM, 1996a). The concerns of these groups, expressed in the political process, are already being heard, especially with respect to the effects of downsizing and restructuring on the nursing profession (IOM, 1996b). These concerns may be a limiting factor on the rate of the changes described above.

6. *Role of the patient in determining the pace and nature of changes in the patterns of medical care.* An increasingly well-informed patient is an important force in determining the future course of medical care, including primary care. Some changes in the patterns of medical care disrupt long-established physician-patient relationships and established patterns of care that patients perceive as desirable. For example, when employers change health plans offered to employees, or when clinicians lose their affiliations with health plans and are no longer included in the panel of clinicians available to patients, then clinician-patient relationships are likely to be interrupted. Some patients resent being cut off from direct access to their established clinicians or to specialists of their choice.

Patients also express resistance to patterns of care established by managed care plans in the interest of cost containment. A current example is the controversy over lengths of hospital stay for obstetric care; pressures for shorter stays are being resisted by both women and clinicians, and state legislative actions are being taken or proposed that would impose length-of-stay requirements on managed care plans. In many of these situations, patients' concerns are augmented by clinicians' concerns about limitations on their freedom to make clinical decisions in the interests of their patients (or to provide patients with all appropriate information necessary for adequate decision making). In the United States, changes in arrangements for a service as basic as medical care are unlikely to endure without the support of patients. If such support is to be achieved, it will need to be based on better understanding of the potential benefits of the changes in terms of the values that patients and their families hold dear.

7. *Effects of changes on academic health centers.* Academic health centers are under pressure to place more emphasis on primary care in their educational and patient care programs. At the same time, the aggressive competition of managed care plans and current and potential declines in federal and state support for their educational missions are making response to change even more difficult for these institutions. Their complex governance patterns make rapid change difficult under any circumstances, but their increasing dependence on clinical income, most of which is derived from highly specialized services, to subsidize their educational and research missions puts these institutions at a competitive disadvantage relative to health care plans that do not have these missions. Furthermore, an emphasis on primary care is at variance with the traditional clinical base of specialized, tertiary care services found in many institutions.

8. *Continued growth of knowledge and technologies for improved medical care.* The results of the continued rapid growth in biomedical knowledge—new diagnostic and therapeutic modalities—will continue to influence the nature and costs of health care. The potential benefits of these advances continue to be exciting and popular, but in a cost-constrained medical environment new technologies are being subjected to more examination of their costs and effectiveness. New technologies have, over the years, prompted increased specialization, but the environment of managed care is leading to more explicit decisions about the introduction and appropriate use of technologies and the roles of primary care clinicians in determining their use.

Advances in information technologies also have considerable potential for shaping the future of health care and the role of primary care. Computer-based patient records and decision assists have the potential to change the roles and functions of primary care clinicians and improve the participation of patients and consumers in making informed decisions about their own care.

Growth in knowledge and techniques for outcomes-based accountability in health care is also shaping the future of primary care. Although cost has been a principal engine of change in health care arrangements, including the shift toward primary care, better techniques for measuring outcomes, including measures that reflect the perceptions of the patient about the outcomes of care, are changing the nature of accountability in health care. Clinicians and health care organizations and institutions will be under more pressure to justify their activities and their use of scarce resources in terms of results—both clinical outcomes and measures of patient functioning and satisfaction. Primary care will face difficult challenges in developing and using appropriate outcome measures that will convince patients, health care systems, and payers that a primary-care-based health system can benefit patients as well as constrain costs. Because of the breadth of primary care and its longitudinal nature, and because of the difficulties of measuring outcomes attributable to the care process over the long time periods often required in ambulatory care, the technical challenges in developing appropriate outcomes-based accountability will be substantial.

ORGANIZATION OF THE REPORT

All the forces outlined above—and indeed others not yet perceived—will shape primary care in ways that this committee cannot fully anticipate. They constitute, however, an important context for the information presented and the findings and recommendations offered in the remainder of this report.

Chapter 2 incorporates much of the committee's interim report defining primary care (IOM, 1994). Chapter 3 discusses the value of primary care as viewed from the perspective of the individual and the policymaker, and it makes extensive use of illustrative vignettes. The nature of primary care, using the committee's definition as an organizing framework and drawing from its workshop on the scientific basis of primary care, is explicated in Chapter 4. Chapter 5 addresses the organization and delivery of primary care from the perspective of several current trends: changes in organization and financing; rising use of teams; growing needs of underserved populations; increasing recognition of the need for strong relationships between primary care and public health, mental health, and long-term care; the increasingly complex and fragile role of academic medical centers; and the emerging emphasis on information about quality of care.

Chapter 6 describes the primary care workforce and calls attention to the need to address all components of that workforce in concert, and Chapter 7 focuses on education and training issues for primary care clinicians. Chapter 8 identifies high priority research topics and documents the need for developing the infrastructure to support research efforts in this field. Finally, Chapter 9 discusses critical steps in implementation of the committee's recommendations.

REFERENCES

Alpert, J.J., and Charney, E. *The Education of Physicians for Primary Care.* Publ. No. (HRA) 74-3113. Washington, D.C.: U.S. Department of Health, Education, and Welfare, 1973.

CCMC (Committee on the Costs of Medical Care). *Medical Care for the American People: The Final Report of the Committee on the Costs of Medical Care.* Publ. No. 28. Chicago: University of Chicago Press, 1932.

Coggeshall, L.T. *Planning for Medical Progress Through Education.* Washington, D.C.: American Association of Medical Colleges, 1965.

COGME (Council on Graduate Medical Education). *Third Report. Improving Access to Health Care Through Physician Workforce Reform: Directions for the 21st Century.* Rockville, Md.: Health Resources and Services Administration, Public Health Service, 1992.

IOM (Institute of Medicine). *A Manpower Policy for Primary Health Care: Report of a Study.* Washington, D.C.: National Academy Press, 1978.

IOM. *Defining Primary Care: An Interim Report.* M. Donaldson, K. Yordy, and N. Vanselow, eds. Washington, D.C.: National Academy Press, 1994.

IOM. *The Nation's Physician Workforce: Options for Balancing Supply and Requirements.* K.N. Lohr, N.A. Vanselow, and D.E. Detmer, eds. Washington, D.C.: National Academy Press, 1996a.

IOM. *Nursing Staff in Hospitals and Nursing Homes: Is It Adequate?* G.S. Wunderlich, F. Sloan, and C.K. Davis, eds. Washington, D.C.: National Academy Press, 1996b.

Journal of Family Practice 42:113–203, 1996.

Millis, J.S. *The Graduate Education of Physicians.* Report of the Citizens' Commission on Graduate Medical Education. Chicago: American Medical Association, 1966.

Starfield, B. Primary Care and Health: A Cross-National Comparison. *Journal of the American Medical Association* 266:2268–2271, 1991.

Starfield, B. *Primary Care: Concept, Evaluation, and Policy.* New York: Oxford University Press, 1992.

White, K.L., Williams, T.F., and Greenberg, B.G. The Ecology of Medical Care. *New England Journal of Medicine* 265:885–893, 1961.

Willard Committee. *Meeting the Challenge of Family Practice: The Report of the Ad Hoc Committee on Education for Family Practice of the Council on Medical Education.* Chicago: American Medical Association, 1966.

2

Defining Primary Care

Since its introduction in 1961, the term *primary care*[1] has been defined in various ways, often using one or more of the following categories to describe what primary care is or who provides it (Lee, 1992; Spitz, 1994). These categories include:

- The *care provided by certain clinicians*—Some proposed legislation, for example, lists the medical specialties of primary care as family medicine, general internal medicine, general pediatrics, and obstetrics and gynecology. Some experts and groups have included nurse practitioners and physician assistants (OTA, 1986; Pew Health Professions Commission, 1994);
- A *set of activities* whose functions define the boundaries of primary care—such as curing or alleviating common illnesses and disabilities;
- A *level of care or setting*—an entry point to a system that includes secondary care (by community hospitals) and tertiary care (by medical centers and teaching hospitals) (Fry, 1980); ambulatory versus inpatient care;
- A *set of attributes,* as in the 1978 IOM definition—care that is accessible, comprehensive, coordinated, continuous, and accountable—or as defined by Starfield (1992)—care that is characterized by first contact, accessibility, longitudinality, and comprehensiveness;

---

[1]This chapter is based on the study committee's interim report, *Defining Primary Care: An Interim Report* (IOM, 1994b). The definition of primary care set forth here is the same as that in the interim report.

- A *strategy for organizing the health care system* as a whole—such as community-oriented primary care, which gives priority to and allocates resources to community-based health care and places less emphasis on hospital-based, technology-intensive, acute-care medicine (IOM, 1984).

No one category incorporates all the dimensions that people believe are denoted by the term, and this has resulted in a lack of clarity and consensus about the meaning of the term. A clue to the difficulty lies in an ambiguity of the word *primary*, as noted in a background paper prepared for this report by Safran (1994). If *primary* is understood in its sense of first in time or order, this leads to a relatively narrow concept of primary care as "first contact," the entry point, or ground floor of health care delivery. This meaning of primary can connote only a triage function in which patients are then passed on to a higher level of care. If, on the other hand, primary is understood in its sense of *chief, principal,* or *main,* then primary care is better understood as central and fundamental to health care. This latter idea of primary care supports the multidimensional view of primary care envisioned by this IOM committee.

This IOM committee thus reaffirms the importance of continuing to define primary care as multidimensional; it cannot be defined on the basis of a single dimension, as attractive as this might be for policymakers who formulate workforce policy and must decide who does or does not provide primary care. This exigency, faced by policymakers, has led to reliance on criteria based on, for example, residency training, care setting, or level of care (e.g., first contact). While fully acknowledging the need for a clearer sense of primary care to guide policymaking at the national and state level, the committee believes a careful but multidimensional view of primary care will permit a far richer discussion of organizational opportunities, professional development and satisfaction, health curricula reform, and improved health care than any single-dimension definition. Given this belief, the committee draws on an extensive literature that includes a number of key articles on primary care.

EARLY DEFINITIONS

The notion of the *primary physician* providing continuing and comprehensive care was introduced very early. According to what became known as the Millis Commission report (1966), the primary physician

> will serve as the primary medical resource and counselor to an individual or a family. When a patient needs hospitalization, the services of other medical specialists, or other medical or paramedical assistance, the primary physician will see that the necessary arrangements are made, giving such responsibility to others as is appropriate, and retaining his own continuing and comprehensive responsibility (Millis, 1966, p. 37).

The report also emphasized the need to focus "not upon individual organs and systems but upon the whole man, who lives in a complex social setting. . . ." (Millis, 1966, p. 35).

From 1966 to the late 1970s variations and refinements of this concept appeared. In a classic monograph, Alpert and Charney (1973) described the three fundamental characteristics of *primary medicine* (defined as the personal health system of individuals and families, as distinguished from public health): Its clinicians (1) provide first-contact care (as compared to that based on referral), (2) assume responsibility for the patient over time regardless of the presence or absence of disease, and (3) serve as the "integrationist" (serve a coordinating role). They also believed that it was preferable that all family members be cared for by the same physician.

THE FIRST IOM DEFINITION

In 1978, the IOM published a report entitled *A Manpower Policy for Primary Health Care: Report of a Study* (IOM, 1978). The second chapter, which had been released a year earlier as an interim report, defined the essence of primary care as it should and could be practiced: "accessible, comprehensive, coordinated and continual care delivered by accountable providers of personal health services." That definition has been widely quoted and used. It has also proved useful as a touchstone for guiding the assessment of primary care.

DISTINGUISHING PUBLIC AND PERSONAL HEALTH SERVICES

Meanwhile, work by McKeown (McKeown and Lowe, 1966) and others led to a better understanding of socioeconomic, environmental, and behavioral factors affecting the health of individuals and populations. In a 1974 report, Canadian Minister of Health Marc Lalonde emphasized the importance of health promotion and disease prevention (Lalonde, 1974). Subsequently, the notion of primary care was expanded to the point where the World Health Organization conference at Alma-Ata defined *primary health care* as

essential health care . . . made universally accessible to individuals and families in the community . . . through their full participation and at a cost that the community and country can afford (WHO, 1978, p. 3).

This definition takes the notion of primary care beyond what this IOM committee intends. The committee therefore distinguishes between two terms: (1) *primary health care* as defined by WHO, which includes such public health measures as sanitation and ensuring clean water for populations; and (2) this committee's term *primary care*, which focuses on the delivery of personal health services. For this reason, this report addresses personal health services in a context of family and community health and not population-based, public health services.

There are, however, vital and important linkages that must be developed between primary care and public health programs, which are addressed in Chapter 5 and Appendix F of this report. The committee notes the increasing intersections and changing connections between public health and personal health care delivery. Two examples are childhood immunization and tuberculosis outreach services that are now provided in the public health sector to individuals and communities.

THE 1984 REPORT ON COMMUNITY-ORIENTED PRIMARY CARE

Abramson and Kark (1983) pioneered an emphasis on communities and their connections with health practitioners. They viewed community-oriented primary care (COPC) as "a strategy whereby elements of primary health care and of community medicine are systematically developed and brought together in a coordinated practice" (p. 22) to facilitate community diagnosis, health surveillance, monitoring, and evaluation. They pointed out that such an approach requires knowledge of the demographic, socioeconomic, and cultural characteristics of communities.

A study completed by the IOM in 1984 addressed COPC. That report described *community-oriented primary care* operationally as

> the provision of primary care services to a defined community, coupled with systematic efforts to identify and address the major health problems of that community through effective modifications in both the primary care services and other appropriate community health programs (IOM, 1984, p. 2).

According to that report, primary care practitioners strive to deliver to their active patients (the "numerator" in a COPC context) effective and appropriate health services. The word *community* as used by the COPC committee meant any group of people that the practice or program might reasonably expect to cover, the denominator in this COPC context. That is, the study directed its attention toward communities that included both users *and* nonusers of primary care services and did *not* mean the community defined solely in terms of the practice's active patients.

An operational COPC model must satisfy three criteria. There must be (1) a primary care practice, (2) an involved and definable community, and (3) a set of activities that systematically address the major health issues of the community. In its case studies at that time, the IOM COPC committee found no fully developed example of COPC. However, efforts to implement COPC continue in many countries, including the United States, with varying degrees of success. In the meantime, broad-scale changes in health delivery have refocused attention on the delivery of personal health care services in this country.

CHANGES IN HEALTH CARE DELIVERY TODAY

The health care system, health policy, and health professional curricula in the United States are undergoing a period of rapid change. These shifts, particularly those that involve integrated delivery systems (Shortell et al., 1994), could not have been reflected in the Millis Commission report, Alpert and Charney's 1973 monograph, or the earlier IOM reports. The development of integrated delivery systems means that primary care cannot be defined or assessed in isolation from the overall system of which it is a part. Such systems involve physicians and other clinicians and the facilities they use to deliver a full array of services, for a given price, to a defined population, in settings that are most appropriate to patients' needs. The committee's first task in considering the future of primary care was to reexamine the 1978 IOM definition and other definitions in light of the current and anticipated health care environment. In doing so, the committee supported the essential features of the earlier definition but also believed that a new definition was needed to reflect the dramatic health system changes that have occurred in the past 18 years and to anticipate and to guide future change. After release of its recent interim report (IOM, 1994b), the committee invited public comment on its definition at conferences, in a published article (Vanselow et al., 1995), and in a public hearing that specifically requested comment on its definition. After considering all comments and letters that the committee received, it concluded that the new definition was well accepted, and it was adopted for this report. The definition is described below.

THE NEW DEFINITION AND AN EXPLANATION OF TERMS

The definition of primary care adopted by the IOM Committee on the Future of Primary Care follows:

> **Primary care is the provision of** *integrated, accessible health care services* **by clinicians who are** *accountable* **for addressing a large** *majority of personal health care needs*, **developing a** *sustained partnership* **with** *patients*, **and practicing in the** *context of family and community*.

Each term in the definition is summarized in Box 2-1 and is explained in the text following the box.

Although the new definition is based on the 1978 IOM definition, it recognizes three additional important perspectives for primary care: (1) the patient and family, (2) the community, and (3) the integrated delivery system. The 1978 IOM report addressed the first perspective, and the 1984 COPC report addressed the second. In recognizing the increasing importance to primary care of the integrated delivery system, this report addresses all three. The new definition thus stresses the importance of the patient-clinician relationship (a) as understood

---

BOX 2-1 **Definition of Primary Care**

Primary care is the provision of *integrated, accessible health care services* by *clinicians* who are *accountable* for addressing a large *majority of personal health care needs*, developing a *sustained partnership* with *patients*, and practicing in the *context of family and community.*

Integrated is intended in this report to encompass the provision of *comprehensive, coordinated,* and *continuous* services that provide a seamless process of care. Integration combines events and information about events occurring in disparate settings, levels of care and over time, preferably throughout the life span.

> *Comprehensive.* Comprehensive care addresses any health problem at any given stage of a patient's life cycle.
>
> *Coordinated.* Coordination ensures the provision of a combination of health services and information that meets a patient's needs. It also refers to the connection between, or the rational ordering of, those services, including the resources of the community.
>
> *Continuous.* Continuity is a characteristic that refers to care over time by a single individual or team of health care professionals ("clinician continuity") and to effective and timely communication of health information (events, risks, advice, and patient preferences) ("record continuity").

Accessible refers to the ease with which a patient can initiate an interaction for any health problem with a clinician (e.g., by phone or at a treatment location) and includes efforts to eliminate barriers such as those posed by geography, administrative hurdles, financing, culture, and language.

Health care services refers to an array of services that are performed by health care professionals or under their direction, for the purpose of promoting,

---

in the context of the patient's family and community, and (b) as facilitated and augmented by health care teams and integrated delivery systems.

Figure 2-1 illustrates this committee's view that the patient-clinician relationship is central to primary care. The patient and primary care clinician interact with one another as appropriate and also with others in the community and the health care delivery system. The shaded areas in the figure are fields this committee newly emphasizes in this report. On the patient side, the family and community provide the context in which to understand and assist the patient. On the health care delivery side, the team and integrated delivery system provide the means for extending and improving the delivery of primary care. One challenge that faces health care clinicians, policymakers, and administrators is how to foster and maintain such patient-clinician relationships in a complex, integrated delivery system. A correlative challenge is how to realize the potential benefits of

maintaining, or restoring health (Last, 1988). The term refers to all settings of care (such as hospitals, nursing homes, clinicians' offices, intermediate care facilities, schools, and homes).

Clinician means an individual who uses a recognized scientific knowledge base and has the authority to direct the delivery of personal health services to patients.

Accountable applies to primary care clinicians and the systems in which they operate. These clinicians and systems are responsible to their patients and communities for addressing a large majority of personal health needs through a sustained partnership with a patient in the context of a family and community and for (1) quality of care, (2) patient satisfaction, (3) efficient use of resources, and (4) ethical behavior.

Majority of personal health care needs refers to the essential characteristic of primary care clinicians: that they receive all problems that patients bring—unrestricted by problem or organ system—and have the appropriate training to diagnose and manage a large majority of those problems and to involve other health care practitioners for further evaluation or treatment when appropriate. *Personal health care needs* include physical, mental, emotional, and social concerns that involve the functioning of an individual.

Sustained partnership refers to the relationship established between the patient and clinician with the mutual expectation of continuation over time. It is predicated on the development of mutual trust, respect, and responsibility.

Patient means an individual who interacts with a clinician either because of illness or for health promotion and disease prevention.

Context of family and community refers to an understanding of the patient's living conditions, family dynamics, and cultural background. *Communities* refers to the population served, whether they are patients or not. Community can refer to a geopolitical boundary (a city, county, or state), or to neighbors who share values, experiences, language, religion, culture, or ethnic heritage.

these organizations and the interdependent work of health professionals in improving patients' health. The committee addresses these issues in Chapter 5 of this report.

Recommendation 2.1 To Adopt the Committee's Definition

This committee has defined primary care as the provision of *integrated, accessible health care services* by *clinicians* who are *accountable* for addressing a large *majority of personal health care needs*, developing a *sustained partnership* with *patients*, and practicing in the *context of family and community*. The committee recommends the adoption of this definition by all parties involved in the delivery and financing of pri-

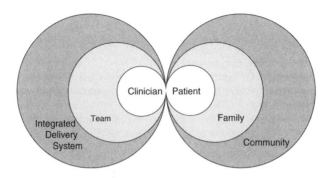

FIGURE 2-1 The interdependence of the constitutents of primary care showing the centrality of the patient-clinician relationship in the context of family and community and as furthered by teams and integrated delivery systems.

mary care and by institutions responsible for the education and training of primary care clinicians.

The committee has recommended that health policymakers, professional groups and academic health centers adopt this definition for use in all relevant activities within their scope of responsibility. The committee believes that the adoption of a common definition will lead to greater clarity in health care delivery and program planning and in policy debate. If those involved in service, education, financing, and research in primary care use the same starting point in discussions, then substantive differences can be better understood and resolved and the field moved forward. Consistent with this objective, this report uses the committee's definition as a reference for framing its discussion about the content of primary care and research priorities.

Patient

By the term *patient*, this committee means an individual who interacts with a clinician either because of disease or illness or for health promotion and disease prevention. In primary care systems not all people are patients. People are usually patients at one time or another, but most of the time they are simply individuals going about their lives. They may need advice, information, or periodic physical examinations for preventive care. Wherever the term patient is used in this report, it is intended to mean individuals who seek care, whether or not they are ill at a given time.

Family

Use of the term *families* in this report acknowledges the care-giving roles, the concerns of family members, and the impact of family dynamics on health and illness. The phrase *context of family and community* in the definition refers to an understanding of the circumstances and facts that surround a patient, such as the patient's living conditions, family dynamics, work situation, and cultural background. This committee uses the term family broadly to include a unit of individuals in a household and not necessarily a traditional nuclear family. Often a family member is a care giver—a parent caring for a child or an adult child caring for a parent. Unless clinicians can understand the nature of these relationships, they can miss opportunities to provide effective care of individual health care needs.

Community

The community refers to the population potentially served, whether its members are patients or not. Community can refer to a social group residing in a defined geopolitical boundary (a city, county, or state), or to neighbors who share values, religion, experiences, language, culture, or ethnic heritage. The use of the term *community* draws attention to the different perspectives that need to be addressed. On the one hand, primary care needs to be concerned with the care that primary care clinicians deliver to individuals. This more traditional and familiar area of primary care addresses the care and outcomes of individual patients. In its broadest sense, primary care must also be linked to the larger community and environment in which people work and live. This also requires that primary care clinicians know the major causes of mortality and morbidity for the community served and that they be aware of what may be happening in the community—such as occupational dangers, patterns of childhood injuries, patterns of lead poisoning or other environmental hazards, homicides, issues of domestic violence, and epidemics. Health care needs and objectives may not be the same for individuals and communities or for different individuals or different communities. Individuals have particular health care needs; the community has a broader perspective that emphasizes improving health status[2] and reforming the way care is delivered. An integrated delivery system has the potential for melding both perspectives.

Prevention of illness and promotion of healthful lifestyles are critical components of good health. The benefit gained from these elements and from broader

---

[2]*Health status* refers broadly to physical, mental, and social function. Although health status is largely determined by environmental and personal variables, health services should, to the extent possible, contribute to improved health status.

public health activities as compared to medical care can vary. For example, 10- to 24-year-olds are likely to gain much more in improved health and rates of survival by preventing injuries and damage due to violence, motor vehicle accidents, or substance abuse than they are from direct, episodic, medical care (IOM, 1994a).

Many barriers to better health are related to socioeconomic status, education, and cultural and behavioral components. At times these factors extend far beyond health care or health promotion and disease prevention in their usual sense. Primary care clinicians are not "responsible" for the environment, jobs, housing, or violence. Primary care clinicians do, however, need to be knowledgeable about the context of their patients' lives and problems and need to be knowledgeable about the resources in their communities. Health promotion activities within the primary care setting should (a) incorporate information about the needs of the community and its health problems, (b) provide information to the community and those involved in its public health efforts, and (c) help to coordinate the public health, social services, mental health services, and other appropriate services needed by patients.

Clinician

The term *clinician* refers to an individual who uses a recognized scientific knowledge base and has the authority to direct the delivery of personal health services to patients. A clinician has direct contact with patients and may be a physician, nurse practitioner, or physician assistant. For most families, this clinician is a physician. Additionally, primary care clinicians might turn to a variety of other individuals—both with and without health care training—for their assistance and skill in particular areas. Examples of individuals other than primary care clinicians who can contribute to primary care are dentists, pharmacists, physical therapists, nutritionists, and social workers. Among many cultural groups, traditional healers may also provide primary care, for instance, the *promotoras* for Latino communities.

This committee has chosen to use the term *clinician* in contrast to other familiar terms such as *provider*. Provider is commonly used not only to refer to individuals who deliver care but also to denote facilities or organizations that provide health care, such as hospitals or health plans. In medical centers, clinician refers to someone with direct patient care responsibilities; in using the term clinician, then, this report underscores the importance of a relationship between a patient and an individual who uses judgment, science, and legal authority to diagnose and manage patient problems.

Partnership

The term *sustained partnership* refers to the relationship established between the patient and clinician with the mutual expectation of continuation over time. It is predicated on the development of mutual trust, respect, and responsibility. A bond to someone you trust may be healing in and of itself. This relationship is essential when guiding patients through the health system. As an ideal, primary care occurs within the context of a personal relationship between a patient and clinician that extends beyond an episode of illness. Such a relationship, developed over time, fosters a sense of trust and confidence. The partnership facilitates tailoring a specific intervention or specific advice to the needs and the circumstances of a particular person.

Although it denotes participation by both clinician and patient, the term *partnership* does not necessarily imply equal roles for clinicians and patients. The term *partnership* means that the patient and clinician agree on goals and the ways to reach them. It also implies that the patient's values and preferences are taken into account. In some cases patients desire and should have a large role in identifying health problems to be addressed or deciding how they should be addressed. In other cases a patient may prefer a relatively small role and may delegate most decisionmaking to a clinician.

The committee that developed the 1978 IOM definition viewed the primary care clinician as a manager for a specific episode of care. The current IOM committee broadens that view considerably. It emphasizes the need for the primary care clinician not only to manage a given health concern and address issues of preventive health care, but also to act as an advocate for the patient in a larger health system so that the patient knows who is directing and coordinating his or her care.

This personal relationship is more important to some people in some circumstances than it is to others. Although in many circumstances patients may feel quite comfortable knowing that information is in their medical record where all those involved in their care can find it, patients often prefer (when they can) to see a particular clinician. Challenges remain, however, about how to structure a team so that personal relationships are supported, and these challenges are addressed later in this report.

Health Care Needs and Health Care Services

The term *personal health care needs* includes reference to physical, mental, emotional, and social concerns that involve the functioning of an individual. The term *health care services* refers to an array of services that are performed by health care professionals or under their direction, for the purpose of promoting, maintaining, or restoring health (Last, 1988). The term refers to all settings of care (e.g., hospitals, nursing homes, clinicians' offices, community sites, schools, and homes). Health care services address physical, mental and emotional, and social functioning. The last concept pertains to any health condition that impedes an individual's ability to fulfill his or her social roles, such as ability to attend school, work at gainful employment, or perform as a parent.

Integrated

A key term used in this definition is *integrated*. It can be defined as "combining separate and diverse elements or units so as to provide a harmonious, interrelated whole" (see Merriam-Webster, 1981; Random House, 1983). *Integrated* as used in this report describes health care that coordinates and combines into an effective whole all of the personal health care services a patient needs over an extended period of time—that is, the provision of *comprehensive, coordinated*, and *continuous* services. Those three terms from the 1978 IOM definition—comprehensive, coordinated, and continuous—are described below. When using the term *integrated* this committee refers to all the office visits and phone calls, tests, procedures, and encounters that individuals have, regardless of setting such as clinic, hospital emergency room, doctor's office, hospital admission, or rehabilitation unit. It refers to services and information about the services of all the clinicians and other health professionals—pharmacists, nurse midwives, physical therapists, and so forth—over an extended period of time.

The committee's use of the term *integrated* when describing personal health care services should not be confused with the widely used term as applied to horizontal and vertical integration in integrated delivery systems. To integrate primary care fully, however, primary care clinicians are likely to practice in teams and in such integrated delivery systems.

Some care settings are very small systems, for example, a solo clinician, nurse, one administrative person, and referrals as needed for specialty care. One can envision, however, the development of primary care networks that use computers to link smaller systems of care into broader ones that are facilitated by information networks (IOM, 1991). Although such primary care networks might not include a full range of services, such developments would move small systems toward the sort of integration envisioned by the committee.

Integration might be fostered in other ways. An example would be linking specialist (e.g., dermatology, psychiatry) or subspecialist (e.g., gastroenterology, pulmonology, cardiology) services for a patient with a chronic illness with a primary care clinician (either within the subspecialty practice or elsewhere) who continues to provide primary care.

Comprehensive

First contact. One element of primary care is sometimes referred to as *first contact*. In a well-developed and functioning system, primary care is the usual and preferred route for entry into the health care system (although not necessarily in all circumstances). In the simplest model, the primary care clinician receives patients regardless of the disease or organ system involved and addresses a given patient's problem. This function may require sorting out a mixture of ill-defined symptoms, or it may call for fairly straightforward treatment. This simplest of models, however, should be flexible enough to allow patients to enter at various points or to skip given steps (e.g., authorizations) based on their needs and safety as well as on efficiency considerations. The model is not intended to describe a regimented or restrictive processing system, and indeed such a system would be antithetical to the committee's future vision of primary care.

First contact with a primary care clinician may lead to referrals to other resources—for example, to a nurse practitioner for diabetic counseling or to a cardiologist for subspecialty care. In some cases, self-referral by a patient may be appropriate—for example, for recurrent problems previously treated by another specialist or subspecialist or refractions for eyeglass prescriptions. Information about these encounters should be provided to the primary care clinician.

The descriptor *first contact* is not, however, a sufficient or unique attribute for defining primary care. It is not unique because some first contact events do not represent primary care—for example, those that occur through an occupational health service, an emergency room, or at a health fair booth for cholesterol screening. Such encounters can be integral to the patient's health care, and information gathered should be communicated to the primary care practice.

First contact is not adequate to define primary care. Insofar as it has come to imply the restriction of primary care to a triage function, it neglects the other characteristics of primary care included in this report, specifically, comprehensiveness.

A derivative term is *gatekeeper*. In many circles, the term *gatekeeper* has been used to describe the function of using the experience and judgment of the primary care clinician to determine whether diagnostic tests are necessary, whether a patient's problem can be handled by the primary care practice, or whether a person needs to be evaluated or treated by another specialist or subspecialist. The primary care clinician's important role in helping the patient to obtain appropriate care in a complex health system requires a high level of skill and judgment. This judgment involves both clinical and economic decision-making.

Patients may view gatekeeping with suspicion because they fear that efforts to control use of services and to manage costs may have subtle effects on clinicians and ultimately work to the detriment of their health. By contrast, many managers, benefits officers, and policymakers view gatekeeping with enthusiasm because they see it as a way of rationalizing, if not restricting, the use of health care resources. The term *gatekeeper*, therefore, has come to have a pejorative connotation when primary care is reduced to the function of managing costs and especially when it implies that the gate is kept closed most of the time. This committee categorically rejects the view that the primary care clinician acts mainly or exclusively as a gatekeeper.

The scope of primary care. Comprehensive care is intended to mean care of any health problem at a given stage of a person's life. It includes ongoing care of patients in various care settings (e.g., hospitals, nursing homes, clinicians' offices, community sites, schools, and homes). Ideally, the primary care clinician listens to the patient, makes diagnoses, manages, and screens for other health care problems. The clinician educates and communicates with the patient and others who may be involved including other specialists when appropriate. He or she assumes ongoing responsibility for maintaining contact with and care of the patient and assuring that the care provided is suitable.

The IOM definition refers to *a large majority of personal health care needs.* That phrase refers to the essential characteristic of primary care clinicians. Primary care clinicians receive all problems that people bring—unrestricted by problem or organ system—and have the appropriate training to manage a large majority of those problems, involve other health professionals for further evaluation or treatment when appropriate, and continue to act as advocates for their patients.

Primary care addresses a mixture of health problems along the spectrum of disease as they occur singly or in combination within a single individual. Ideally, primary care clinicians elicit the full range of patient concerns, whether physical or psychosocial, and are sensitive to the concerns and circumstances that accompany a patient's symptoms.

Not all patient problems represent deviations from normal health that require medical action. Thus, primary care clinicians have a special responsibility to be sensitive to those concerns that are appropriately labeled health problems and those that are not or that could be made worse by medical intervention.[3]

Some portion of patient problems—based on a particular individual's needs, on safety, or on efficiency considerations—may not be manageable by the primary care clinician. Some portion may require the expertise of other health professionals, other specialists, or subspecialists. The following categories of service are within the scope of primary care as defined by the committee:

1. Acute care.[4]   (a) The primary care clinician evaluates a patient with a symptom or symptoms sufficient to prompt him or her to seek medical attention. Health concerns may range from an acute, relatively minor, self-limited illness, to a complex set of symptoms that could be life threatening, to a mental problem. The clinician arranges for further evaluation by specialists or subspecialists when

---

[3]The term *undifferentiated* is sometimes used to describe a patient whose symptoms and preventive care needs have not been given diagnostic labels—the kind of patient often seen in primary care. Such a term expresses the complexity of the primary care task, but it is not otherwise a particularly useful or attractive term.

[4]The usual distinction between acute and chronic is not always exact. Duodenal ulcers and depressive disorder are examples of conditions that may be neither clearly acute nor clearly chronic.

appropriate. (b) The clinician manages acute problems or, when beyond the scope of the particular clinician, arranges for other management of the problem.

2. Chronic care. A primary care clinician (a) serves as the principal provider of ongoing care for some patients who have one or more chronic diseases, including mental disorders, with appropriate consultations, and (b) collaborates in the care of other patients whose chronic illnesses are of such a nature that the principal provider of care[5] is another specialist or subspecialist. The primary care clinician manages intercurrent illnesses, provides preventive care (e.g., screening tests, immunization, counseling about life style), and incorporates knowledge of the family and the patient's community. An example would be managing the dermatitis, hypertension, or upper respiratory infection of a patient who is under the care of a rheumatologist for rheumatoid arthritis.[6]

3. Prevention and early detection. The primary care clinician provides periodic health assessments for all patients, including screening, counseling, risk assessment, and patient education. Periodic health assessments are a natural part of primary care. Primary care must reflect an understanding of risk factors associated with these illnesses, including genetic risks, and of the early stages of disease that may be difficult to detect at their outset.

4. Coordination of referrals. The clinician coordinates referrals to and from other clinicians and provides advice and education to patients who are referred for further evaluation or treatment.

Coordinated

Coordination ensures the provision of a combination of health services and information that meets a patient's needs and specifically means the connection

---

[5]The term *principal provider* or *principal physician* is sometimes used to describe clinicians who may be specialists or subspecialists and from whom some patients receive most of their health care because of a major ongoing illness or medical condition—e.g., cancer, heart disease, rheumatoid arthritis, chronic renal failure, or chronic obstructive pulmonary disease. When they act as the principal physician for a patient, these specialists may provide primary care (as defined by this committee) to these patients; on the whole, however, the committee believes that most patients should obtain such primary care—e.g., preventive screening and counseling and care for episodes of injury or illness not clearly related to their major condition—from primary care clinicians.

[6]In medicine, the term *generalist* is sometimes used to denote the medical disciplines of family practice, general pediatrics, and general internal medicine—i.e., clinicians whose roles are focused on a wide spectrum of health-related problems and ambulatory care but often include hospital care, including care provided in specialized hospital units such as intensive care.

The terms *generalist* and *primary care clinician* are both sometimes used to describe specialists who provide a broad spectrum of care *within their own specialty*, for example, generalist orthopedist, primary care ophthalmologist, or generalist obstetrician. The committee emphasizes, however, that general care of an organ such as the eye or of an organ system does not constitute primary care as the committee defines it.

within and across those services and settings—putting them in the right order and appropriately using resources of the community. The goal is to focus on interactions with patient and family and their health concerns, clarify clinical care decisions, advise hospitalized patients and their families, and help patients and their families cope with the social and emotional implications of disease or illness.

The primary care clinician will often be the principal clinician of inpatient care for certain conditions that require hospitalization (e.g., pneumonia). He or she follows hospitalized patients, even those whose principal clinician may be another specialist or a subspecialist. The primary care clinician brings knowledge of a patient and family history and social perspectives to bear on that episode of care. He or she may also manage other aspects of the patient's care during hospitalization, for example, by continuing to manage the diabetes of a patient who is hospitalized for a hip fracture. The primary care clinician also coordinates a patient's transition between health care settings—for example, hospital and home, home and nursing home, or between clinicians' offices.

Teams. An individual may need a set of activities that entail an array of services. The sorts of tasks required are varied and require efficient management of both care and available resources. The emphasis in this report on primary care teams acknowledges that we need not depend on a single person to organize and provide all expertise and care. Much primary care is rendered by single clinicians, but increasingly teams are managing the health problems presented to primary care practices.

A team is a group of people organized for a particular purpose. It may be organized to subdivide tasks, increase accessibility, extend the expertise of a health professional by drawing on several disciplines, or delegate tasks that do not require a clinician's level of training. The organization of health services for a defined population can be greatly facilitated by using teams with a mix of practitioners who together are best suited to meet the range of needs of a given patient or of a population. A pediatric practice may, for instance, have a group of pediatricians, a pediatric nurse practitioner, and a receptionist who work together giving general pediatric care. Other multidisciplinary groups might be organized for the care of those with particular problems, for instance, children who have been abused. Yet another case in point is a geriatric practice team that includes a social worker, dietitian, physical therapist, geriatric nurse practitioner, and geriatrician. Team composition may vary by specialty, subspecialty, clinician interest, expertise, and resource availability. The population served by a team may vary by gender, age, health concerns, and social problems.

As indicated in Figure 2-1, the committee views the team as an extension of the patient-clinician relationship, not as an alternative to it. Although primary care can be delivered by teams, exemplary primary care requires that one or more members of that team develop a close one-on-one relationship with the patient.

Interaction with Communities

The effective coordination of health care services requires an intimate knowledge of the communities in which those services are delivered. Such coordination requires:

- knowledge of other health care agencies, resources, and institutions within the community (e.g., the availability of classes teaching cardiopulmonary resuscitation or of smoking cessation support groups);
- an understanding of the financial concerns of patients and communities;
- an understanding of the cultural, nutritional, and belief systems of patients and communities that may assist or hinder effective health care delivery;
- an understanding of day-to-day lifestyle patterns of patients and in communities that may enhance or diminish coordination efforts (e.g., work, transportation, school, child care); and
- effective information systems.

Continuous

The term *continuous* means "uninterrupted in time, without cessation; being in immediate connection or spatial relationship" (Random House, 1983). In this report, continuity is a characteristic that refers to care over time by a single individual or team of health professionals ("clinician continuity") and to effective and timely communication of health information (about events, risks, advice, and patient preferences) ("record continuity"). It applies to both space and time. It combines events and information about events occurring in disparate settings, at different levels of care, and over time, preferably throughout a person's life span. Continuity encompasses patient and clinician knowledge of one another and the effective and timely communication of health information that should occur among patients, their families, other specialists, and primary care clinicians.

Clinician continuity, when achieved, is an effective way to provide continuity in primary care. The patient record is essential, but it does not substitute for clinician continuity. Information such as family, sexual, or emotional problems is often intentionally excluded from the record because of concern that the information might not be kept confidential. Knowledge of a patient's usual ways of dealing with symptoms such as pain is another example of how care can be dramatically altered by sustained personal relationships between clinicians and patients. A patient's story is dynamic, not static, and a primary care clinician who knows a patient understands when it is appropriate to use or disregard medical information in the patient's record because it is outdated, irrelevant, or wrong.

Given our propensity in the United States for moving from place to place, for changing employers and health insurance plans, and for changing household composition, such a goal of clinician continuity is not likely to be perfectly realized. At an earlier time in our nation's history, a general practitioner might care for a couple, deliver their babies, and see those children grow, marry, and have children of their own. Physicians knew their patients and their families, and record keeping was modest. Now the amount and complexity of information that must be recorded about patients is steadily increasing. If continuity is to be an element of primary care, it will likely be achieved by ensuring that relevant, accurate information is available to all clinicians, even when the relevance of data is not immediately apparent; this reflects the goal of record continuity.

Increasingly sophisticated clinical (as opposed to financial) information systems are being developed rapidly, and the progress of computer technology has led to efforts to aggregate health data from many sources such as hospitals, offices, pharmacies, and laboratories. Such data aggregation has tremendous potential for ensuring the continuity of medical information. Two IOM reports, *The Computer-Based Patient Record: An Essential Technology for Health Care* (1991) and *Health Data in the Information Age: Use, Disclosure, and Privacy* (1994c), have explored the benefits and risks of computer-based patient records and community-level information databases. Meeting the need for continuity of care is a significant element of computer-based patient records. Continuity can apply to an integrated delivery system, a primary care practice or team, and a single primary care clinician. Although the ideal may be an individual seeing the same clinician at each visit, there may be tradeoffs between continuity and access. Continuity of clinician may be more important for some people and in some circumstances than others. For a patient with hypertension who makes appointments at regular intervals, for example, it is particularly helpful to both the clinician and the patient to ensure continuity over a succession of visits so that progress and the need to adjust medications can be assessed. Continuity can also be a major source of satisfaction both to patients and clinicians, as it fosters the long-term relationships that represent, for many clinicians, a significant reward of medical practice.

Sometimes, however, patients have an acute illness or injury and would prefer quick access to a clinician who might be known to them as a member of a team or practice or might even be a complete stranger at an urgent care center or emergency room. Balancing the competing values of continuity and access represents one of primary care's important challenges and one for which integrated delivery systems may offer some solution.

Comment: Who Is a Primary Care Clinician?

The committee acknowledges that the use of a functional definition of primary care does not provide a definitive answer to those who must count primary care clinicians and develop policies regarding payment for primary care services. Because the definition is normative, the committee hopes that the functions of primary care will increasingly be adopted. The committee preferred not to use the definition to differentiate among clinicians, despite the interest of many that it do so. If pushed to differentiate among clinicians, however, the committee would use as a reference its knowledge of how clinicians are currently trained and what they generally do in their practices. From this perspective, it seems clear that those trained in family medicine, general internal medicine, general pediatrics, many nurse practitioners, and physician assistants are trained in and are generally most likely to practice primary care.

Some physicians in other specialties may also be practicing primary care. For example, obstetrician-gynecologists undoubtedly deliver some primary care, but others are surgically oriented, are not currently trained in primary care, and do not consider themselves primary care clinicians (Leader and Perales, 1995). Subspecialists, particularly in internal medicine, may provide primary care for a subset of their patients with chronic conditions and they may well provide a majority of those patients' care. Specialists in emergency medicine may provide first-contact care, but this care is not usually integrated. It is certainly not continuous, and this care does not comprise the full spectrum of primary care. General dentists may provide general dental care, but they do not provide the full range of health care needs. If other medical specialties and health care disciplines are to provide primary care as defined by this committee, training would have to be modified as described in Chapter 7.

Accessible

The term *accessible* means "easy to approach, reach, enter, speak with or use" (Random House, 1983). It refers to the ease with which a patient can initiate an interaction for any problem with a clinician (e.g., by phone or at a treatment location). It includes efforts to eliminate barriers such as those posed by geography, administrative hurdles, financing, culture, and language.

Accessibility is also used to refer to the ability of a population to obtain care. For example, having public insurance coverage does not guarantee access to care if no local clinicians are willing to see individuals with that form of insurance. Accessibility is also a characteristic of an evolved system of which primary care is a basic unit. Potential enrollees of a health plan want to know whether they have "access" to other specialists or subspecialists, how to obtain that access, and where they would need to go to be seen on a weekend or holiday. Determining the level of accessibility that has been achieved is a judgment that is based on a community's needs and expectations as defined by members of the community and based on their experiences in obtaining the care they desire.

Clearly, no single clinician can be accessible at all times to all patients. Integrated delivery systems seek ways to ensure timely care, to meet patient expectations, and to use resources efficiently. Integrated delivery systems may establish policies regarding maximum waiting times for an urgent appointment, periodic health examinations, coverage when a clinician is out of the office, getting patients into substance abuse treatment programs on a weekend, or handling an out-of-market-area health problem.

Primary care is a key to accessibility because it can provide an entry point to appropriate care. It is the place to which all health problems can be taken to be addressed. People do not have to know what organ systems are affected, what disease they have, or what kind of skills are needed for their care.

Accessibility also involves user friendliness. It refers to the information people have about a health system that will allow them to navigate the system appropriately. Health plan members need directions about where to call for certain information or how to get help in an emergency. Patients need to understand how to get information about self-care or community resources, about the use of computer technologies to obtain information, or about how to obtain their own medical record.

Administrative barriers to accessing health services deserve special attention. Even when individuals have a benefit package that provides coverage for a given service, administrative hurdles may sometimes be so burdensome, whether by intention or not, that the service is effectively denied. For example, the approval process for obtaining mental health care is, in some organizations, so intimidating or personally intrusive that individuals may be unable to get timely assistance or even any adequate care at all.

Accessibility can also be increased by the use of telecommunication and information management technologies. Clinicians in rural practices can use telecommunication to obtain subspecialist consultations in the reading of diagnostic tests for heart function and for reading slides of pathology specimens.

Accountable

The term *accountability* in a general sense means the quality or state of being responsible or answerable. It also means "subject to the obligation to report, explain, or justify" (Random House, 1983). Like all clinicians, primary care clinicians are responsible for the care they provide, both legally and ethically. Primary care clinicians and the systems in which they operate are, in particular, answerable to their patients and communities, to legal authorities, and to their professional peers and colleagues. They can be held legally and morally responsible for meeting patients' needs in terms of the components of value—quality of care, patient satisfaction, efficient use of resources—and for ethical behavior. Primary care clinicians are also accountable to the systems in which they work.

Quality of Care

Primary care practices are accountable for the quality of care they provide.

A 1990 IOM report, *Medicare: A Strategy for Quality Assurance*, defined quality of care in the following way:

> Quality of care is the degree to which health services for individuals and populations increase the likelihood of desired health outcomes and are consistent with current professional knowledge (IOM, 1990, p. 21).

Focusing on outcomes requires clinicians to take their patients' preferences and values into account as together they make health care decisions. The phrase *current professional knowledge* in the above definition underscores the need for health professionals to stay abreast of the knowledge base of their professions and to take responsibility for explaining to their patients the processes and expected outcomes of care. High standards for licensure, certification, and recertification for all individuals and institutions that provide health care must be maintained. In accordance with this definition, primary care practices must be able to address three fundamental quality-of-care issues in their assessments of quality and in the steps they take to improve it (IOM, 1990):

1. *Use of unnecessary or inappropriate care.* This makes patients vulnerable to harmful side effects. It also wastes money and resources that could be put to more productive use.

2. *Underuse of needed, effective, and appropriate care.* This is related to accessibility—that is, whether people get the proper preventive, diagnostic, or therapeutic services; whether they delay seeking care; and whether they receive appropriate recommendations and referrals for care. People may face geographic, administrative, cultural, attitudinal, or other barriers that limit their abilities to seek or receive such care. Within managed care environments, efforts to restrict access to some services may result in underuse of care.

3. *Shortcomings in technical and interpersonal aspects of care.* Technical quality refers to the ways health care is delivered—e.g., skill and knowledge in making correct diagnoses and prescribing appropriate medications. Professional competence is critical to high quality care, and inferior care results when health care professionals are not competent in their clinical areas. Interpersonal aspects of care are of particular importance in primary care. They include listening, answering questions, providing information, and eliciting and including patient (and family) preferences in decisionmaking. Interpersonal skills are also essential to primary care clinicians in their roles as coordinators, as members of a collaborative team, and with other health professionals.

Quality Measurement

Quality assessment involves more than the measurement of a single clinician's performance. The performance of systems—including primary care and entire integrated delivery systems—must also be measured and improved.

Greater attention will need to be focused on the failures of systems of care in which well-trained and well-meaning clinicians work. A shift in focus is occurring—from reviewing records of individual patients and compiling assessments of care by individual clinicians to monitoring the performance of health plans and populations, and this has other implications for quality measurement. Although individual record review will undoubtedly continue to be necessary in some instances (e.g., surgical complications, adverse drug reactions), the creation of reliable, uniform data systems and the collection of consistent data from a variety of sources means that quality assessment may become less dependent on review of individual cases. This change in perspective from individual patients and clinicians to the performance of health plans might also result in less attention being paid to changes in the patient-clinician relationship. As policymakers shift attention toward systems of care, integration, and team approaches to health care delivery, it will be especially important to understand the relative risks and benefits to health outcomes and patient satisfaction of promoting or disrupting personal relationships.

The appropriate unit of assessment. To assess important attributes of primary care such as continuity, coordination, and the outcomes of and satisfaction with primary care, the most appropriate unit of analysis is the *episode of care* whose beginning and ending points are determined, in principle, by the individual. An episode of care refers to all the care provided for a patient for a discrete illness. A particular episode of care begins when a patient brings a problem to the attention of a clinician (or when a clinician brings a problem to the attention of a patient), and that patient accepts the continuing care that may be offered (should it be needed). Multiple episodes (sometimes referred to as comorbidity) may occur at the same time for a given patient. Because the beginning and ending points of an episode of care are defined in practice by a patient, the use of episodes of care to assess quality explicitly incorporates the patient's perspective whether those episodes last for a visit or two, for a year, or over a patient's lifetime. This means that structures for accountability and especially for measuring outcomes of care need to be able to define and measure episodes of care. In particular, an assessment of the outcome of care—both what is measured and the results of the assessment—may be quite different after a single visit than after an episode of care.

Patient Satisfaction

An emphasis on satisfaction and information highlights the importance of patients' and society's preferences and values and implies that they should be elicited (or acknowledged) and taken into account in health care decisionmaking (IOM, 1990). Knowledge about patient and family experiences in the health care system can be derived from patient reports—interviews and surveys of patients about their care. Patient reports on satisfaction can tell much about patient experiences in terms of access to and coordination of care, interpersonal and technical aspects of care, and understanding of instructions and follow-up advice.

Efficiency

In common parlance, efficiency is related to the organization and delivery of services so that waste and cost are minimized. Underuse of needed services (such as tests, therapies, or assistance) or overuse of services that result in unwarranted interventions or exposure to harm can hurt patients and waste resources—the time of patients and clinicians, money, and access for other patients. Tests that must be repeated because results are lost or wrong are examples of inefficiency that are quality of care problems. Good primary care presupposes a careful effort to manage care to ensure the efficient use of resources including the effective use of other health and social services.

Ethical Behavior

A critical part of accountability in primary care concerns the ethical behavior and decisionmaking by primary health care clinicians in relation to their patients, the community, and the health systems in which they practice. Primary care clinicians are responsible for care that respects and protects the dignity of patients and ensures that an individual's presenting complaint is addressed. Although the issues are not unique to primary care, clinicians must be competent in managing events with significant ethical overtones. These may include informed consent, advance directives, avoidance of conflicts of interest in financial arrangements, care of family members when goals are in conflict, reproductive decisionmaking, genetic counseling, privacy and confidentiality, and equitable distribution of resources. Clinicians are accountable first and foremost to their patients. They are also accountable to the health care systems in which they practice, and this may contribute to tension, especially when they must advocate for a patient's use of resources. Primary care clinicians are always ethically accountable for their advice, consultations, and actions, especially when they have financial or other incentives to use or not use certain resources.

Accountability of Patients

Use of the term *partnership* is intended to convey the idea that both clinicians and patients have responsibilities. Clinicians are accountable as described above; patients are responsible for helping to sustain the relationship, for conveying complete and timely information to the primary care clinician, for undertaking reasonable preventive care, for making healthy lifestyle choices, for seeking care as appropriate, and for participating in the management and treatment plan.

Patients are responsible for their own health to the extent that they are capable—that is, to the extent that they have the knowledge and skills that allow them to participate in improving their health. Patients must also be responsible in their use of resources when they need health care.

ACHIEVING THE GOALS OF PRIMARY CARE AS DEFINED

The committee believes that these attributes of primary care are highly desirable and achievable over time. It also believes that the degree to which current primary care practices match these attributes varies considerably. However, the committee did not want to propose a limited definition of primary care that sets goals that might be more immediately achievable by most practices but does not present challenging goals for the future. Neither did the committee want to establish a commendable but ideal definition of primary care that would bear little relationship to current realities.

In the committee's judgment, all practices deserving the primary care label can aspire to many of the attributes in the near term; indeed, some may already be there. In the spirit of continuous quality improvement, however, the committee believes that all primary care activities must strive toward a fuller realization of these attributes. The pace of accomplishment will vary depending on a practice's starting point, its circumstances, and its resources.

The committee has already indicated its belief that the achievement of the desired attributes of primary care will be easier in some form of integrated delivery system serving a defined population than in isolated practices without a defined member population. A major advantage of integration lies in providing infrastructure support for personal health care services and for developing systems of accountability. Such arrangements often do not exist in many primary care settings and may be a long time in coming. In the meantime, every practice can move toward meeting the goals of primary care.

REFERENCES

Abramson, J.H., and Kark, S.L. Community-Oriented Primary Care: Meaning and Scope. Pp. 21–59 in: *Community-Oriented Primary Care—New Directions for Health Services.* Washington, D.C.: National Academy Press, 1983.

Alpert, J.J., and Charney, E. *The Education of Physicians for Primary Care.* Publ. No. (HRA) 74-3113. Washington, D.C.: U.S. Department of Health, Education, and Welfare, 1973.

Fry, J., ed. *Primary Care.* London: Heineman, 1980.

IOM (Institute of Medicine). *A Manpower Policy for Primary Health Care: Report of a Study.* Washington, D.C.: National Academy Press, 1978.

IOM. *Community-Oriented Primary Care: A Practical Assessment. Volume I. The Committee Report.* Washington, D.C.: National Academy Press, 1984.

IOM. *Medicare: A Strategy for Quality Assurance. Volume I.* K.N. Lohr, ed. Washington, D.C.: National Academy Press, 1990.

IOM. *The Computer-Based Patient Record: An Essential Technology for Health Care.* R.S. Dick and E.B. Steen, eds. Washington, D.C.: National Academy Press, 1991.

IOM. *America's Health in Transition: Protecting the Quality of Health and Health Care. A Statement of the Council of the Institute of Medicine.* Washington, D.C.: National Academy Press, 1994a.

IOM. *Defining Primary Care: An Interim Report.* M. Donaldson, K. Yordy, and N. Vanselow, eds. Washington, D.C.: National Academy Press, 1994b.

IOM. *Health Data in the Information Age: Use, Disclosure, and Privacy.* M.S. Donaldson and K.N. Lohr, eds. Washington, D.C.: National Academy Press, 1994c.

Lalonde, M. *A New Perspective on the Health of Canadians.* Ottawa: Ministry of National Health and Welfare, 1974.

Last, J., ed. *A Dictionary of Epidemiology.* 2d ed. New York: Oxford University, 1988.

Leader, S., and Perales, P.J. Provision of Primary Preventive Health Care Services by Obstetrician-Gynecologists. *Obstetrics and Gynecology* 85:391–395, 1995.

Lee, P. The Problem: Assessing the Primary Care Paradigm. In *Proceedings: Volume I. The National Primary Care Conference.* Washington, D.C., March 29–31, 1992. Rockville, Md.: U.S. Public Health Service, Health Resources and Services Administration, 1992.

McKeown, T., and Lowe, C.R. *An Introduction to Social Medicine.* Oxford: Blackwell, 1966.

Merriam-Webster. *Webster's Third New International Dictionary of the English Language. Unabridged.* Springfield, Mass.: Merriam-Webster, 1981.

Millis, J.S. *The Graduate Education of Physicians.* Report of the Citizens' Commission on Graduate Medical Education. Chicago: American Medical Association, 1966.

OTA (Office of Technology Assessment). *Nurse Practitioners, Physician Assistants, and Certified Nurse-Midwives: A Policy Analysis.* Health Technology Case Study 37. Publ. No. OTA-HCS-37. Washington, D.C.: U.S. Government Printing Office, 1986.

Pew Health Professions Commission. *Nurse Practitioners: Doubling the Graduates by the Year 2000.* San Francisco: Pew Health Professions Commission, 1994.

Random House. *The Random House Dictionary of the English Language, 2nd Edition. Unabridged.* New York: Random House, 1983.

Safran, D.G. Defining Primary Care. Paper prepared for the Committee on the Future of Primary Care, Institute of Medicine, 1994.

Shortell, S.M., Gillies, R.R., and Anderson, D.A. The New World of Managed Care: Creating Organized Delivery Systems. *Health Affairs* 13(Winter):46–64, 1994.

Spitz, B. The Architecture of Reform, or How Do We Build Our Health Care System Around Primary Care When We Don't Know Who a Primary Care Provider Is, How Many We Need, or What They Do? Unpublished draft document, 1994.

Starfield, B. *Primary Care: Concept, Evaluation, and Policy.* New York: Oxford University Press, 1992.

Vanselow, N.A., Donaldson, M.S., and Yordy, K.D. From the Institute of Medicine: A New Defintion of Primary Care. *Journal of the American Medical Association* 273:192, 1995.

WHO (World Health Organization). *Alma-Ata 1978: Primary Health Care.* Report of the International Conference on Primary Health Care, Alma-Ata, Union of Soviet Socialist Republics, 6–12 September 1978. Geneva: World Health Organization, 1978.

3

The Value of Primary Care

In setting out its view of the value of primary care, the committee makes two critical assumptions. First, primary care is the logical basis of an effective health care system. Second, primary care is essential to reaching the objectives that constitute value in health care: high quality care (including achieving desired outcomes), good patient satisfaction, and efficient use of resources. If the health care system is to move in the directions identified in this report, the value of primary care must be clear to the American public, policymakers, communities, educators, individual health professionals, and students. All people—adults as well as children, middle-class as well as poor, the healthy as well as the ill—must be seen to benefit.

This chapter addresses the value of primary care from two main perspectives. The first section provides some illustrative examples of the value of primary care for individuals; they are organized by the key elements of primary care in the definition from Chapter 2 and are oriented to primary care as it should be. The second section focuses on the benefits of primary care for populations and for the broader society. In reviewing evidence that primary care improves the quality and efficiency of care as well as access to care for populations, the section focuses, of necessity, on primary care as it is now provided. Because much of the current provision of primary care does not match all of the attributes set out in the definition, the value of primary care may, in our judgment, be understated compared with its potential benefits.

THE VALUE OF PRIMARY CARE FOR INDIVIDUALS

Primary care is valuable to individuals in at least the five ways listed below:

1. It provides a place to which patients can bring a wide range of health problems for appropriate attention—a place in which patients can expect, in most instances, that their problems will be resolved without referral.

2. It guides patients through the health system, including appropriate referrals for services from other health professionals.

3. It facilitates an ongoing relationship between patients and clinicians and fosters participation by patients in decisionmaking about their health and their own care.

4. It provides opportunities for disease prevention and health promotion as well as early detection of problems.

5. It helps build bridges between personal health care services and patients' families and communities that can assist in meeting the health needs of the patient.

These key components of high quality and efficient health care for individuals are illustrated in vignettes throughout this section of the chapter.[1] Reflecting the nature of primary care, the vignettes include situations in which a variety of seemingly routine or simple problems may be embedded in the possibility of a patient's having conditions that could have serious consequences for his or her health. They illustrate the need for excellent primary care training that underlies clinicians' ability to distinguish among simple, serious, and complex conditions and to provide care for all.

Addressing Most Problems That Patients Bring

Most of the problems that people bring to the health care system are appropriately resolved at the level of primary care. Having the capacity to address "a large majority of personal health care needs" also means that primary care offers patients a sensible and convenient route to appropriate care, which may involve referrals or coordination of services by others; patients do not need to guess for themselves what is causing a symptom or concern to be able to enter the health care system at the right place.

---

[1] Although fictitious composites, the vignettes are drawn from the clinical experience of the committee members to illustrate the terms in the definition and a variety of settings, practitioners, patients, and problems.

Jan Anderson, a 28-year-old woman, visits her doctor because her lower back has been hurting for a week. She has been a patient of Dr. Bloch, a family physician, since she was 10 years old, for a variety of problems. Dr. Bloch has been involved in treating her scoliosis (when she was a young girl) and in managing, over the years, a recurrent kidney infection, irritable bowel syndrome, and, before she used contraceptive pills, painful menstrual cramps, all possible sources of her pain. Dr. Bloch also knows that Ms. Anderson is an avid exercise enthusiast. Dr. Bloch evaluates the low back pain to determine if it is related to one of the earlier problems or to exercise. After he has diagnosed her problem, he treats her and makes arrangements for follow-up care.

Helping patients sort out and resolve such symptoms and dilemmas is an essential feature of primary care. Sometimes evaluation may reveal that, in addition to the patient's stated reason for a visit, an even more important problem or concern lies unspoken and perhaps unacknowledged or unrecognized by the patient.

Caroline Clark is a 40-year-old married woman who manages her own business. She visits her primary care team and sees the nurse practitioner, Donna Washington, complaining of insomnia. Ms. Washington knows that in the past year, Mrs. Clark has had a severe allergic reaction to a bee sting and lithotripsy for a kidney stone; she also knows that Mrs. Clark's 10-year-old son is being treated for leukemia in a nearby medical center, which causes many trips to the hospital, repeated difficult laboratory tests, and frequent school absences; she is aware that Mr. Clark's profession requires frequent and long trips away from home. Ms. Washington prescribes Mrs. Clark a mild sleeping pill, renews her prescription for adrenalin in case she suffers any bee sting in the future, and advises Mrs. Clark about what she may expect in the future regarding kidney stones. Ms. Washington also provides support in coping with these personal and family stresses that may affect her current and future health, including information about how she can, if she wishes, arrange an appointment with a clinical psychologist who is part of her health plan.

These vignettes illustrate that in addressing the "large majority of health needs" the primary care clinician and the patient benefit from the characteristics of primary care, including integration, the development of a sustained partnership, and attention to the context of family and community.

Guiding Patients in Using the Health Care System

A major element of good primary care is the ability of primary care clinicians to diagnose and manage their patients' health care problems. In many cases, this may require considerable understanding of the local health care scene and how best it might be navigated. When patients (or family) are new to an area or otherwise lacking in knowledge of the full range of resources open to them, the primary care team can play a significant role in ensuring that those individuals move through the system efficiently and comfortably. For example, for patients with frightening symptoms such as acute dizzy spells upon awakening, a major question is where to go for help. Is this a problem that requires the services of a specialist, such as a neurologist? Is the problem related to other health problems for which the patient is being treated by a medical subspecialist and a psychiatrist, both of whom have prescribed prescription drugs? A primary care clinician can evaluate the problem and either manage the problem or arrange the appropriate referrals.

More generally, with its complex array of personnel, facilities, technologies, and other components, the health care system can confuse and intimidate patients. Primary care clinicians who know how the health system operates and have the expertise to evaluate information can provide instructions that patients can understand and help patients and families to make appropriate decisions and use the health care system to best advantage. In pediatrics, this concept is known as a "medical home";[2] it is an appealing concept for all ages.

The tasks involved include: coordinating referrals to other specialists and sorting out the sometimes conflicting advice these clinicians give; arranging and overseeing care provided in different settings (e.g., hospitals or nursing homes); and finding and helping to secure ancillary resources such as physical therapy. To be sure, some patients can coordinate much of their own care; all too often, however, this responsibility falls to patients or their families who lack full knowledge of available health care resources. When patients are frail, lack family support, are faced with several difficult options, or have a problem that is complex and not well understood, they need help. Primary care teams can carry out these formidable tasks of coordination on behalf of the patient, drawing on their knowledge of the range of the patient's health problems, family or other social supports, and living arrangements.

Mary Ellerbee, herself elderly, lives with her 83-year-old husband who is being treated for hypertension, diabetes, and poor eyesight. She has moderate dementia and frequently wanders. The couple is cared for by a primary care team; in particular, Robert Griffith, a general internist, and Linda Fuentes, a nurse practitioner, who alternate in seeing the Ellerbees. All of the office staff

---

[2]The American Academy of Pediatrics (AAP, 1992, p. 251) describes the "medical home" (with respect to care for infants, children, and adolescents) as: "accessible, continuous, comprehensive, family centered, coordinated, and compassionate"; "delivered or directed by well-trained physicians who are able to manage or facilitate essentially all aspects of pediatric care"; and involving physicians who "should be known to the child and family and able to develop a relationship of mutual responsibility and trust with them." The IOM committee on pediatric emergency medical services (EMS) strongly endorsed the idea of a medical home, and the contributions of primary care providers, in the context of EMS for children (IOM, 1993b).

are familiar with the couple and their health problems, so that calls can be referred appropriately to Ms. Fuentes and Dr. Griffith. Ms. Fuentes has arranged for a home health aide to assist the couple and has located respite services, and at Mr. Ellerbee's request, Dr. Griffith has been in touch with their only son to give him updates on his parents' health.

Mr. Ellerbee experiences chest pain; in response to a neighbor's call to 9-1-1, he is hospitalized under Dr. Griffith's care, who arranges a consultation by a cardiologist. Ms. Fuentes helps the son find temporary care for his mother and, at the time of Mr. Ellerbee's discharge, Dr. Griffith assesses both Mr. Ellerbee's needs and those of his wife. Other health professionals are involved in their care as needed and to ensure that the couple can remain at home and that both receive appropriate medical care.

Providing an Ongoing Relationship Between Patient and Clinician

Continuity

An important feature of primary care is the continuity that results from an ongoing relationship with clinicians who know their patients and their patients' health histories. Such relationships open opportunities for patients to disclose sensitive problems and for clinicians to discover favorable moments to provide counsel and advice.

Some problems are clearly related one to another; some are not clearly related but, when concurrent, may influence each other. Over the years, primary care clinicians will see patients through waves of episodes of care—some spells of illness and treatment stop, others begin, and others overlap. Periods of wellness are interspersed with problems that are chronic, acute, or intermittent. Some patients have only occasional acute problems that can be treated in isolation—a cough, a sprained ankle—and may seek only assured and rapid access to care. Other patients have problems that are recognized only because of patterns of illness that occur over months and years as opposed to hours or days—such as work-related asthma, or depression that results in many physical complaints. All in all, viewing health care as a continuum of interrelated episodes presents a very different picture of health and health care from one in which illness and disease are considered in isolation.

John Williams is an overweight 48-year-old bank executive who comes to his health plan because of his wife's complaints about his snoring. He wonders whether he has a serious condition called sleep apnea and has heard about multiple options for the ailment—diagnostic tests in a sleep disorders laboratory or neurologic testing, and therapies in the form of nasal surgery by an ear, nose, and throat specialist or laser surgery on the uvula by a plastic surgeon. Dr. Xanthos, his general internist, reviews his medical history, probes especially into Mr. Williams's current lifestyle and responsibilities, and orders a preliminary set of tests. His aim is to understand to what extent the condition is serious and may require surgery, is caused or influenced by Mr. Williams' obesity, his heavy business and social schedule that often involves drinking alcohol in the evening, his sleeping position, or some other problem. Upon the return of the laboratory tests, Dr. Xanthos and Mr. Williams will discuss whether any further evaluations are needed, but in the meantime Mr. Williams is counseled about healthier lifestyle choices he might make in the area of exercise, diet, and alcohol intake.

Time—in effect an element of continuity—is an excellent diagnostic tool. Because of ongoing relationships with patients, primary care clinicians can better evaluate the importance of a patient's symptoms than can practitioners who do not know the patient. This may in turn mean that extensive diagnostic testing for ill-defined symptoms or complaints can be postponed or avoided altogether, because the patient will be assured of follow-up care in person and by telephone.

Another aspect of continuity is having relevant, up-to-date information about a patient available when it is needed. Although this information can reside in paper records and the memories of physicians or others with long-standing relationships to patients, ideally the record will reside on a computer-based patient record that can, with proper authority and passwords and due attention to privacy and confidentiality, be accessed by all clinical members of the primary care team (IOM, 1991; IOM, 1994).

Larry Jones calls his health plan during the weekend because he believes he is experiencing a side effect from his new heart medicine. Although the physician who is on call is not his usual primary care clinician (Dr. Kelly), a list of the patient's current medications, problems, and allergies is available on-line and can be accessed by the on-call physician. Knowing Mr. Jones' diagnosis, the type of medication he has begun and its dosage, the physician changes the dose, assures Mr. Jones that Dr. Kelly will be notified of the change, and advises him to call back if he has further problems.

Accountability

Accountability reflects the degree to which clinicians or health plans take responsibility for the care they provide and the extent to which they are legally and morally answerable for important attributes of that care, such as quality, patient satisfaction, and efficient use of services. Accountability also involves continuing oversight of the patient's condition and placing occasional acute events in the context of a patient's problems. Being accountable also implies some obligation to maintain adequate, accurate, and retrievable records on patients. As implied above with respect to computer-based patient records, primary care can serve as the hub of an integrated health information system; clinicians can increase the accountability of the system by maintaining patient records of, among other things, medications, allergies, laboratory test results, and family medical histories. Such information serves a variety of purposes. For example, by reviewing test results, tracking abnormal findings, and making sure patients know about these results, members of a primary care team can ensure that the health system is accountable for follow-up when it is needed. All such information can help patients avoid the problems that sometimes result when they see many different health practitioners, no one of whom has all the relevant information.

> *Myron Laramie, now 70 years of age, had triple bypass surgery 10 years ago. His current medical problems include diabetes, which he controls with diet; benign prostate enlargement, which his general internist, Dr. Mishalani, checks periodically; and recurrent depression, for which he sometimes takes medications. Recently, he had a cataract operation in his left eye. In all, Mr. Laramie takes six different medications—some several times a day, some daily, and some only when needed—each of which, taken one by one, is effective for a given condition. Mr. Laramie finds it hard to keep track of doses and to recognize side effects and interactions among these medications. Dr. Mishalani knows that overuse of medication in older patients is an important clinical issue and that, if possible, it is preferable to reduce the number of medications a patient must take. Dr. Mishalani cautiously starts a program of carefully withdrawing medications that may not be absolutely necessary. He monitors these medications and helps Mr. Laramie know how to recognize and manage potential side effects and interactions that may arise in the future. The doctor also tracks changes in Mr. Laramie's overall health status and his ability to function independently and confers with specialists who are also treating Mr. Laramie.*

Preventing Illness and Detecting Diseases Early

At all ages, patients benefit from the proactive stance that primary care physicians, nurse practitioners, and physician assistants can take to listen, ask questions, and provide information. Indeed, primary care is often considered the front line for many aspects of health promotion and disease prevention.

> *Annette Nilsson, now 15 years old, has been followed by Dr. O'Brien, a pediatrician, since childhood; she now comes for a visit for treatment of mild acne. This visit presents an opportunity for Dr. O'Brien, who otherwise rarely sees this healthy young woman, to discuss Ms. Nilsson's understandable concerns about changes in her body and to offer appropriate personal guidance concerning smoking, alcohol, sexual activity, and other risk-taking behaviors.*

Primary care fosters early detection of various disorders (including those that begin insidiously). The benefits include earlier and less onerous health care interventions, better and less hurried decisionmaking between the primary care clinicians and patients and their families, and likely lower costs of an episode of care.

> *In a primary care clinic, Dr. Renfroe sees a new patient, Betty Simms, for a sore throat. He also identifies high blood pressure and obesity and learns from Mrs. Simms that she has a two-pack-a-day history of cigarette smoking. Dr.*

Renfroe evaluates her sore throat, determines that it is not bacterial in origin, and suggests some useful remedies; in addition, he counsels her about the dangers of her smoking addiction. With Mrs. Simms's agreement, he arranges to follow up her high blood pressure. Finally, he enlists the assistance of the clinic's receptionist to arrange for Mrs. Simms to have a nutrition consultation concerning her weight problem, noting the interactions between her smoking and eating habits and her hypertension.

Bridging Personal Health Care, Family, and Community

Primary care clinicians can establish links with communities and their resources, including those that patients on their own may not be aware of or be able to gain access to. In this way, they can create valuable bridges between what is done to and for patients and their families within the personal health care system and the preventive health or social services that may be available in the area in which patients reside. Knowledge of the family and community may also help the primary care clinician understand better the health problems and health risks faced by the patient. In addition, personnel in primary care teams and settings may often be able to act on behalf of their patients in settings and circumstances outside the traditional health care environment.

Primary Care and the School

Schools are among the settings most amenable to certain types of primary care, at least for persons from school age through late adolescence or early adulthood.[3] Obviously, schools are environments in which acute illness, emotional stress, and violence all can occur. They are also windows onto health-related problems whose etiology may not, in the first instance, be obvious to school personnel. Primary care outreach may, therefore, be a useful tool for identifying and managing health-related problems before they irreparably damage a person's educational experience and accomplishments.

Johnny Torres, who is eight years old, has been a good student. Midway through the third grade, however, his teacher reports that he is having difficulty

---

[3]A current IOM committee is exploring issues related to a "comprehensive school health program," which consists of health services, education, counseling, nutrition, school policies, and related activities (IOM, 1995). With respect to "school health services," the committee is working with a concept of "a coordinated system that ensures a continuum of care from school to home to community health care provider and back." According to this study (IOM, 1996, in press), the most commonly provided services include first aid and administering medications, screening and referral (immunization, height, weight, vision, and hearing), and services mandated by law for children with disabilities and special health care needs. That committee has found a great deal of interest exists in school-based health centers that provide primary care, especially in disadvantaged areas where students have great needs and limited access to care.

in reading and is "hyperactive" and disruptive in class; she wonders if Johnny has an attention deficit disorder and would benefit from drug therapy. At the teacher's urging, the family calls Dr. Ursini, their pediatrician, who has cared for Johnny since birth. Dr. Ursini knows that a new baby sister is occupying much of Mrs. Torres's time and that the family is under economic stress because Mr. Torres's firm is anticipating layoffs following a corporate merger. At a quickly arranged visit, Dr. Ursini confirms that Johnny is reacting to stress; during a call to the school shortly thereafter, the pediatrician explains to Johnny's teacher and the school principal that no testing or medication is indicated right now but that Johnny would benefit from extra support and attention. Arrangements are made for a follow-up conference in six weeks.

Primary Care and the Elderly

Consistent aspects of caring for elderly patients include how the aging process affects health problems, the provision of care across different institutional settings, the need to involve family and community, and the benefit of working in a sustained relationship. Families of these patients need to be involved in planning for transportation, for direct care, for managing emergencies, and for issues of advance directives.

Assistance with buying groceries, cooking, managing finances, and personal care can be critical, because mobilizing these home or community services may enable elderly persons to stay in their homes or independent living situations rather than be moved to a nursing home. A primary care team can work closely with older persons and their families (or close friends or members of other social support systems, such as churches) to sustain these connections between personal health care services and long-term-care and social services.

Anthony Villarreal, now 88, has been discharged from the hospital following treatment for an episode of severe congestive heart failure, kidney failure, and paralysis caused by a recent stroke; his prognosis is not encouraging. Mr. Villarreal, his family, and his primary care physician, Dr. Young, have agreed that Mr. Villarreal will end his days at home without rehospitalization. His care is then orchestrated by Dr. Young with the help of Susan Zall (a visiting nurse), social services, and the office receptionist. Mrs. Zall obtains needed laboratory tests on a routine basis and sees that oxygen therapy and other services are arranged through social services; the office receptionist directs phone calls from home. Overall assessment of the patient's condition is based on reports from the family and occasional home visits by Dr. Young and Mrs. Zall, who also have advised the family about procedures they will need to take at the time Mr. Villarreal dies, which happens several months later at home.

Primary Care and Public Health

Links between primary, community, and public health functions are important parts of primary care. Although primary care clinicians typically cannot intervene to solve public health problems that require community action, their awareness of infections, risks, and sources of morbidity in communities—in the environment, workplaces, homes, neighborhoods, and schools—can prompt important cooperative relationships with those who can intervene at a community level more effectively.

> *Following a discussion with a teacher, a school-based nurse practitioner, Sarah Aaronson, wonders what might explain the irritable behavior of five-year-old Melissa Edelman. Suspecting lead poisoning, Ms. Aaronson refers Melissa to a community health center. There Jerry Ikle, the center's physician assistant, takes a medical history and does a physical examination and orders appropriate laboratory tests. The lead test result shows elevated levels, and Mr. Ikle notifies his supervising family physician, begins an appropriate protocol-driven treatment, prescribes a follow-up visit with the physician, and alerts the city's medical social worker, Sharon Tang. Mrs. Tang visits Melissa's home, because she has begun to see a pattern of lead poisoning in that part of town, and suspects that it may be caused by old plumbing in many of the houses there. After comparing records, Mr. Ikle and Mrs. Tang alert the local housing authority, the school, and the public health department to both Melissa's case and the broader threat to the community who reside in that area.*

The primary care clinician can also be an effective advocate in the community for needed public health actions. Good examples are the successes pediatricians have had in advancing child health through community actions, e.g., lead abatement, child safety seats, safety caps on medicines, community awareness of child abuse, support of poison control centers, and immunization campaigns.

Comment

These vignettes describe primary care that can be, and is, provided by well-trained, skillful, and dedicated individuals and teams. It would be naive, however, to conclude that the sorts of coordination, continuity, sustained personal relationships, and linkage of services within the health system, the family, and community that have been described here are either easy or inexpensive. Similarly, it would be naive not to recognize the inherent tensions between a drive for efficiency, as reflected in the private-sector reforms in health care delivery, and a desire to maintain strong patient-clinician relationships.

As to the first, the need to assemble, access, and make sense of huge amounts of information is growing. Also rising in intensity is the drive toward more efficient care in a managed care environment, which can sometimes lead to fragmented care that involves many health professionals who work under increasingly stringent time constraints. In the committee's view, however, achieving efficiency by delivering discrete services in this way—care for a sprain by one clinician, management of a serious infection by another, adjustment of chronic medication by a third—cannot be the most important goal of health care delivery; indeed, a "division of labor" approach may not necessarily be the most efficient health care delivery.

Rather, a subtlety exists in patient-clinician relationships that so-called efficient systems cannot replace. An integrative function must be nurtured, and it almost certainly requires sensitivity and judgment on the part of a single, specific individual who knows the patient and the patient's circumstances. A group of clinicians—despite the best of intentions and the best-run team management—cannot replace this function. Moreover, medical records or a computerized summary cannot substitute for verbal and nonverbal communication that is based on an ongoing relationship between patient and clinician.

This tension between organized arrangements that facilitate care and efficient practice, on the one hand, and the intimate and personal relationships that are at the core of health care, on the other, is a central challenge for health care delivery systems. In posing these illustrative scenarios, the committee wishes to draw attention not only to the promise of primary care in pulling these threads together on behalf of the patient but also to the obstacles that opposing trends in health care delivery can place in the path of realizing that promise.

PRIMARY CARE AND COSTS, ACCESS, AND QUALITY

Empirical research, though sometimes indirect, indicates that primary care reduces costs, increases access to appropriate medical services for the population being served, and does not reduce the quality of care, thereby advancing the broader social interests in health care. This section reviews a portion of the literature comparing resource utilization, quality, and access to care among generalists and specialists. Some of this literature is reviewed in greater detail by Bowman (1989), Starfield (1992), Moore (1992), and Blumenthal and Mort (1992) and includes international comparisons of health status and costs as related to a country's primary care orientation, retrospective review of care given to patients in different settings, and randomized studies that assign patients to primary care and non-primary-care arms of a study. Investigators measure and compare the use of resources and the processes and outcomes of care to understand better whether the frequent claims that primary care reduces costs of care and improves quality and access to appropriate care can be justified. As noted at the start of this chapter, such empirical research is based on primary care as it has been or is now delivered in a number of settings. Demonstration of the full benefits of primary care as this committee has defined it will require prospective studies.

As noted by a preeminent researcher in this area, the effectiveness of primary care can be assessed by measuring each attribute of primary care and determining the impact on outcomes such as health status, satisfaction, use of services, and costs of care (Starfield, 1992). Some comparisons are based on structural features that permit or facilitate the provision of primary care and on the performance of that system. Many studies, however, assume that if the structural features of primary care are present (for example, "a usual source of care"), then primary care is being provided. Other studies use the provision of care by health maintenance organizations (HMOs) as a proxy for primary care without estimating the extent to which primary care is actually provided. Readers need to consider these issues when reviewing assertions in the literature about quality and costs of primary care. They must also keep in mind that primary care is a moving target, evolving in response to social, economic, and professional factors as it is being studied.

Costs of Care

The primary care model is widely believed to be less expensive than specialty medicine, in part because payments to primary care clinicians are lower and in part because primary care clinicians tend to use fewer resources than other specialists.

Several studies suggest that primary care physicians tend to deliver less intensive care than specialists, particularly in hospital settings. Manu and Schwartz (1983) studied procedures ordered in a medical service ward of a teaching hospital. When the ward team was headed by a subspecialist, substantially more procedures were ordered, including more colonoscopies, bone marrow biopsies, and exercise treadmill tests. Since then Cherkin et al. (1987) found that recent graduates of internal medicine programs, which included many individuals headed for careers in subspecialties, were twice as likely as recently graduated family physicians to order blood tests, blood counts, chest x-rays, and electrocardiograms for their patients.

The Medical Outcomes Study (MOS) is a major observational study of more than 20,000 patients conducted in the late 1980s and into the 1990s.[4] Greenfield et al. (1992) compared use of resources in specialty practice (cardiology and endocrinology) and generalist practice (family practice and general internal medicine) in five different systems of care that included both fee-for-service and prepaid practice. Adjusting for patient mix and comparing hospital admission rates, annual office visits, prescription drugs, and common tests and procedures, the authors concluded that specialty training as well as payment system and practice organization had independent effects on resource use.

----

[4]Among the analyses from the MOS are those involving primary care performance in fee-for-service and prepaid health care systems (Safran et al., 1994); patient ratings of outpatient visits (Rubin et al., 1993); and diagnosis-specific investigations of hypertension and non-insulin-dependent diabetes mellitus (Greenfield et al., 1995) and depression (Wells et al., 1989; Rogers et al., 1993). A description of the MOS can be found in Tarlov et al. (1989) and Stewart and Ware (1992).

In particular, cardiologists and endocrinologists had higher rates of hospitalization than did family practitioners and general internists. With respect to office visits, endocrinologists had significantly higher rates than the other physician groups. For prescription drugs, the rates for family practice and general internal medicine were "considerably lower" than the rates for the subspecialties, and the proportion of patients having tests and procedures and the mean number of tests and procedures per visit and per year were generally lower for the generalists than for the subspecialists. Overall differences across the four specialties were highly significant statistically.

Another study compared expenditures for Colorado Medicaid patients who were and were not enrolled in a primary care physician program using as outcome variables the use of emergency department and inpatient services (Fryer, 1991). Fryer found a slight increase in expenditures for physician services, but this was more than offset by decreases in inpatient and emergency department expenditures. Overall, there was a 15 percent decrease in costs for the group enrolled in the primary care physician program as compared to usual costs in the Medicaid program in which patients did not have access to a usual primary care physician.

Evidence demonstrating that primary care providers are more efficient in their use of resources has led managed care organizations to use "networks" of primary care physicians. Premiums for managed care plans have been about 7 percent lower than they are for more traditional indemnity insurance plans (Barents Group, 1995). Whether these cost savings can be attributed to better management of care, economies of scale realized through administrative efficiencies, selection bias, or all three, remains unresolved. What cannot be disputed is the rapid growth of managed care based on primary care as a principal way to moderate increases in health care costs.

The supply of primary care physicians in a geographic area also appears to be associated with the level of costs. Dor and Holahan (1990) reported that Medicare physician expenditures were lower in areas with higher numbers of general practitioners (GPs) and family physicians (FPs). Total Medicare expenditures per beneficiary—adjusted for the prevailing charge index—decreased by 1 percent for every 10 percent increase in the supply of GPs and FPs. Similarly, according to Welch et al. (1993), expenditures for the delivery of physicians' services to Medicare beneficiaries are higher in areas of the country with a lower proportion of primary care practitioners. A recent study (Mark et al., 1995) found that U.S. urban counties with higher population densities of family practice and general internal medicine physicians have lower total Medicare Part B reimbursements per beneficiary.

Although evidence indicates that organizational models that emphasize primary care are less expensive than organizational models emphasizing specialty medicine, skeptics may still ask whether such savings come at the expense of good quality care.

The early work of the Ambulatory Sentinel Practice Network (ASPN, 1988) (see Chapter 8), a practice-based research network, included a study that suggested that excellent results can be attained in primary care with less intensive use of services than are indicated by specialty-based practice standards. In a study of usual care of miscarriage as managed in primary care practices, for about half of patients, management departed from textbook recommendations (in which all patients should be hospitalized), but results at follow-up were no different among patients treated according to standard teaching and those who were not. The primary care physicians were evidently able to discriminate on the basis of clinical presentations those women who would do well with less intensive treatment than recommended.

The same network later reported a series of investigations concerning the evaluation of headache and the detection of intracranial tumors, subarachnoid hemorrhages, and subdural hematomas in primary care patients (Becker et al., 1993a, 1993b). Becker and his colleagues found that primary care clinicians used computed tomography (CT) scanning very selectively and that more extensive use of CT scans would be a weak strategy to improve detection of these serious disorders because increased use would lead to higher health care costs and to unintended adverse effects, but they provide little if any benefit. Although these studies are not conclusive, they suggest that policies directed toward the use of low-cost providers will not necessarily lead to a deterioration in the quality of care.

Access to Care

According to an IOM report on access (IOM 1993a), access is the timely receipt of appropriate care. The concept is relevant to primary, specialty, and even exotic or experimental care, but in all cases, access to appropriate care is influenced by the number and distribution of primary care clinicians.

To cite cases in point, when individuals do not have a usual source of primary care because of geographic, financial, or other barriers, the care they receive through emergency departments may be both costly and inefficient (Shea et al., 1992). Lack of health insurance or gaps in insurance can mean loss of a source of primary care (Berman, 1995; Kogan et al., 1995). Having a "regular source of care" is sometimes used as a proxy for availability of primary care and of continuity. The Rand Health Insurance Study demonstrated the benefit of access to primary care services, in particular for the poor, that resulted in improved vision, more complete immunization, better blood pressure control, enhanced dental status, and reduction in estimated mortality in comparison to low-income individuals and their children who had financial barriers to access consisting of cost sharing (Lohr et al., 1986; Goldberg and Newhouse, 1987; Newhouse and the Health Insurance Group, 1993).

Some patients identify the emergency department as their regular source of care (Baker et al., 1994), but this cannot be considered primary care, and as a regular source of care it may not be appropriate to their needs. Hurley et al. (1988) randomized Medicaid patients into two groups: those with a primary care physician and those without. Patients who were assigned to a primary care physician had substantially fewer emergency department visits without an accompanying increase in office visits to a primary care physician.

With respect to hospital admissions, Parchman and Culler (1994) showed that, even after controlling for per capita income, preventable hospitalization rates among adults and children were significantly lower where the ratio of family and general practice physicians to population was greater. Bindman et al. (1995a) and Starfield (1995) report evidence suggesting that preventable hospitalizations are associated with a lack of primary care. Communities in which residents reported lower access to medical care (meaning principally primary care) had higher rates of preventable admissions for chronic medical conditions such as asthma, hypertension, congestive heart failure, chronic obstructive pulmonary disease, and diabetes.

Lurie et al. (1984, 1986) studied the effects of termination of Medi-Cal benefits for California's 270,000 medically indigent adults. They found that access to care and health status of those who lost their health coverage worsened. One year after their benefits were ended, only half of these low-income adults could identify a regular doctor, indicating a lack of access to primary care, and only two in five thought they could obtain care when they needed it. Sixty-eight percent of the group reported a specific episode in which they had not obtained care that they believed they needed; of those patients, 78 percent listed cost as a reason for not obtaining care. The percentage of medically indigent adults satisfied with their care decreased from 97 percent before termination to 40 percent one year after termination of benefits. While these findings extend beyond primary care, the finding of loss of a regular doctor for many would indicate that access to primary care was an important casualty of the loss of health benefits.

Quality of Care

General Observations

How might we know if primary care produces equivalent or better outcomes and increases patient satisfaction compared to other health care delivery arrangements for serving populations with similar needs? Measures can include the classic triad of structure, process, and outcome described by Donabedian (1966, 1980, 1982, 1985). One can quantify underuse and overuse of services as well as technical and interpersonal quality in primary care settings, offices of medical subspecialists, and other settings such as emergency departments. To make such comparisons, one needs, first, to know how to measure primary care and, second, to determine which settings are providing primary care.

Measurement of primary care is made more difficult because the committee's definition emphasizes characteristics of primary care that extend well beyond the competence with which a specific medical service is performed. Both process and outcome data need to relate to the objectives of integration (continuity, comprehensiveness, and coordination), accessibility of services, sustained partnership with patients, the scope of services and the pattern of referrals, and knowledge of relationships to family and community relevant to the provision of primary care.

An important task in comparing the quality of care in primary care and non-primary-care settings is the need to control for variation in the kinds of patients seen in each setting—that is, to account accurately for demographic characteristics and severity and type of illness or injury. As Bindman (1994) notes, the extensive literature comparing generalist and specialist practice is difficult to interpret because of such differences. Studies that have avoided selection bias or adjusted for differences in patient populations have found that primary care physicians use fewer technologies and admit patients to the hospital less frequently.

Outcomes

A primary care orientation has been an important variable in improving health status. It enables individuals to obtain services for illnesses before they become severe (Gonnella et al., 1977). It can improve health by controlling chronic conditions and thereby reducing preventable hospitalizations and what is usually thought to be inefficient utilization of nonemergency services provided by emergency departments. For example, Shea et al. (1992) determined that patients who had uncontrolled hypertension and did not have any primary care physician were more likely to seek emergency department care or to be admitted to a hospital than those with primary care physicians, even after controlling for patients' insurance status and compliance with medical therapy.

Higher levels of primary care in a geographic area are associated with lower mortality rates. Shi (1992) showed a consistent relationship between the availability of primary care physicians and positive health status in 50 states and the District of Columbia, as assessed by age-adjusted and standardized overall mortality, mortality associated with cancer and heart disease, neonatal mortality, and life expectancy; the association held even after controlling for the effect of urban-rural differences, poverty rates, education, and lifestyle factors. His results confirmed an earlier study by Farmer et al. (1991), which found that the ratio of primary care physicians to population was the only consistent predictor of age-specific mortality rates, even when considering such other characteristics as rurality, percentage of female-headed households, education levels, minority status, and poverty rates.

Information from countries with strong systems of primary care is illuminating as well. For example, in the 11 European, Scandinavian, and North American countries studied by Starfield (1994), countries whose health systems are more oriented toward primary care generally realize better population outcomes. They achieve better health status (based on 14 indicators such as low birthweight ratio, neonatal mortality, age-adjusted life expectancy, and years of potential life lost), higher satisfaction with health services among their populations, lower expenditures per capita, and lower medication use.

The only study to compare outcomes of care in general and subspecialist practice is the Medical Outcomes Study. Outcomes of care for primary care and specialty care for patients with hypertension and diabetes mellitus were compared in an observational study with follow-up at three periods. Measured outcomes included mortality, disease-specific physiological markers, and measures of physical and emotional health. The authors found that clinicians in medical subspecialties (cardiology and endocrinology) used more services than did clinicians in family medicine and general internal medicine for patients with cardiac disease and diabetes mellitus, even after controlling for patient mix (patients' sociodemographic characteristics and severity of their illness). The research team also determined that the number of office visits, percentage of patients tested per visit, and the percentage of patients admitted to the hospital were higher for medical subspecialists than for clinicians in family medicine or general internal medicine (Greenfield et al., 1995).

In terms of outcomes, no meaningful differences were found in the mean health outcomes (including 7-year mortality) for moderately-ill patients with hypertension or non-insulin-dependent diabetes mellitus. Without further research, MOS conclusions based on the care of patients with diabetes mellitus cannot be extrapolated to the management of other conditions, but the evidence from this study indicates that care for these conditions by specialists does not result in better outcomes than care provided by generalists.

Attributes of Primary Care

Comprehensiveness. Certain attributes of primary care, including comprehensiveness, continuity, and coordination of care, are associated with better health outcomes and patient satisfaction. Hochheiser et al. (1971) compared the number of emergency department visits by children in 1967, before and after the opening of a neighborhood health center in Rochester, New York. They reported a 38 percent decrease in emergency department visits by center-area children from 1967 to 1970. For routine care of these children, the primary care setting can be presumed to be more appropriate and less expensive than alternative settings, such as emergency departments or hospitals.

Alpert et al. (1976) compared the effectiveness of comprehensive family-focused pediatric care with the episodic pediatric care provided at hospitals and public clinics. The patients with comprehensive care had fewer hospitalizations, operations, illness visits, and "no-show" appointments; they had more health supervision visits and used more preventive services; and they reported higher patient satisfaction.

Continuity. Continuity, in the primary care context, has several meanings. It refers to care over time by a single individual or team of health professionals, but it can also refer to continuity of information about the patient.

Starfield and others have reviewed research evidence that continuity of care is "associated with more indicated preventive care, better identification of patients' psychosocial problems, fewer emergency hospitalizations, fewer hospitalizations in general, shorter lengths of stay, better compliance with appointments and taking of medications, and more timely care for problems" (Starfield, 1986, p. 194). Research has linked continuity of care to improved health outcomes. For example, Shear et al. (1983) used pregnancy as a tracer condition to analyze the association between clinician continuity and the quality of ambulatory care. Utilizing a retrospective cohort study design, they examined two groups of pregnant women—one cared for in family practice centers and the other in obstetric clinics. The newborn infants of women in the family practice group, who had much higher clinician continuity, were of higher birthweight, even after controlling for race, income, education, and parity of their mothers.

Using a double-blind randomized trial of elderly men assigned to either a "provider-continuity group" or a "provider-discontinuity group," Wasson et al. (1984) found that patients in the continuity group had fewer emergency admissions and shorter hospital lengths of stay. These patients also viewed their providers as more knowledgeable, thorough, and interested in patient education. Billings and Teicholz (1990) reported that patients with a single individual whom they considered to be in charge of their care experienced much lower rates of preventable hospital admissions.

Coordination. When patient care is well coordinated, it reflects an appropriate range of services that are orchestrated in a rational, cost-effective manner. Coordinated care can lower the risk of harmful complications of unnecessary tests and procedures (Franks et al., 1992). Furthermore, because coordination of care can often reduce the numbers of tests and procedures performed, it can lower the overall costs of care. Although several authors have expressed concern about the risks that undertreatment might pose for patient outcomes (Hillman, 1987; Reagan, 1987; Stephens, 1989), little if any evidence indicates that coordination of care might be associated with unfavorable outcomes, once confounding factors are taken into account (Franks et al., 1992).

Computer-based information systems lie in the future for primary care and are an important element of both continuity and coordination. For example, in one randomized controlled trial, Rogers and Haring (1979) found that computerized feedback of certain types of information enhanced patient care by facilitating coordination. Summaries with information about patients—including a problem list, medications, results of laboratory tests, and suggested courses of action for care—were given to some physicians before their patient visits. Those patients whose doctors received such summaries had more completed procedures and referrals, more designated diets, and more discovery of new problems. These patients also spent, on average, fewer days in the hospital.

Management of Referrals

An important tenet of primary care is that self-referral defeats coordination of care, risks picking the wrong type of clinician and receiving less than optimum care, may result in additional and sometimes inappropriate referrals by specialists to other specialists, and increases the cost of medical care. Most managed care plans insist that the primary care clinician be the pathway to specialty care. Some empirical work supports this principle in terms of its effect on quality. For example, Roos (1979) found that the appropriateness and outcomes of tonsillectomy and adenoidectomy were better when patients had been referred to specialists by primary care physicians than when they were self-referred.

Specialists tend to refer to other specialists less appropriately than generalists (Rothert et al., 1984; Flood et al., 1993). Self-referral may be associated with other quality-of-care problems. For instance, although specialists seem to achieve better results than primary care physicians when treating patients with problems within their specialty, they do less well outside their specialty area (Rhee et al., 1981).

When referrals by primary care physicians are required before visits to specialists, use of specialty services and emergency room visits drops. Martin et al. (1989) randomized patients into two groups; one required a referral for specialty services and the other did not. The patients in the plan with the referral requirement had an average of 0.3 fewer visits to a specialist over a one-year period. These findings have obvious implications for costs of services as well as for the appropriateness of care, illustrating how cost and quality considerations are often intertwined.

Preventive Care

Studies show conflicting evidence about the comparative levels of preventive services provided by generalists and specialists, though Dietrich and Goldberg (1984) found that *both* generalists and specialists were well below preventive services guidelines in providing these services to their patients. More recently, a telephone survey in urban California found that having a regular source of primary care has several positive features (Bindman et al., 1995b); compared to individuals who did not have a regular source of care, those who did (after controlling for differences in health insurance status) received more preventive care services.

THE LIMITS OF PRIMARY CARE
IN IMPROVING POPULATION HEALTH

What are the limits of medical care—in particular, of primary care—in improving health status? Chapter 2 defined primary care and differentiated it from primary *health* care as defined by the World Health Organization (1978, p. 3). As noted there, primary *health* care includes population-oriented services such as sanitation and safe drinking water. By contrast, primary care as defined by this committee includes personal health services but not population-based, public health services.

The distinction between public and personal health services is not the only boundary of interest, however. Those who emphasize community-oriented primary care (COPC) view COPC as a strategy for focusing attention on community determinants of health, especially socioeconomic determinants (Abramson and Kark, 1983; IOM, 1984). COPC proponents and others recognize that health care by itself, whether primary or specialty-based services, will have a limited impact on health status until or unless these determinants of public and social health are addressed.

The aggregate benefits in health status to be gained from increasing income or education greatly outweigh the gains from medical intervention. For example, health status has been demonstrated repeatedly to have a direct, positive relationship to per capita income and to level of education. Similarly, preventing injuries from violence, child neglect, or motor vehicle crashes and deterring the adverse health effects of teenage pregnancy, substance abuse, and sexually transmitted diseases are critical to the health of the community.

Despite diligent efforts by individual clinicians to assist individual patients, these broader influences on health may outweigh the contributions of traditional personal health services. During the committee's site visit to one rural area, a primary care clinician described the community's poverty, illiteracy, lack of transportation, and lack of knowledge about self-care, all of which made caring for acutely ill children and the elderly with common chronic problems particularly difficult and discouraging. She depicted her primary care services as "a cup bobbing on a sea of social problems."

High levels of teenage pregnancy, perinatal mortality, substance abuse, or occupational illness all signal factors far beyond the capacity of individual health care or even health promotion and disease prevention programs to cope with successfully. Primary care clinicians do, however, form an important bridge between the health and public health realms—that is, between personal and population health services. They have knowledge of community and environmental conditions and understand how their particular patients may be affected by those conditions. Clearly, primary care clinicians are not "responsible" for the lack of prenatal care, substance abuse, outbreaks of infectious disease, or malnutrition, and they cannot alone shoulder the burdens of social dysfunction. They can and do, however, promote collaborative working relationships that include community resources, employer- or school-based initiatives, lay workers, and volunteer support groups. As discussed in Chapter 5, primary care is an arrangement well suited to forming these relationships.

Finally, most primary care interventions are undertaken at the level of personal health services. Nonetheless, the committee believes that such interventions—whether counseling, referral, or active listening—are made more effective by a sustained and personal relationship with patients' families and knowledge of their communities. In this way, an important conceptual and practical link between personal and population health services is both maintained and enhanced.

SUMMARY

The value of primary care to individuals is found in all the core elements of the definition of primary care. The vignettes in this chapter illustrate that primary care provides a place to which patients can bring a wide range of health problems for appropriate attention; guides patients through the health system; facilitates an ongoing relationship between patients and clinicians in which patients participate in decision making about their health and their own care; provides opportunities for disease prevention and health promotion as well as early detection of problems; and helps build bridges between clinicians and patients' families and communities. Empirical research also indicates the merits of primary care as a means of improving the overall performance of the health care system, by improving the quality and efficiency of care and expanding access to care. The chapter comments on the relationships between personal health care services (i.e., primary care) and public health services focused on the population. Chapter 4 explores in more detail the nature of primary care.

REFERENCES

AAP (American Academy of Pediatrics). Ad Hoc Task Force on Definition of the Medical Home. The Medical Home. In *Emergency Medical Services for Children: The Role of the Primary Care Provider.* J. Singer and S. Ludwig, eds. Elk Grove Village, Ill.: American Academy of Pediatrics, 1992.

Abramson, J.H., and Kark, S.L. Community-Oriented Primary Care: Meaning and Scope. Pp. 21–59 in: *Community-Oriented Primary Care—New Directions for Health Services.* Washington, D.C.: National Academy Press, 1983.

Alpert, J.J., Robertson, L.S., Kosa, J., et al. Delivery of Health Care for Children: Report of an Experiment. *Pediatrics* 57:917-930, 1976.

ASPN. Spontaneous abortion in Primary Care. A Report from ASPN. *Journal of the American Board of Family Practice.* 1:15–23, 1988.

Baker, D.W., Stevens, C.D., and Brook, R.H. Regular Source of Ambulatory Care and Medical Utilization by Patients Presenting to a Public Hospital Emergency Department. *Journal of the American Medical Association* 271:1909–1912, 1994.

Barents Group. *The Role of Primary Care Physicians in Controlling Health Care Costs: Evidence and Effects.* Prepared for the American Academy of Family Physicians. Washington, D.C.: Barents Group, 1995.

Becker, L.A., Green, L.A, Beaufait, D., et al. Use of CT Scans for the Investigation of Headache: A Report from ASPN, Part 1. *Journal of Family Practice* 37:135–141, 1993a.

Becker L.A., Green L.A., Beaufait D, et al. Detection of Intracranial Tumors, Subarachnoid Hemorrhages, and Subdural Hematomas in Primary Care Patients: A Report from ASPN, Part 2. *Journal of Family Practice* 37: 135–141, 1993b.

Berman, S. Uninsured Children. An Unintended Consequence of Health Care System Reform Efforts. *Journal of the American Medical Association* 274:1472–1473, 1995.

Billings, J., and Teicholz, N. Data Watch. Uninsured Patients in District of Columbia Hospitals. *Health Affairs* 9(Winter):158-165, 1990.

Bindman, A.B. Primary and Managed Care: Ingredients for Health Care Reform. *Western Journal of Medicine* 161:78-82, 1994.

Bindman, A.B., Grumbach, K., Osmond, D., et al. Preventable Hospitalizations and Access to Health Care. *Journal of the American Medical Association* 274:305-311, 1995a.

Bindman, A.B., Grumbach, K., Osmond, D., et al. Primary Care and Receipt of Preventive Services. Unpublished document. San Francisco: Bindman, San Francisco General Hospital and the Institute for Health Policy Studies, University of California, San Francisco, 1995b.

Blumenthal, D., and Mort, E. Primary Care for the Uninsured: A Review of the Literature. Draft of a paper prepared under contract for the Office of Technology Assessment, U.S. Congress. Boston: Massachusetts General Hospital and Harvard Medical School, 1992.

Bowman, M.A. The Quality of Care Provided by Family Physicians. *Journal of Family Practice* 28:346–355, 1989.

Cherkin, D.C., Rosenblatt, R.A, Hart, L.G., et al. The Use of Medical Resources by Residency-Trained Family Physicians and General Internists. *Medical Care* 25:455–468, 1987.

Dietrich, A.J., and Goldberg, H. Preventive Content of Adult Primary Care: Do Generalists and Subspecialists Differ? *American Journal of Public Health* 74:223–227, 1984.

Donabedian, A. Evaluating the Quality of Medical Care. *Milbank Memorial Fund Quarterly* 44:166–203, July (part 2), 1966.

Donabedian, A. *Explorations in Quality Assessment and Monitoring.* Vols. 1–3. Ann Arbor, Mich.: Health Administration, 1980, 1982, 1985.

Dor, A., and Holahan, J. Urban-Rural Differences in Medicare Physician Expenditures. *Inquiry* 27:307–318, 1990.

Farmer, F.L., Stokes, C.S., Fiser, R.H., and Papini, D.P. Poverty, Primary Care and Age-Specific Mortality. *Journal of Rural Health* 7:153–169, 1991.

Flood, A.B., Fremont, A.M., Bott, D.M., et al. Comparing Disease-Specific Practice Patterns of Generalists and Specialists. Presentation at the annual meeting of the Association for Health Services Research, Washington, D.C., June 1993.

Franks, P., Clancy, C.M., and Nutting, P.A. Gatekeeping Revisited—Protecting Patients from Overtreatment. *New England Journal of Medicine* 327:424-429, 1992.

Fryer, G.E. Evaluation of the Primary Care Physician Program. Unpublished report to the Colorado Department of Social Services, November, 1991.

Goldberg, G.A., and Newhouse, J.P. Effects of Cost Sharing on Physiological Health, Health Practices, and Worry. *Health Services Research* 22:279–306, 1987.

Gonnella, J., Cattani, J., Louis, D., et al. Use of Outcome Measures in Ambulatory Care Evaluation. In: G. Giebink, N. White, and E. Short, eds. *Ambulatory Medical Care—Quality Assurance 1977.* La Jolla, Calif.: La Jolla Health Science Publications, 1977.

Greenfield, S., Nelson, E.C., Zubkoff, M., et al. Variations in Resource Utilization Among Medical Specialties and Systems of Care: Results from the Medical Outcomes Study. *Journal of the American Medical Association* 267:1624–1630, 1992.

Greenfield, S., Rogers, W., Mangotich, M., et al. Outcomes of Patients With Hypertension and Non-Insulin-Dependent Diabetes Mellitus Treated by Different Systems and Specialties: Results from the Medical Outcomes Study. *Journal of the American Medical Association* 274:1436–1444, 1995.

Hillman, A.L. Financial Incentives for Physicians in HMOs: Is There a Conflict of Interest? *New England Journal of Medicine* 317:1743–1748, 1987.

Hochheiser, L.I., Woodward, K., and Charney, E. Effect of the Neighborhood Health Center on the Use of Pediatric Emergency Departments in Rochester, New York. *New England Journal of Medicine* 285:148-152, 1971.

Hurley R.E., Freund, D.A., and Taylor, D.E. Emergency Room Use and Primary Care Case Management: Evidence from Four Medicaid Demonstration Programs. *American Journal of Public Health* 79:843–846, 1988.

IOM (Institute of Medicine). *Community-Oriented Primary Care: A Practical Assessment. Volume I. The Committee Report.* Washington, D.C.: National Academy Press, 1984.

IOM. *The Computer-Based Patient Record: An Essential Technology for Health Care.* R.S. Dick and E.B. Steen, eds. Washington, D.C.: National Academy Press, 1991.

IOM. *Access to Health Care in America.* M. Millman, ed. Washington, D.C.: National Academy Press, 1993a.

IOM. *Emergency Medical Services for Children.* J.S. Durch and K.N. Lohr, eds. Washington, D.C.: National Academy Press, 1993b.

IOM. *Health Data in the Information Age: Use, Disclosure, and Privacy.* M.S. Donaldson and K.N. Lohr, eds. Washington, D.C.: National Academy Press, 1994.

IOM. *Defining a Comprehensive School Health Program: An Interim Statement.* D. Allensworth, J. Wyche, E. Lawson, and L. Nicholson, eds. Washington, D.C.: National Academy Press, 1995.

IOM. *Schools and Health: Our Nation's Investment.* D. Allensworth, J. Wyche, E. Lawson, and L. Nicholson, eds. Washington, D.C.: National Academy Press, in press.

Kogan, M.D., Alexander, G.R., Teitelbaum, M.A., et al. The Effect of Gaps in Health Insurance on Continuity of a Regular Source of Care Among Preschool-Aged Children in the United States. *Journal of the American Medical Association* 274:1429–1435, 1995.

Lohr, K.N., Brook, R.H., Kamberg, C.J., et al. Use of Medical Care in the Rand Health Insurance Experiment: Diagnosis- and Service-Specific Analyses in a Randomized Controlled Trial. *Medical Care* 24:(9 Suppl.):S1–S87, 1986.

Lurie, N., Ward, N.B., Shapiro, M.F., and Brook, R.H. Termination from Medi-Cal—Does It Affect Health? *New England Journal of Medicine* 311:480–484, 1984.

Lurie, N., Ward, N.B., Shapiro, M.F., et al. Special Report. Termination of Medi-Cal Benefits: A Follow-Up Study One Year Later. *New England Journal of Medicine* 314:1266-1268, 1986.

Manu, P., and Schwartz, S.E. Patterns of Diagnostic Testing in the Academic Setting: The Influence of Medical Attendings' Subspecialty Training. *Social Science and Medicine* 17:1339-1342, 1983.

Mark, D.H., Gottleib, M.S., Zellner, B.B., et al. Medicare Costs and the Supply of Primary Care Physicians. Unpublished document. Milwaukee, Wisc.: D.H. Mark, Medical College of Wisconsin, 1995.

Martin, D.P., Diehr, P., Price, K.F., and Richardson, W.C. Effect of a Gatekeeper Plan on Health Services Use and Charges: A Randomized Trial. *American Journal of Public Health* 79:1628–1632, 1989.

Moore, G.T. The Case of the Disappearing Generalist: Does It Need to Be Solved? *The Milbank Quarterly* 70:361–379, 1992.

Newhouse, J.P., and the Health Insurance Group. *Free for All? Lessons from the RAND Health Insurance Experiment.* Cambridge: Harvard University Press, 1993.

Parchman, M.L., and Culler, S. Primary Care Physicians and Avoidable Hospitalization. *Journal of Family Practice* 39:123–128, 1994.

Reagan, M.D. Sounding Board. Physicians as Gatekeepers: A Complex Challenge. *New England Journal of Medicine* 317:1731–1734, 1987.

Rhee, S.-O., Luke, R.D., Lyons, T.F., and Payne, B.C. Domain of Practice and the Quality of Physician Performance. *Medical Care* 19:14–23, 1981.

Rogers, J.L., and Haring, O.M. The Impact of a Computerized Medical Record Summary System on Incidence and Length of Hospitalization. *Medical Care* 17:618–630, 1979.

Rogers, W.H., Wells, K.B., Meredith, L.S., et al. Outcomes for Adult Outpatients with Depression Under Prepaid or Fee-for-Service Financing. *Archives of General Psychiatry* 50:517–525, 1993.

Roos, N.P. Who Should Do the Surgery? Tonsillectomy-Adenoidectomy in One Canadian Province. *Inquiry* 16:73-83, 1979.

Rothert, M.L., Rovner, D.R., Elstein, A.S., et al. Differences in Medical Referral Decisions for Obesity Among Family Practitioners, General Internists, and Gynecologists. *Medical Care* 22:42–55, 1984.

Rubin, H.R., Gandek, B., Kosinski, M., et al. Patient Ratings of Outpatient Visits in Different Practice Settings. Results from the Medical Outcomes Study. *Journal of the American Medical Association* 270:835–840, 1993.

Safran, D., Tarlov, A.R., and Rogers, W. Primary Care Performance in Fee-for-Service and Prepaid Health Care Systems. Results from the Medical Outcomes Study. *Journal of the American Medical Association* 271:1579–1586, 1994.

Shea, S., Misra, D., Ehrlich, M.H., et al. Predisposing Factors for Severe, Uncontrolled Hypertension in an Inner-City Minority Population. *New England Journal of Medicine* 327:776-781, 1992.

Shear, C.L., Gipe, B.T., Mattheis, J.K., et al. Provider Continuity and Quality of Medical Care: A Retrospective Analysis of Prenatal and Perinatal Outcome. *Medical Care* 21:1204-1210, 1983.

Shi, L. The Relationship Between Primary Care and Life Chances. *Journal of Health Care for the Poor and Underserved* 3:321–335, 1992.

Starfield, B. Primary Care in the United States. *International Journal of Health Services* 16:179–198, 1986.

Starfield, B. *Primary Care: Concept, Evaluation, and Policy.* New York: Oxford University Press, 1992.

Starfield, B. Is Primary Care Essential? *The Lancet* 344:1129–1133, 1994.

Starfield, B. Editorial. Access—Perceived or Real, and to What? *Journal of the American Medical Association* 274:346–347, 1995.

Stephens, G. Can the Family Physician Avoid Conflict of Interest in the Gatekeeper Role? An Opposing View. *Journal of Family Practice* 28:701–704, 1989.

Stewart, A.L., and Ware, J.E., eds. *Measuring Functioning and Well-Being: The Medical Outcomes Study Approach.* Raleigh-Durham, N.C.: Duke University Press, 1992.

Tarlov, A.R., Ware, J.E., Greenfield, S., et al. The Medical Outcomes Study: An Application of Methods for Monitoring the Results of Medical Care. *Journal of the American Medical Association* 262:925–930, 1989.

Wasson, J.H., Sauvigne, A.E., Mogielnicki, P., et al. Continuity of Outpatient Medical Care in Elderly Men: A Randomized Trial. *Journal of the American Medical Association* 252:2413-2417, 1984.

Welch, W.P., Miller, M.E., Welch, H.G., et al. Geographic Variation in Expenditures for Physicians' Services in the United States. *New England Journal of Medicine* 328:621-627, 1993.

Wells, K.B., Hays, R.D., Burnam, M.A., et al. Detection of Depressive Disorder for Patients Receiving Prepaid or Fee-for-Service Care: Results from the Medical Outcomes Study. *Journal of the American Medical Association* 262:3298–3302, 1989.

World Health Organization. *Alma-Ata 1978: Primary Health Care.* Report of the International Conference on Primary Health Care, Alma-Ata, USSR, 6–12 September 1978. Geneva: World Health Organization, 1978.

4

The Nature of Primary Care

Primary care can be a rewarding and challenging enterprise. Its position in relation to the body of health care was characterized in 1961 in the now classic paper "The Ecology of Medical Care." This report by White and his colleagues (White et al., 1961) found that for every 1,000 adults, 750 people perceived a personal illness of some sort in a given month and 250 people sought care from a health care professional. Few of these patients were seen by specialists or hospitalized, and only a tiny fraction made their way to academic centers where most medical teaching and research take place. Primary care could be considered the care provided to these 250 individuals—care that is positioned between self-care and the remainder of the clinical enterprise. Primary care also includes carefully defined efforts to promote health and prevent disease in the entire population in coordination with public health activities.

On the one hand, the problems presented to primary care physicians are sufficiently important for patients to seek help. On the other hand, most of the problems are resolved at the level of primary care and typically do not result in referral, consultation, or hospitalization. Indeed, problems that can be resolved at the primary care level are known to constitute the bulk of the contemporary clinical enterprise.

The committee learned through site visits, public testimony, and workshops that primary care is neither so easy that anyone can do it, nor so difficult that no one can do it. The knowledge base required in primary care includes elements from the biomedical, behavioral, and social sciences, clinical epidemiology, and biostatistics, but the base required in primary care is not merely the sum of existing specialty knowledge found in medicine and nursing. Some of these elements are shared with public health (e.g., epidemiology and biostatistics), and many are shared with other fields of medicine. Primary care practice uses a unique blend of these knowledge bases, skills, and communication style. This chapter, without attempting to be exhaustive, describes further the content and characteristics of primary care.

CONTENT OF PRIMARY CARE

The Large Majority of Health Care Needs

The committee's definition of primary care stresses that primary care clinicians address a large majority of the problems people bring to the health care system. The content of primary care has been described in multiple ways, and the committee examined data from national surveys conducted in the United States and other countries. Glimpses of primary care can be appreciated by considering reasons for visits and the range of problems addressed by various clinicians.

The National Ambulatory Medical Care Survey (NAMCS) samples office visits to physicians and provides information on type of physician, the patient's stated reason for visit, the diagnosis, interventions, and so forth. Rosenblatt et al. (1995) using NAMCS data from 1989 and 1990 has characterized the content of nonreferred ambulatory visits to office-based physicians in the United States as diagnostic clusters. These clusters incorporate the problems people choose to bring to the health care system. They have remained stable over time and approximate the content of primary care practice.

The 20 diagnostic clusters shown in Table 4-1 (in rank order by frequency) incorporate just over half of nonreferred visits to U.S. physicians. They cover a spectrum of conditions that are not confined to a particular organ system, gender, or age group. They include acute and chronic problems, diseases and syndromes, mental health concerns and trauma, and visits focused on prevention. All of the clusters reflect problems whose solutions could have a considerable impact on the health of individuals and for which people expect expert care. They are neither trivial in their importance nor simple in terms of their diagnosis and management.

Figure 4-1 shows the portion of care for these clusters that is provided by three types of physicians: family physicians, internists, and pediatricians. Other physicians provide the remaining 10 percent or so of visits associated with a given diagnostic cluster. These specialties include orthopedists for sprains, strains, low back pain, and degenerative joint disease, and obstetricians for general medical examinations and urinary tract infections.

Although the NAMCS data display the most common diagnostic clusters, the distribution of visits by cluster cannot convey the level of complexity or severity of problems seen in primary care. Some indication of this complexity has been provided by Barondess (1982), who reviewed consecutive visits to his practice of

TABLE 4-1 Diagnosis Clusters That Make Up the Majority of Nonreferred Ambulatory Visits to U.S. Office-Based Physicians, NAMCS, 1989–1990

Rank	Cluster Title	Percent	Cumulative Percent
1.	General medical examination	7.2	7.2
2.	Acute upper respiratory tract infection	6.2	13.4
3.	Hypertension	4.4	17.8
4.	Prenatal care	4.3	22.1
5.	Acute otitis media	3.5	25.6
6.	Acute lower respiratory tract infection	2.7	28.3
7.	Acute sprains and strains	2.7	31.0
8.	Depression and anxiety	2.5	33.5
9.	Diabetes mellitus	2.1	35.6
10.	Lacerations and contusions	1.9	37.5
11.	Malignant neoplasms	1.7	39.2
12.	Degenerative joint disease	1.7	40.9
13.	Acute sinusitis	1.6	42.5
14.	Fractures and dislocations	1.6	44.1
15.	Chronic rhinitis	1.5	45.6
16.	Ischemic heart disease	1.4	47.0
17.	Acne and diseases of sweat glands	1.3	48.3
18.	Low back pain	1.2	49.5
19.	Dermatitis and eczema	1.2	50.7
20.	Urinary tract infection	1.1	51.8

*The estimated number of visits for 1989–1990 (the denominator) is 1,297,334 (in thousands). This is based on 74,390 survey visits. All relative standard errors are less than 30%.

SOURCE: Rosenblatt et al., 1995.

general internal medicine over a 20-day period. He divided the clinical problems that he saw into several broad categories—cardiovascular, psychiatric, gastrointestinal, infectious, and so forth. Barondess concluded that about 10 percent of patients seen in each category of problems had major and often life-threatening disease, some acute and some chronic, some with complications and some without. In addition, within each organ system, some patients had an unusually complex disorder. Overall, he reported that a large number of these patients required sophisticated and complex clinical judgments "related to the identification, clinical course, potential complications, and management of a large number of major organic diseases" (p. 736). Such problems may require the judicious use of available technologies and efforts to enhance comfort and functional status and to forestall hospitalization.

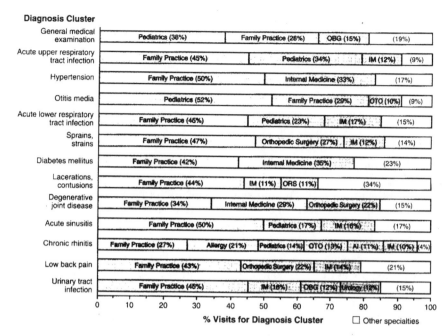

FIGURE 4-1 Physician specialties providing care for generalist-dominant diagnosis cluster, NAMCS 1989–1990 (all specialties are listed that accounted for ≥ 10% of visits for that condition). All relative standard errors are ≤ 30%. AI = allergy and immunology; Internal Medicine (IM) = general internal medicine; OBG = obstetrics and gynecology; ORS = orthopedic surgery; OTO = otolaryngology; Pediatrics = general pediatrics. Unlabeled cells represent other specialties. SOURCE: Rosenblatt et al., 1995.

Episodes of Primary Care

To measure accurately the effects of primary care, data systems and research methods must be able to reflect the co-occurrence of health problems and the longer time frames needed to evaluate the integrative functions of primary care—comprehensiveness, continuity, and coordination. However, in primary care, recording the content of care using standard coding systems such as the International Classification of Diseases or the Diagnostic and Statistical Manual (for mental health) is inadequate because of the complex interplay among diagnostic categories and other clinical or social problems a patient may often simultaneously experience. Current U.S. databases, such as those provided by NAMCS, are by design cross-sectional analyses of single visits and thus cannot capture episode information.

These databases compile diagnostic data from the point of view of visits to clinicians reflecting the practitioner perspective rather than the perspective of the patient in terms of the variety of problems that a given patient brings to the health care system and the services of clinicians who care for those problems over a period of time.

Because of such limitations in coding, attempts have been made to describe primary care in terms of episodes. The term *episode of care* refers to a problem or illness in a patient during the time from its first presentation to a clinician until the completion of the last encounter for that same problem or illness, whether this covers a short period of, for example, several weeks or a much longer time (Lamberts et al., 1993). The concept of episodes of care is discussed in more detail in Chapter 8 with respect to research applications.

The Netherlands Transition Project, which uses the International Classification of Primary Care (ICPC), provides detailed information on the content of family practice in the form of episodes of care for age- and sex-specific groups (Lamberts and Wood, 1987; Lamberts et al., 1993; Lamberts and Hofmans-Okkes, 1996). By distinguishing reasons for encounter, diagnoses, and interventions and displaying them for such groups, the Project provides a wealth of information about the distribution of interventions, comorbidities, and rates of referral in enrolled primary care populations. The committee undertook data analyses using both national databases and data provided by several large HMOs to see whether the European approach could be used to understand how primary care is delivered in the United States.

The use and sequencing of interventions and the complex interplay in primary care of comorbidities can be understood using ICPC and methods that are well suited to primary care. This methodology is now used in several European countries; however, the committee found very little comparable work in the United States to elucidate primary care in this promising manner (Klinkman and Green, 1995). The committee undertook a data exercise using U.S. data from national surveys and data collected from several large integrated health care delivery systems to approximate the Dutch analyses as a means of understanding what range of personal health care needs appear to be met here by primary care. This effort is briefly reviewed in the Appendix.

CHARACTERISTICS OF PRIMARY CARE

The complexity of primary care requires that its description include a variety of attributes. Participants at a workshop organized by the Institute of Medicine (IOM) committee in January 1995 explored the science base of primary care and described research needed to strengthen that knowledge base (Appendix C). The six aspects of primary care were emphasized.

1. Excellent primary care is grounded in both the biomedical and the social sciences.

2. Clinical decisionmaking in primary care frequently differs from that in referral specialties.

3. Primary care has at its core a sustained personal relationship between patient and clinician.

4. Primary care does not consider mental health separately from physical health.

5. Opportunities to promote health and prevent disease are intrinsic to primary care practice.

6. Primary care is information intensive.

Biomedical and Social Sciences

Biomedical Sciences

Biomedical knowledge is as important in primary care as it is in secondary or tertiary care. Primary care draws from biology to provide diagnostic, prognostic, and therapeutic services to help acutely and chronically ill patients. Biomedicine incorporates a range of sciences including physics, chemistry, molecular and cellular biology, and clinical epidemiology. Few conditions are now completely understood at all levels ranging from the molecular to the behavioral, although such understanding seems achievable in the future.

Social Sciences and the Humanities in Primary Care

Beyond the knowledge of disease is knowledge of the patient as a human being. Humanism is a core area of primary care practice. Defined knowledge, skills, and attitudes contribute to a good clinical process in several core areas: the medical interview, behavioral medicine, and medical ethics.

Behavioral sciences. The management of many primary care problems, especially in the context of family and community, leans heavily on the social sciences. Theories of behavior change help primary care clinicians to

- involve individuals in their own care,
- improve compliance with therapeutic regimens,
- understand causes and utilize effective interventions to reduce substance abuse, and
- integrate the family in dealing with illness and health.

Knowledge from the social sciences and theories regarding social support and confidence in one's ability to change behavior in dealing with a particular problem—called self-efficacy—can also be applied to many primary care conditions. Such knowledge and theories include those relating to occupationally related problems and disorders emanating from the stresses of living and to the adoption of health-promoting behaviors.

Communication. A core skill for the primary care clinician is expertise in communication and, in particular, the medical interview. The behavioral sciences can contribute to effective skills in sequencing the interview, organizing information, eliciting and responding to patients, understanding verbal and nonverbal communication, and engaging the patient's participation as an ally in the therapeutic plan (Lipkin et al., 1984).

Medical ethics. The primary care clinician is an agent of the patient and his or her welfare, but ethical dilemmas often present themselves. Such issues require working skills in applying sometimes conflicting ethical precepts related to bringing about benefit, avoiding harm, enhancing patient autonomy, and increasing the aggregate well-being of a panel of patients under the clinician's care as well as that of an individual patient. As is true for clinicians in any field of medicine, these issues require not only compassion but also skills drawn in part from the humanities. They include a range of concerns such as accommodating or resisting end-of-life decisions; assisting and intervening when necessary with problems involving patients and their families; adopting appropriate roles when disagreements arise about insurance coverage or the confidentiality of patient information; using genetic and diagnostic tests; and deciding to use or not use life-sustaining technologies.

Evidence-Based Medicine

Biomedical knowledge in primary care requires that research evidence be applied to individual patients using an approach that has come to be called evidence-based medicine. A large portion of the research evidence comes from basic research and from randomized clinical trials. Applying such information in the primary care setting is particularly challenging because such studies typically restrict their choice of subjects to those who do not have multiple problems or are of a specific age or gender.

In addition to knowledge derived from the basic and biomedical sciences and randomized clinical trials, primary care clinicians use results of population-based epidemiological studies that examine risk factors for disease and information from outcomes and effectiveness studies of treatments used by community-based clinicians. Clinicians supplement their knowledge of mechanisms of disease and therapies and their clinical experience with information about the probabilities that (a) particular screening or diagnostic tests will be useful, (b) a patient has a given illness, and (c) such an illness will progress or improve. This, in the aggregate, is evidence-based medicine, and it requires that clinicians be proficient in searching the literature and in critically appraising that literature using formal rules of evidence (Evidence-Based Medicine Working Group, 1992).

Clinical Decisionmaking

General Observations

Rosser (1996) and Sox (1996) have suggested that primary care clinicians differ from specialists in their approach to clinical decisionmaking. The additional information available to primary care clinicians but not to specialists affects the development of hypotheses to explain conditions, influences the ordering of probabilities, and either enlarges or constrains the options for response. Primary care clinicians, in contrast to referral specialists, must consider a very broad range of possibilities, often at an earlier time in the natural history of their patients' problems, and they must tolerate unavoidable uncertainty when diagnosis is not possible. Some problems never resolve, some are never diagnosable, and some never require further intervention; they simply persist as part of the environment in which a patient-clinician relationship continues. What may appear as a lack of precision in diagnosis by primary care clinicians is often appropriate, given the nature of the problems presented to primary care clinicians.

Influence of Different Clinical Roles

The overall care process. According to Sox (1996), different clinical roles in primary care and referral practice affect decisionmaking throughout the care process. The specialist is often asked to focus on a single problem, whereas the primary care clinician is often required to deal with multiple problems simultaneously. Indeed, comorbidity is virtually a constant in primary care practice; a typical primary care patient has an active problem list of about six problems. This factor often precludes assignment of causal relationships with any certainty, and it constrains therapeutic options that would otherwise be available to manage a single disease or problem.

Furthermore, the referral specialist often sees patients for a single visit and has only limited knowledge of the patient's background or history; by contrast, the primary care clinician often has an ongoing relationship with the patient and has relevant knowledge of the patient's history and situation. The specialist is frequently expected to reach an immediate and definitive resolution of a health concern; the primary care clinician can observe the patient over time, watching for evolution that indicates greater (or lesser) importance or urgency. Common concerns such as fatigue, headache, or insomnia require that the primary care clinician assess the situation, estimate its immediate seriousness, and, in many instances, provide reassurance to the patient even if a diagnosis of disease cannot be made at that time. Prognosis in primary care requires a knowledge of the person, community, and family as well as the importance of the symptom or concern. Utilizing this information enables the primary care clinician to determine whether early action can do more harm than good and whether watchful waiting is indicated.

Use of diagnostic tests and procedures. Sox (1996) compares the reasoning by both kinds of clinicians to explain why primary care clinicians may order fewer diagnostic tests than referral physicians. If primary care clinicians tend to refer when tests are equivocal or symptoms do not resolve with observation or treatment, a referral practice would be enriched with patients who have intermediate probabilities of disease—that is, the diagnostic puzzles of medicine. Said differently, referral practice consists of patients with a higher probability of having particular diseases than would be expected in primary care practices.

This circumstance may lead both to a different approach to testing and to a different frequency and selection of tests in primary care as compared to the patterns in referral practice. For one thing, diagnostic tests and procedures have different performance characteristics depending on the prevalence of conditions in the tested population. Tests that could be of great help to a primary care clinician might lack the precision required in specialty practice, and tests that help a specialist might cause more harm than good in primary care practice.

Consequently, the choice and interpretation of tests in primary care practice would logically be expected to differ from testing in specialty practice. For example, a test that measures the sedimentation rate of red blood cells is relatively nonspecific, but it helps to rule out significant disease if the result is negative. This is of more value in primary care than in specialty care. By contrast, invasive tests that carry some risk of morbidity and even mortality may be of more value in specialty practice where the probability of disease is higher.

Personal Aspects of Primary Care

Primary care has at its core a partnership between patient and clinician; that partnership is meant to encourage active patient participation, sharing of information and responsibility, and joint goal setting and decisionmaking. The contributions of primary care to effective health care systems are not achievable in the absence of trust between primary care clinicians and their patients.

Patients' views of primary care are expressed through their decisions about whether and when to bring a problem to the attention of clinicians. The reasons people give for seeking care—the symptom or concern—and the degree to which these problems are addressed during a patient visit are negotiated during the encounter between clinician and patient. This negotiation may be direct or unspoken. Some questions may be left unanswered, some problems unexplored.

When addressing patient health problems, diagnosis may be critically important or irrelevant to the care that is given, and diagnostic codes often fail to capture the content of a visit and the important contributions of primary care. For example, providing emotional support, information, and accurate assessment of a condition may be of great importance. At times, the most important task is simply to listen as a patient shares his or her burden, and the most powerful intervention may be the interest shown in the patient and the problem the patient is concerned about.

Health care choices can be critical for a patient. From the patient's perspective health care is complex and perplexing, both in terms of how to navigate the system to obtain appropriate care and in terms of what choices exist and how to go about making them. Considerations such as whether to act now or wait, choose a surgical procedure, or embark on a lifetime course of medication are fraught with uncertainty.

Surveys have repeatedly shown that patients want information about diseases, treatments, and their benefits and risks. For clinicians to be able to frame risks and benefits accurately and to recommend interventions also requires them to have good knowledge of their patients and their patients' goals and preferences.

The fields of decision analysis, risk communication, and health behavior have all contributed to a better understanding of how to assess and convey information in primary care practice; work by Mulley, Wennberg, and others in the area of shared decisionmaking has been especially influential (Mulley, 1991; Kasper et al., 1992). Mort (1996) reported on the use of interactive laser disc technology as a decision support tool for patients. This technique combines narrative and patient testimonials in ways that permit viewers to hear from patients who have made different choices and experienced different outcomes. The narrative tailors estimates of risk and benefits to help patients consider difficult decisions such as hormone replacement therapy, prostate surgery, and surgical alternatives for early-stage breast cancer.

Patients come to primary care with their own belief systems, however, based in the context of their family, community, and culture. A lack of awareness or insensitivity to the patient's background reduces the likelihood that the goals of primary care will be achieved. Two recent studies demonstrate this point.

Western clinicians typically view informed consent and advanced care planning as having great importance and potential to benefit their patients; moreover, their patients usually expect such information and input into decisionmaking. Carrese and Rhodes (1995) documented the potential of cross-cultural misunderstanding involving beliefs that speech itself has the power to help or to harm. Among traditional Navajo, discussing and thinking about negative information is viewed as potentially harmful. Understanding this cultural preference has clear implications for how a clinician should discuss with Navajo patients the need for prenatal care or immunizations, the options and risks for a treatment or surgical procedure, or advance directives concerning life-sustaining therapies. In a second example, Blackhall et al. (1995) found that Korean Americans and Mexican Americans were less likely than European Americans to believe that patients should be told of a terminal prognosis. They suggested that physicians ask their patients if they wish to receive such information and make decisions themselves or if they prefer that their families handle such matters. Primary care clinicians must be aware of these preferences on the part of their patients and insofar as possible act accordingly. The personal aspects of primary care also include the important area of self care. Most symptoms are self-evaluated and self-treated without the help of health professionals (White et al., 1961), and a vital function of primary care is to increase self-care competence so that patients can become active partners in health care (Sobel, 1994; Vickery and Lynch, 1995). By providing information, answering questions, and helping patients find other resources for help, primary care clinicians can foster knowledgeable and confident self care.

Mental Health and Physical Health

In a paper prepared for the IOM committee deGruy has documented the inability to separate mental and physical health states (see Appendix D).[1] Mental distress, symptoms, and disorders are usually embedded in a matrix of explained or unexplained physical symptoms as well as acute and chronic medical illnesses. When a patient with a mental disorder presents to a primary care clinician, it is usually by means of a physical complaint. Primary care patients with mental diagnoses—whether or not they meet formally defined diagnostic criteria—show profound functional impairment. Wells and colleagues (1989) demonstrated, for example, that depressed patients had functional impairments comparable to patients with chronic medical conditions such as chronic obstructive pulmonary disease, diabetes, coronary artery disease, hypertension, and arthritis (see also Wells and Sturm, 1995). Patients with mental diagnoses also have consistently higher medical utilization rates than their unaffected counterparts.

Primary care clinicians frequently are required to deal with mental symptoms as part of a physical problem. For example, two-thirds of primary care patients with a psychiatric diagnosis have a significant physical illness that precedes the psychiatric diagnosis. Chronic medical illnesses increase the likelihood of depression by two- to threefold. Primary care patients do not view their mental diagnoses as something apart from their general health, and they frequently will not tolerate clinicians' doing so. One-third to one-half of primary care patients refuse referral to a mental health professional even when a diagnosis of an important mental illness is present. The future of primary care obviously requires

---

[1]Material included in this section is referenced in Appendix D, Mental Health Care in the Primary Care Setting.

learning more about the utility of recognizing and managing mental health problems as an inseparable component of practice.

Recognized biases in recording mental health problems often occur because of reimbursement disincentives for clinicians and stigmatization of patients. These biases, whether attributable to underrecognition or underreporting by primary care clinicians, produce remarkable underestimates of mental health problems and subsequent care for these problems in primary care; for example, the diagnostic cluster of depression and anxiety accounts for only about 2.5 percent of nonreferred ambulatory visits according to the NAMCS data (see Table 4-1). By contrast, other sources estimate that 10 to 20 percent of the general population will consult a primary care clinician for a mental health problem in the course of a year. The proportions of pediatric primary care patients with significant psychosocial or psychosomatic problems are about 15 percent and 8 percent, respectively. Overall, 10 to 40 percent of primary care patients have a diagnosable mental disorder (this does not imply, however, that it would be desirable to recognize or treat all of these).

All in all, the committee views the indivisibility of mental and physical health as very significant for the future of primary care and for the ultimate health and well-being of patients and populations. The topic is addressed in more depth in the following chapter.

Health Promotion and Disease Prevention

Although society has long espoused the need for preventive as well as curative medicine, only recently has prevention been incorporated into primary care on a scientific basis. In 1974 the Lalonde report, *A New Perspective on the Health of Canadians*, estimated the burden of disease and concluded that about 40 percent of this burden was the result of personal behaviors and modifiable risk factors (Lalonde, 1974). Thus, effective screening programs aimed at well-designed preventive care were recognized as potentially fundamental components of primary care. The immediate responses to this report were twofold: (1) to examine modifiable risk factors more systematically, especially those attributable to personal behaviors; and (2) to develop strategies that could detect problems at the level of primary care, where early intervention could lead to superior results for patients and the population as a whole.

Given the large number and variety of possible preventive services that primary care clinicians might offer their patients, a systematic approach to selection is essential. The principles of screening applicable to the primary care setting have been carefully crafted and include such considerations as seriousness and prevalence of possible target conditions, the value of early detection, and the availability of adequate, acceptable, and affordable tests and treatments. The U.S. Preventive Services Task Force (1989, 1996) has continued the systematic evaluation of clinical prevention strategies, and now primary care clinicians have a host of scientifically supported recommendations to forward to their patients and implement in their practices.

Another goal of prevention is to maintain function in the presence of unavoidable impairment in children and adults of all ages. Accomplishing this often involves dealing with complex problems that require clinicians to coordinate care across different settings, to involve family and community in meaningful ways, and to develop and pass along anticipatory guidance for children and families.

Increased opportunities to develop preventive strategies in primary care and to coordinate them with public health efforts using a systems approach are elucidated by Welton et al. (Appendix F). Currently, the interface between primary care and public health is irregular and undefined, but achievable linkages exist that could improve community and population health and lead to the achievement of public health goals. As with the issues of mental health noted above, the coordination of primary care personal services with public health programs is examined in more detail in Chapter 5.

The Power of Information

The knowledge base that is relevant to a large majority of the problems that people bring to their primary care clinicians is large and constantly evolving. Similarly, the databases that ought to be developed and maintained for patients registered and seen in primary care practices are sizeable and expanding. In the past, many clinicians interested in primary care declined to enter primary care practice because of the intimidating prospects of not being able to manage the information challenges. That situation is changing.

The computer revolution has matured to the point that useful applications of information systems and computer-based patient records—technologies not previously available in any meaningful way—are now poised for wide implementation into primary care practice; indeed, computer-based systems and telecommunications are likely to become key elements of the primary care infrastructure. Management functions of such electronic information technologies include those related to registering patients, making appointments, and handling financial elements of practice. More important, however, are the growing numbers of clinically useful applications, which provide profiles of practice patterns, produce reminders for needed services, and open up access to support systems of various kinds. Although these advances are relevant for both primary and specialty care, they hold special promise for primary care, where the information and coordination needs are greater.

SUMMARY

No health care system can be complete without primary care, the nature of which has been examined in this chapter in terms of the large majority of personal health care needs of patients and with respect to several key characteristics. In the United States, the time is right for primary care, as understood by this committee, to undergo more systematic and creative development and to expand as the foundation of health care delivery. Primary care is amenable to improvement through the methods of science, the implementation of key supporting infrastructures such as information systems, and the use of relevant principles of management and organization.

What has been described about the nature of primary care in this chapter has implications for the actual delivery of primary care (discussed in Chapter 5), for the existing supply of primary care clinicians (Chapter 6), and for health professions education (Chapter 7). An understanding of the nature of primary care also raises questions that cannot now be answered because of the inadequacy of the current knowledge base. These topics are the basis of the committee's conclusions and recommendations about needed research in primary care that are described in Chapter 8.

APPENDIX:
DATA ON THE MAJORITY OF PERSONAL HEALTH CARE NEEDS

As noted in the main text, the Netherlands Transition Project of the Department of Family Practice at the University of Amsterdam (Lamberts et al., 1993; Lamberts and Hofmans-Okkes, 1996) uses episodes of care to characterize age- and sex-specific patterns of care. These data yield considerable insights into the types of conditions, diagnoses, and reasons for visit for the Dutch population. The information and the episode-based approach can also provide insights for the U.S. population, notwithstanding the fact that the Dutch population is both considerably smaller and far more homogeneous than that in the United States. Apart from the value of the information with respect to indicating the incidence and prevalence of conditions seen by primary care practitioners, the Netherlands Project data point the way to using a form of episode analysis that may be useful here for both epidemiologic and research purposes.

To explore this possibility, the committee engaged in a data collection and analysis effort based on national survey information and specially generated information from selected health maintenance organizations and managed care entities (Hofmans-Okkes and Lamberts, 1995). This appendix presents a brief explanation of the Netherlands Transition Project approach and gives an illustrative set of data on one age-sex cohort (women ages 25 to 44); it also includes a short discussion of the analyses done using U.S. data.

Description of Data

The Netherlands Transition Project

The Dutch data shown in the first set of tables in this appendix include episode-oriented information for 15,158 enrolled women between the ages of 25 to 44 (of whom 11,570 had visited their family physician at least once in the relevant year). The information here is given for illustrative purposes; similar data are available on women in all other age categories (e.g., 75 years or older), on men of all age groups, and children.

For making inferences about diagnoses, reasons for encounter, and other specific elements of episodes of care, the Transition Project uses the International Classification of Primary Care (ICPC); the ICPC is specifically designed by the World Organization of Family Doctors to characterize primary care episodes (Lamberts and Wood, 1987; Lamberts et al., 1993). This classification scheme uses three main elements: (1) the patient's reason(s) for encounter; (2) the diagnostic label assigned to the episode of care; and (3) the diagnostic and therapeutic interventions by the primary care clinician, including referrals to specialists. It maps well to the International Classification of Diseases (ICD) tenth edition and reasonably well to the ICD-9-CM, which is the ninth edition with clinical modifications.

The tables in this appendix present data in terms of the "top 20s," that is, the first (or top) 20 diagnoses or reasons for encounter among women in this age group. Typically, analyses involving the top 20s will account for a proportion of episodes of care that exceed, often by wide margins, 30 percent of all episodes. Thus, the top 20 new episodes give a global impression of the magnitude and diversity of acute personal health care needs; the top 20 old episodes indicate the burden of chronic illness and long-term episodes or follow-up (including for health maintenance and preventive care). The information on interventions reflects the processes of care; for enrolled populations in plans or health care systems that rely heavily on primary care practitioners, the information on referrals suggests what portion of care cannot be or customarily is not handled by those in primary care.

The Dutch data are presented for the following types of enumerations:

1. diagnostic labels—for "new" episodes—i.e., episodes of care for reasons that have not surfaced previously for these patients (Table 4A-1);

2. diagnostic labels for "old" episodes—i.e., episodes of care that have been ongoing for some period of time (Table 4A-2);

3. patients' reasons for encounter at the start of a new episode (Table 4A-3);

4. patients' reasons for encounter during follow-up (Table 4A-4);

5. diagnostic and therapeutic interventions (Table 4A-5); and

6. referrals to specialist care (Table 4A-6).

TABLE 4A-1 Top 20 New Episodes for Women Ages 25–44 Years

New Episodes	N	Inc[a]	%
Pap smear	1,313	86.6	3.6
URI (head cold)	1,299	85.7	3.6
No disease	1,295	85.4	3.6
Sinusitis acute/chron	788	52.0	2.2
Pregnancy confirmed	730	48.2	2.0
Family planning/oral contraceptive	703	46.4	1.9
Low back complaint excl radiation	654	43.1	1.8
Urogenital candidiasis proven	556	36.7	1.5
Contact dermatitis/other eczema	520	34.3	1.4
Muscle pain/fibrositis	517	34.1	1.4
General weakness/tiredness	512	33.8	1.4
Excessive ear wax	439	29.0	1.2
Adverse effect med agent proper dose	388	25.6	1.1
Cystitis/other urin infect NOS	379	25.0	1.0
Acute bronchitis/bronchiolitis	351	23.2	1.0
Menstruation excessive/irregular	347	22.9	1.0
Vaginitis/vulvitis NOS	344	22.7	1.0
Dermatophytosis	334	22.0	0.9
Acute laryngitis/tracheitis	321	21.2	0.9
Neck sympt/complaint excl headache	320	21.1	0.9
Total top 20	12,110		33.5

[a]Inc = incidence per 1,000 patients per year; NOS = not otherwise specified.

SOURCE: Hofmans-Okkes and Lamberts, 1995.

Data on the 15,158 women studied are presented in three ways. First are given the raw counts (labeled N) of episodes, interventions, or referrals. Second appears information on incidence (Inc) or *rates* per 1,000 enrolled persons per year for episodes, interventions, or referrals. Third are percentages (%), which show how much of the entire health care experience is accounted for by the 20 episodes, reasons for encounter, interventions, or referrals. Other information includes the total number of episodes (interventions, etc.) in the top 20 listing and the total percentage of all episodes represented by the top 20; from these two figures, the grand total of episodes (interventions, etc.) can be calculated.

The U.S. Data

The committee examined information from the National Ambulatory Medical Care Survey (NAMCS) (Schappert, 1994) and the National Health Interview Survey (NHIS) (Adams and Benson, 1992) in much the same way for the same

TABLE 4A-2 Top 20 Old Episodes for Women Ages 25–44 Years

Top 20 Old Episodes for Women 25–44	N	Rate[a]	%
Family planning/oral contraceptive	1,440	95.0	17.4
Pap smear	378	24.9	4.6
Family planning/IUD	276	18.2	3.3
Pregnancy confirmed	170	11.2	2.1
Contact dermatitis/other eczema	152	10.0	1.8
Uncomplicated hypertension	148	9.8	1.8
Irritable bowel syndrome	133	8.8	1.6
Hayfever/allergic rhinitis	129	8.5	1.6
Migraine	116	7.7	1.4
Asthma	110	7.3	1.3
No disease	102	6.7	1.2
Depressive disorder	101	6.7	1.2
Feeling anxious/nervous/tense	96	6.3	1.2
Abnormal Pap smear	94	6.2	1.1
Relation problem partners	91	6.0	1.1
Complaints of infertility	88	5.8	1.1
Low back complaint excl radiation	84	5.5	1.0
Acne	76	5.0	0.9
Other diseases female genital system	75	4.9	0.9
Hyperventilation	74	4.9	0.9
Total top 20	3,933		47.5

[a]Rate = per 1,000 patients per year; IUD = intrauterine device.

SOURCE: Hofmans-Okkes and Lamberts, 1995.

sex-age cohort for years during the late 1980s and early 1990s. In this case, however, the top 40 diagnoses are used. In addition, the committee requested and received special episode data runs from three managed care organizations (of six approached; these three were the only ones able to produce the requested episode-oriented information from their internal records). The NHIS and NAMCS data were used to provide baseline indicators of episodes per person per year and the diagnoses, conditions, and reasons for seeking health care that relate to those episodes. In this sense, they provide a proxy for "the large majority of personal health care needs" as understood by this committee. NHIS information cannot be subdivided into new and follow-up episodes; information from NAMCS and the private managed care organizations can be so classified. None of these data sets employs the ICPC approach to labeling diagnosis or reason for encounter, so information is not strictly comparable to the Dutch data.

TABLE 4A-3 Patient Reason for Encounter for New Episodes for Women Ages 25–44 Years

Reason at Start of Episode	N	Rate[a]	%
Cough	1,395	92.0	3.5
Pap smear	1,349	89.0	3.4
General weakness/tiredness	1,089	71.8	2.7
Headache	1,000	66.0	2.5
Sympt/complaint throat	933	61.6	2.3
Local swelling/papul/lump/mass	900	59.4	2.3
Low back complaint excl radiation	836	55.2	2.1
Other localized abdominal pain	792	52.2	2.0
Local redness/erythema/rash	681	44.9	1.7
Sympt/complaint pelvis	543	35.8	1.4
Neck sympt/complaint excl headache	512	33.8	1.3
Fever	495	32.7	1.2
Question of pregnancy	479	31.6	1.2
Ear pain/earache	473	31.2	1.2
Pruritis	451	29.8	1.1
Menstruation excessive/irregular	429	28.3	1.1
Other sympt/complaint vagina	426	28.1	1.1
URI (head cold)	411	27.1	1.0
Sympt/complaint sinus (incl pain)	405	26.7	1.0
Feeling anxious/nervous/tense	403	26.6	1.0
Total top 20	14,002		35.3

[a]Rate = per 1,000 patients per year.

SOURCE: Hofmans-Okkes and Lamberts, 1995.

Results

The Netherlands Transition Project

Because these data are presented mainly for illustrative and heuristic reasons, they are not discussed in detail. The information in Table 4A-1 indicates that, among women of child-bearing age in this Dutch study cohort, the top 20 diagnoses account for one-third of all new episodes for this cohort of patients. Thus, they had, on average, 2.4 new episodes per year (total of 36,150 episodes among 15,158 women). Among the top 20 entries, as might be expected, pregnancy and family planning episodes appear frequently, as do certain health maintenance diagnoses (e.g., Pap smears); other important diagnoses involve infectious disease (e.g., upper respiratory and genitourinary tract). For example, the incidence of upper respiratory infections was almost 86 per 1,000 persons; by

TABLE 4A-4 Patient Reason for Encounter for Follow-up Care for Women Ages 25–44 Years

Reason During Follow-up	N	Rate[a]	%
Med exam/health evaluation/partial (reproductive functions)	3,051	201.3	10.7
Family planning/oral contraceptive	1,100	72.6	3.9
Med exam/health evalua/partial (cardiovascular problems)	872	57.5	3.1
Medication/prescript/injection (reproductive functions)	836	55.2	2.9
Medication/prescript/injection (psychological problems)	599	39.5	2.1
Pap smear	509	33.6	1.8
Feeling anxious/nervous/tense	420	27.7	1.5
Provide initial episode ongoing (psychological problems)	417	27.5	1.5
Therap counseling/listening	399	26.3	1.4
General weakness/tiredness	392	25.9	1.4
Headache	389	25.7	1.4
Other localized abdominal pain	378	24.9	1.3
Low back complaint excl radiation	357	23.6	1.3
Med exam/health, evaluation/partial (musculoskeletal problems)	314	20.7	1.1
Provide initial episode ongoing (female genital)	278	18.3	1.0
Advice/health education (psychological problems)	276	18.2	1.0
Provide initial episode ongoing (reproductive functions)	274	18.1	1.0
Advice/health education (reproductive functions)	264	17.4	0.9
Cough	259	17.1	0.9
Med exam/health evaluation/partial (skin problems)	259	17.1	0.9
Total top 20	11,643		41.0

[a]Rate = per 1,000 patients per year.

SOURCE: Hofmans-Okkes and Lamberts, 1995.

TABLE 4A-5 Top 20 Diagnostic and Therapeutic Interventions for Women Ages 25–44 Years

Interventions	N	Rate[a]	%
Med exam/health evalua/partial	42,248	2,787.2	39.4
Medication/prescript/injection	21,621	1,426.4	20.2
Advice/health education	18,300	1,207.3	17.1
Therap counseling/listening	3,742	246.9	3.5
Referral to other physician/specialist	3,251	214.5	3.0
Blood test	3,117	205.6	2.9
Urine test	2,661	175.6	2.5
Histology/cytology	2,601	171.6	2.4
Referral to nurse, physical therapist	2,303	151.9	2.1
Diagnostic radiology/imaging	1,512	99.7	1.4
Microbio/other immunol test	962	63.5	0.9
Excision/biopsy/removal/cautery	646	42.6	0.6
Incision/drainage/aspiration	553	36.5	0.5
Repair/suture/cast/prosthet. device	537	35.4	0.5
Dressing/compression/packing	517	34.1	0.5
Administrative procedure	350	23.1	0.3
Local injection/infiltration	299	19.7	0.3
Cathet/intubat/dilat/instrument	251	16.6	0.2
Other diagnostic procedures	235	15.5	0.2
Other laboratory test NOS	209	13.8	0.2
Total top 20	105,915		98.8

[a]Rate = per 1,000 patients per year; NOS = not otherwise specified.

SOURCE: Hofmans-Okkes and Lamberts, 1995.

contrast, the incidence of acute laryngitis and tracheitis was only about 21 per 1,000 individuals.

A comparison of information in Tables 4A-1 and 4A-2 indicates that the annual rate of continuing episodes drops by almost four-fifths (to about 0.54 old episodes per woman per year, based on 8,280 episodes among 15,158 women). Thus, women in the age group had, on average, 2.9 episodes overall in one year (2.4 new and 0.5 follow-up episodes).

The top 20 episodes of care account for nearly one-half of the continuing care for this group. Several of the diagnoses appear in both new and ongoing episodes. Among them are family planning and pregnancy (which have rates of 95.0, 18.2, and 11.2 per 1,000 enrolled women); Pap smears and abnormal Pap smears (rates of 24.9 and 6.2 per 1,000, respectively); and "no disease." More striking, however, is the substantial change in the frequency of certain episodes, in particular a move away from acute infections and a shift toward a variety of

TABLE 4A-6 Top 20 Types of Referrals to Specialist Care for Women Ages 25–44 Years

Referrals	N	Rate[a]	%
Gynecologist	893	58.9	27.6
Surgeon	381	25.1	11.8
Dermatologist	354	23.4	10.9
Ophthalmologist	225	14.8	7.0
E.N.T. surgeon	223	14.7	6.9
Neurologist	176	11.6	5.4
Internist	170	11.2	5.3
Orthopedic surgeon	133	8.8	4.1
Ambulatory mental health	131	8.6	4.0
Plastic surgeon	113	7.5	3.5
Psychiatrist	99	6.5	3.1
Other referrals	71	4.7	2.2
Abortion clinic	65	4.3	2.0
Cardiologist	40	2.6	1.2
Urologist	34	2.2	1.1
Pulmonologist	26	1.7	0.8
Rheumatologist	22	1.5	0.7
Dental surgeon	16	1.1	0.5
Gastroenterologist	15	1.0	0.5
Allergist	12	0.8	0.4
Total top 20	3,199		98.9

[a]Rate = per 1,000 patients per year.

SOURCE: Hofmans-Okkes and Lamberts, 1995

chronic conditions. Among the latter are hypertension, irritable bowel syndrome, and asthma; quite notable is the rate of affective mental disorders (depressive disorders and anxiety, nervousness, and tension, which have rates of 6.7 and 6.3, respectively).

"Reasons for encounter," shown in Tables 4A-3 and 4A-4, are different from the diagnoses enumerated in Tables 4A-1 and 4A-2. They reflect the issues that brought these women to their primary care practitioner, and thus they are couched less in diagnostic terms than in terms relating to symptoms or signs. (The exception are Pap smears in Table 4A-3 for new episodes and Pap smears as well as a variety of specific services such as medications and health education in Table 4A-4 for follow-up.)

The top 20 entries account for about one-third and two-fifths, respectively, of the reasons for which patients seek new or follow-up care. Reasons for encounter involving follow-up comprise large numbers of requests for interventions (Table 4A-4). Clinically and epidemiologically, patterns similar to those for episodes can be seen in Tables 4A-3 and 4A-4. For instance, there is a shift from acute symptoms (for new episodes) to either chronic conditions or health maintenance services (for old episodes).

Finally, Tables 4A-5 and 4A-6 are concerned with the interventions used to manage the conditions presented by women in the age group. Of a total of about 107,200 discrete diagnostic and therapeutic interventions recorded, the top 20 shown in Table 4A-5 constituted nearly 99 percent; said differently, for all intents and purposes, these 20 classes of interventions describe the content of primary care. By far the most frequent involved examination, medications, and health education and counseling (see Table 4A-5), with incidence rates, per 1,000 enrolled women in this age group, of more than 2,787 examinations, 1,426 medication prescriptions or injections given, and 1,207 instances of health education and advice. Various laboratory tests were the next most common types of interventions, together with referrals to other types of physicians or primary care providers.

The referrals away from primary care to specialist care (which totaled 3,235) are shown in Table 4A-6. The top 20 entries here account for virtually all possible referrals. By far the most frequent specialty was gynecology, with a referral rate of about 59 per 1,000 women. Other commonly used specialists were surgeons of various types (including general surgery; ophthalmology; ear, nose, and throat; orthopedics; and plastic surgery) and mental health specialists.

The U.S. Data

Table 4A-7 provides information on the new and follow-up "episodes" for U.S. women 25 to 44 years of age, based on the various sources of U.S. information available to the committee (Hofmans-Okkes and Lamberts, 1995). The order of types of episodes is somewhat arbitrary, in that it groups preventive services, various types of gynecologic or obstetric services, a broad set of acute upper respiratory conditions, widely prevalent chronic conditions, and a wide array of other conditions that proved to be important in at least one of these data sets. The data are shown as rates per 1,000 women.

The NHIS data suggest that women in this age group have a total of 2.8 episodes per year on average, although the breakdown between new and follow-up care cannot be done with these data. By contrast, the NAMCS data are lower, suggesting that, overall, 2.1 episodes per woman occur per year (0.9 new, 1.2 follow-up). This split does not map to that seen in the Dutch data, but doubtless the narrower emphasis in the NAMCS data (essentially only physician offices) and differences in data recording and coding account for some of the discrepancy.

Information from the three managed care organizations is about as diverse as that from the two U.S. national surveys. The total rate of episodes from Organization A appears to be nearly 3.7 per enrolled woman per year, with a rate of *new* episodes approximating that of the total for the Transition Project or the NHIS.

TABLE 4A-7 Rates of Episodes of Care per 1,000 Women Ages 25–44 Years, by Diagnosis

Reason for Encounter	NHIS[a] Episodes	NAMCS[b] Rates of Episodes		Organization A Rates of Episodes		Organization B Rates of Episodes		Organization C Rates of Episodes	
		New	Follow-up	New	Old	New	Old	New	Old
Checkup	801	60	140	291	213	168	68	76	33
Pregnancy		68	350	106	81	54	66	12	5
Contraception		17	23	35	9	12		5	
Abortion	23								
Vaginitis/candidiasis	20	17	12	25	8	18	14	10	3
Menstrual problems	16			41	14	5		3	
Breast problems	25	9	12	17	6	5		2	
Other female genital problems	122	68	105						
Upper respiratory and viral infections	346	94	35	223	74	94	37	85	35
Sinusitis (acute and chronic)		26	23	77		36	23	58	16
Bronchitis (acute)	42	17	12	52	18	16	10	44	8
Otitis media	28	9		17	7			18	

Condition									
Chronic obstructive pulmonary disease, including asthma	15		12			5		10	3
Hypertension	57*	9	23	9				4	2
Diabetes	29		12	4				4	2
Thyroid problems	20							1	2
Obesity			23						
Low back conditions	75	9	35	3	36	12	8	22	4
Rheumatism	44	9	12	8	59	5		17	3
Injuries, dislocations, sprains, fractures	112	9			73			35	
Dermatitis		9			29	10	8	10	
Other skin conditions	108	26			53	26		24	
Headache (nonmigraine)					28	6		10	3
Migraine			12			5		9	2
Refraction problems			12		44	24	6		
Other central nervous system disorders	48	9		39					
Allergy and allergic rhinitis		9	12		20	7		14	4
Weakness, fatigue					16			5	
Depression			12			20			
Other psychiatric or psychologic conditions	30		12				17	2	

Continued

TABLE 4A-7 Continued

Reason for Encounter	NHIS[a] Episodes	NAMCS[b] Rates of Episodes		Organization A Rates of Episodes		Organization B Rates of Episodes		Organization C Rates of Episodes	
		New	Follow-up	New	Old	New	Old	New	Old
Cystitis	29	9					17	42	6
Other urinary systems conditions	54	17	12	45	19	16	11	30	9
Other gastrointestinal conditions	51	9		44				12	
Adverse effects of medications		9	12					2	
All listed conditions	2,780	850	1,165	2,856	806	903	660	1,103	196

NOTE: Rates are for episodes of care for 1,000 persons per year; conditions include the top 40 diagnoses in at least one dataset; some groupings have been made.

[a]NHIS = National Health Interview Survey.

[b]NAMCS = National Ambulatory Medical Care Survey.

SOURCE: Hofmans-Okkes and Lamberts, 1995; NHIS and NAMCS data originate from unpublished information made available to the committee by Peter Franks, Carolyn Clancy, Paul Nutting and analyzed by Inge Hofmans-Okkes and Henk Lamberts. Organizational data from three managed care plans were analyzed by Inge Hofmans-Okkes and Henk Lamberts.

Total episodes rates for Organizations B and C are considerably lower and different in the split between new and follow-up episodes.

In terms of diagnosis, the "top 20" approach used for the Dutch data could not be applied entirely, as the specifics differ considerably. Not surprisingly, of course, the basic classes of problems that appear to be prevalent in this cohort are the same—for example, in the case of new episodes, pregnancy and family planning issues and an array of infectious disease symptoms. The NAMCS data also indicate something of the shift in problems between new episodes and follow-up care.

Comment

This data exercise had two purposes. One was to determine what information on episodes of care pertinent to the entire U.S. population might be gleaned from various federal (public sector) sources and from private sector health care organizations. The other was to shed some light, if possible, on the epidemiology of "the great majority of health care needs" that the committee points to in its definition of primary care. The data from the Netherlands Transition Project were used as a analytic prototype. Inferences about the U.S. population should be made only cautiously from the Dutch data for two reasons: (1) the considerable differences in the racial, ethnic, and other characteristics of the two populations, and (2) the more advanced methods used in the project to classify episodes and code them in terms of diagnosis or reason for encounter.

Several lessons might be drawn. First, the available information in the United States does not lend itself at present to episode-of-care analysis. To the extent an episode orientation will be important in the future for research, policy, health care delivery, or population statistics purposes, this may be a drawback to appropriate data collection, analysis, and decisionmaking. In that regard, therefore, the committee was of the view that high priority might well be given to developing structures and computer-based methods (e.g., computer-based patient records) that would permit either the public sector (for national statistics or for its own health care programs) and the private sector to create and analyze episodes of care in adequate detail. Second, the "great majority of health care needs" is broad indeed, especially when *both* new and follow-up episodes are considered. Third, according to the Dutch data, diagnostic labels for episodes and reasons for visit or encounter as provided by patients differ considerably. This underscores the significance of adequate and complete communication between patient and practitioner, an aspect of care related to the committee's notion of a "sustained partnership" and a cornerstone of the traditional "art of care" element of high quality of care.

REFERENCES

Adams, P.F., and Benson, V. Current Estimates from the National Health Interview Survey, 1991. *Vital and Health Statistics, Series 10* 184(Dec.):1-232, 1992.

Barondess, J.A. Content and Process in Ambulatory Care. *American Journal of Medicine* 73:735–739, 1982.

Blackhall, L.J, Murphy, S.T., Frank, G., et al. Ethnicity and Attitudes Toward Patient Autonomy. *Journal of the American Medical Association* 274:820–825, 1995.

Carrese, J.A. and Rhodes, L.A. Western Bioethics on the Navajo Reservation: Benefit or Harm? *Journal of the American Medical Association* 274:826–829, 1995.

Evidence-Based Medicine Working Group. Evidence-Based Medicine: A New Approach to Teaching the Practice of Medicine. *Journal of the American Medical Association* 268:2420–2425, 1992.

Hofmans-Okkes, I., and Lamberts, H. Episodes of Care and the Large Majority of Personal Health Care Needs: Is the New IOM Definition of Primary Care Reflected in U.S. Primary Care Data? Paper commissioned by the Institute of Medicine Committee on the Future of Primary Care, 1995.

Kasper, J.F., Mulley, A.G., and Wennberg, J.E. Developing Shared Decision-making Programs to Improve the Quality of Health Care. *Quality Review Bulletin* 18:183–190, 1992.

Klinkman, M.S., and Green, L.A. Using ICPC in a Computer-based Primary Care Information System. *Family Medicine* 27:449–456, 1995.

Lalonde, M. *A New Perspective on the Health of Canadians.* Ottawa: Ministry of National Health and Welfare, 1974.

Lamberts, H., and Hofmans-Okkes, I. Characteristics of Primary Care. Episode of Care: A Core Concept in Family Practice. *Journal of Family Practice* 42:161–167, 1996.

Lamberts, H., and Wood, M., eds. *International Classification of Primary Care (ICPC).* Oxford: Oxford University Press, 1987.

Lamberts, H., Wood, M., and Hofmans-Okkes, I.M., eds. *The International Classification of Primary Care in the European Community With a Multilanguage Layer.* Oxford: Oxford University Press, 1993.

Lipkin, M., Jr., Quill, T.E., Napodano, R.J., et al. The Medical Interview: A Core Curriculum for Residencies in Internal Medicine. *Annals of Internal Medicine* 100:277–284, 1984.

Mort, E.A. Clinical Decision-making in the Face of Scientific Uncertainty: Hormone Replacement Therapy as an Example. *Journal of Family Practice* 42:147–151, 1996.

Mulley, A.G., Jr. A Patient Outcomes Orientation: The Committee View. Pages 63–72 in *Medicare: New Directions in Quality Assurance. Proceedings.* M.S. Donaldson, J. Harris-Wehling, and K.N. Lohr, eds. Washington, D.C.: National Academy Press, 1991.

Rosenblatt, R.A., Hart, J., Gamliel, S., et al. Identifying Primary Care Disciplines by Analyzing the Diagnostic Content of Ambulatory Care. *Journal of the American Board of Family Practice* 8:34–45, 1995.

Rosser, W.W. Approach to Diagnosis by Primary Care Clinicians and Specialists: Is There a Difference? *Journal of Family Practice* 42:139–144, 1996.

Schappert, S.M. National Ambulatory Medical Care Survey: 1991 Summary. *Vital and Health Statistics, Series 13* 116(May):1–110, 1994.

Sobel, D.S. Partners in Health: Empowering the Patient in Health Care. Presented at the Annual Convention of the American Hospital Association and Texas Hospital Association, Dallas, August 8–10, 1994.

Sox, H.C., Jr. Decision-making: A Comparison of Referral Practice and Primary Care. *Journal of Family Practice* 42:155–160, 1996.

U.S. Preventive Services Task Force. *Guide to Clinical Preventive Services: An Assessment of the Effectiveness of 169 Interventions.* Baltimore: Williams and Wilkins, 1989.

U.S. Preventive Services Task Force. *Guide to Clinical Preventive Services: An Assessment of the Effectiveness of 169 Interventions.* 2d ed. Baltimore: William and Wilkins, 1996.

Vickery, D.M., and Lynch, W.D. Demand Management: Enabling Patients to Use Medical Care Appropriately. *Journal of Occupational and Environmental Medicine* 37:551–557, 1995.

Wells, K.B., Stewart, A., Hays, R.D., et al. The Functioning and Well-Being of Depressed Patients: Results from the Medical Outcomes Study. *Journal of the American Medical Association* 262:914–919, 1989.

Wells, K.B., and Sturm, R. Care for Depression in a Changing Environment. *Health Affairs* 14(3):78–89, 1995.

White, K.L., Williams, T.F., and Greenberg, B.G. The Ecology of Medical Care. *New England Journal of Medicine* 265:885–893, 1961.

5

The Delivery of Primary Care

The definition of primary care (Chapter 2) is a normative definition; that is, it defines what the committee believes the function of primary care should be. Whether the elements of this definition can be achieved and whether primary care can assume its proper role in the delivery of health care will be determined in a world of health care that is being reshaped by the forces described in Chapter 1. Although some of those forces are favorable to aspects of primary care, the committee is not convinced that the current health care market, by itself, will shape primary care to match all aspects of the definition. Further actions will need to be taken to provide the financial incentives and infrastructure that will help the health care system overcome barriers. This chapter includes recommendations for such actions. In addition to barriers that are specific to primary care, the committee notes that the lack of universal entitlement to health care benefits will continue to raise special problems for the uninsured and underinsured in obtaining access to primary care.

The committee is under no illusion that it can, or should, prescribe a single path for delivering primary care in an environment that is so diverse and changing so rapidly. Nevertheless, the definition presents clear guideposts for actions by the many actors in health care: health professions, health plans and organizations, payers for group coverage who set many of the standards within which health care is organized, and government regulators. Diversity in the means of achieving the committee's primary care objectives may be desirable, but the key elements of the definition should be the criteria by which actions to advance primary care are judged.

This chapter is presented in two sections. The first section outlines the committee's observations about the current trends and characteristics of U.S. health care that form the current context for the delivery of primary care. The second section contains the committee's conclusions and recommendations about changes needed to improve the delivery of primary care in order to realize more fully the potential of primary care to improve the health and satisfaction of patients.

CURRENT PATHWAYS FOR PRIMARY CARE

The rapid pace of change and the diversity of local circumstances are striking characteristics of current health care. Descriptive evidence about current directions of health care, augmented by the committee's five site visits, confirms the magnitude and rapidity of those changes. Ours is a health care system going through a major transition. From an era of growth in expensive services supported by open-ended financing, wide choice of clinicians and hospitals, and almost complete freedom for clinical judgment, the U.S. health system is moving quickly into an era of limits on resources, cost-based competition among health plans and providers, financial risk-sharing by providers, and constraints on patient choice of clinician. No one can predict accurately where the health care system will be in 5 years, let alone 10 or 20 years. Simple generalizations informed by past studies, even studies only a few years old, are limited in their ability to describe or explain current directions in health care. Yet we believe that broad pathways for that change can be identified and need to be taken into consideration.

Some studies have identified stages of the health care market that imply a progression toward "mature" markets (University Hospital Consortium, 1993)— essentially those dominated by a handful of large, fiercely competitive health plans. The committee is wary, however, of any interpretation that such a progression is an orderly one. In visiting several areas of the country that are usually considered more mature health care markets (e.g., Minnesota and southern California), committee members observed that the pace of change continues to be rapid. Wherever these markets are going, they are not there yet.

With these cautions and caveats, we do see broad themes, both in what is happening and in what has not happened.

Spread of Managed Care

The term *managed care* has come to have many meanings. This committee uses managed care to refer to health plans that have a selective list of providers, both health professionals and hospitals, and that include mechanisms for influencing the nature, quantity, and site of services delivered. Many of these plans have focused initially on using their market power to obtain discounts from physicians, hospitals, and other providers in an oversupplied market. They are evolving, however, toward more organized arrangements that include some form of involvement of the providers in the risk assumed by the plan. That risk derives from the plan's agreement to deliver a defined package of services for a fixed amount per capita for an enrolled population, such as with the various forms of health maintenance organizations (HMOs). The involvement of providers in the success of the plan is intended to offer incentives for containing costs while maintaining patient satisfaction with the care received.

Bailit (1995) estimates that in 1994, of a total of 180 million insured by private plans, enrollment in managed care totalled about 115 million persons. This estimate uses a definition of managed care that includes HMOs; "point of service" plans that combine HMO enrollment with an option to use providers outside the plan for an additional cost; and PPOs (preferred provider organizations), which offer a less structured arrangement that presents the enrolled person with a financial incentive to choose providers from a preferred list. He estimates that the number of individuals enrolled in managed care in the private market increased about 10 percent from 1993 to 1994.

Enrollment in managed care in the public programs in 1994 was much lower than in private plans, at about 8 percent of Medicare beneficiaries and about 25 percent of those eligible for Medicaid. The rate of increase is greater, however, especially in the Medicaid program. Forty-two states are implementing some form of managed care in their Medicaid programs. Arizona (100 percent), Tennessee (74.9 percent), and Oregon (21.9 percent) lead the way in the percentage of Medicaid dollars spent through managed care arrangements, but many other states are moving aggressively in this direction (Lewin-VHI, 1995). Current congressional deliberations on the future course of the Medicare program may result in further encouragement of enrollment of Medicare beneficiaries in capitated managed care plans.

Of particular significance for this study is that one major objective of most managed care plans is to reduce the use of specialists and to increase the use of primary care clinicians. The path to specialized care in most plans is through the primary care physician or other primary care clinician. Managed care, therefore, enhances the power of the primary care clinician to determine the services provided and by whom. The increasing future opportunities for primary care clinicians and the contrasting decline in the need for specialists have been described by Weiner and others in projecting future physician requirements (Weiner, 1993; COGME, 1995; PPRC, 1995).

The growth of managed care, although substantial, is taking place predominantly in large and medium-sized markets. Those providing services in rural areas are anticipating the move of managed care into their communities, but managed care was not yet evident in the rural areas visited by the committee.

The development of managed care varies widely by region. The most significant market penetration has been in the West, the upper Middle West, and the Northeast. The Southeast and South Central regions have less managed care at this time (GHAA, 1995). In all areas, managed care on the basis of an enrolled, capitated population is not available to the uninsured and many of the under-insured, a growing proportion of the U.S. population (EBRI, 1995).

The growth of managed care plans is blurring the traditional boundaries between the insuring or financing function, with its strong concern for managing risk, and the provision of services and clinical decisions regarding those services. Managing risk is still important; no plan, regardless how efficient, wants to have a disproportionate share of sicker patients unless that risk can be shared. Most managed care plans, however, are also interested in how to improve the efficiency of services and how to maintain or increase patient satisfaction. Sophisticated buyers, such as the business community in the Twin Cities area, are developing performance standards for health plans that include clinical measures (Institute for Clinical Systems Integration, no date). Older staff and group model HMOs, such as Kaiser Permanente and Group Health Cooperative of Puget Sound, have long combined the insurance and patient care functions under a single organizational umbrella.

Development of Integrated Health Care Delivery Systems

A related and overlapping trend is the development of vertically integrated delivery systems that combine physicians and other health professionals, hospitals, rehabilitation units, social services, chronic care capabilities, mental health and substance abuse programs, and health promotion and disease prevention programs into an organized whole that can provide and coordinate a comprehensive array of services. Some of the motivation behind the development of these systems is to increase and protect market share in areas where there is surplus capacity. It is difficult to quantify the extent of systems change because so much is happening so rapidly. Many examples exist, mostly in larger cities but some in more rural areas, often built on preexisting multispecialty groups such as those of the Mayo, Marshfield, and Geisinger clinics.

Based on examples seen in the site visits, these systems at their best provide opportunities for innovations in arrangements for services, in part by breaking down institutional and professional barriers to delivering services more efficiently. They also provide the critical mass and capital needed for the development of infrastructure, such as information and clinical decision systems, telephone triage programs, and training. In the best of these organizations, the functions of primary care move well beyond the gatekeeper function toward a fuller application of the committee's definition.

These systems are not a new phenomenon; some of the older staff and group model HMOs have had many of these characteristics for some time. What may be new is an environment that encourages change rather than one that regards innovations as a questionable deviation from the norm. The pressure for continuing improvement in the cost-effective provision of services is present in older integrated systems with long track records of success as well as in newer systems that have been built by combining previously independent providers.

For our purposes, the important point is that all of these systems are built on, or are building on, foundations of primary care clinicians, often by purchasing existing primary care practices. This primary care base is seen as necessary for both building and protecting market share and for creating a mechanism to control access to specialized services. In a capitated system, specialized services are seen as cost centers, rather than as revenue centers, and the organization has strong incentives to control such costs.

Consolidation of Health Plans and Systems

Both health plans and integrated systems are consolidating into larger organizations. They are driven to do so by several factors, including the need for capital, advantages in marketing, and potential economies of scale in developing and using infrastructure such as clinical information systems. Site visits to urban markets (the Twin Cities, southern California, and Boston) provided multiple examples in each site of major consolidations of health plans and provider organizations.

In communities where this consolidation is far along, characterization of health care as a very local and personalized service—a cottage industry as it has often been called—no longer holds. Becoming part of a larger organization is causing considerable stress for clinicians who value highly the autonomy of their practice and personal relationships with their patients. Some patients are also disturbed if they believe that their relationship with a primary care clinician who is committed to their interests is being compromised by a large, impersonal, and perhaps distant organization.

Growth in For-Profit Health Plans and Delivery Systems

Along with consolidation, health plans and integrated systems are increasingly under for-profit ownership. In addition to the growth of existing for-profit plans and their acquisition of not-for-profit plans, some not-for-profit plans are converting to for-profit forms of ownership. The need to raise capital for expansion is often given as the reason for the growth of for-profit ownership. The long range effects of this trend are not clear, but it raises the possibility of conflict between the desires of the stockholders to maximize profit and the objectives of primary care to ensure adequate care for patients. It also underlines the need to have measures of performance that include the interests of patients, not just the financial interests of group purchasers and stockholders, and that are available to guide patients' health care choices (for a fuller discussion of these issues, which is beyond the scope of this report, see IOM, 1986a, and Gray, 1991).

Diversity Among and Within Markets

As noted, markets vary widely in the extent to which services have moved along the pathways described above. Most rural areas have not yet joined these trends, and some urban areas have much lower rates of managed care penetration. Within markets observed on the site visits, some health plans are developing service innovations that improve the efficiency of care; others are focusing on utilization management, sales efforts to increase market share, and risk-sharing with providers as their means to compete successfully in their markets. Some groups of clinicians are tightly organized, and some are looser confederations of clinicians who remain essentially independent contractors with ownership and control of their own practices.

The clinicians involved in primary care services vary from plan to plan and setting to setting. In some plans extensive use is made of nurse practitioners and physician assistants; in others, much less. Other practices continue to emphasize the traditional role of the physician. Diversity is also seen in the type of primary care physicians involved. For example, in rural areas family physicians are prevalent, whereas in urban areas pediatricians and internists play a more prominent role.

Coordination of Primary Care with Other Services

The focus of most of the large delivery systems remains on more traditional medical services—acute and chronic care and preventive services provided by clinicians. The extent to which plans with enrolled populations are dealing with population-based health issues is not clear, although many examples of health education and behavior change programs exist. Cooperation with the public health agencies also seems weak.

Coordination regarding mental health and substance abuse services may be harder because of the trend toward "carve-outs" for these services into separate benefit packages that are independently managed. This new trend is in addition to the continuing patterns of delivery of many of these services by separate organizations and of limitations on these services in benefit packages.

Financial barriers to long-term care remain a significant problem. Few private plans include long-term care benefits. In the public sector, the Department of Veterans Affairs (VA) is a notable exception. All in all, concern about the lack of involvement of primary care clinicians in the medical care of patients in long-term care settings remains high (IOM, 1986b; 1995).

Vision care and pharmacy services are collocated in some group model plans, and many plans include a dental care benefit. Dental services as an integral part of the primary care delivery system, however, are seen mostly in programs organized for the poor and by the Indian Health Service.

Judgments may differ as to the likely results of these fissures in services for common health problems. Nonetheless, the lack of explicit arrangements for coordinating primary care with other services that are needed on a routine and recurring basis by many patients is striking, especially as integration of other aspects of acute services moves ahead rapidly.

Current and Evolving Professional Roles

There is evidence of the increasing demand for primary care physicians as their incomes are rising relative to those of specialists in many areas (Mitka, 1994a,b; 1995). Further evidence of the rising status of primary care among physicians is the desire of many specialists to be designated as primary care physicians. California has given the primary care label to obstetrics and gynecology through state law, and other specialist groups have staked out a claim to the domain of primary care. This desire to be designated as primary care clinicians is the result of managed care plans' requiring that enrollees choose a primary care clinician, usually a family practitioner, general internist, or pediatrician, who will control access to specialized services.

There is also evidence of increasing demand for the use of nurse practitioners and physician assistants in primary care. Training programs for these professionals are expanding rapidly (see Chapters 6 and 7). The committee saw many examples of the involvement of these professions in primary care during its site visits, nearly always as part of a team that included physicians in a key role. Within integrated systems, the use of teams and delegation of primary care functions is proceeding rapidly (see Appendix E). In some locales, supply constraints, in particular, shortages of nurse practitioners, are impeding their greater use.

During site visits, committee members saw examples of further delegation of clinical functions to registered nurses, licensed practical nurses, and desk clerks. Such delegation was the result of a deliberate decision process that examined how specific clinical problems could be managed more efficiently. In some of these settings, primary care physicians were focusing on more complex clinical problems and taking on managerial roles, thus moving the clinical boundaries between primary care physicians and specialists toward more specialized care.

How widespread these changes are is difficult to document because doing so requires knowledge of the details of how particular functions are carried out, and these are only partially reflected in aggregate data on the numbers and types of professionals. This effort on the part of some of the more advanced integrated systems to redefine professional roles within a team concept may prove very important, however, as a future pathway for improving the efficiency and effectiveness of primary care. It may in turn have significant implications for training programs and for workforce policy. The care delivered by other first contact professionals such as dentists, eye care clinicians, and pharmacists is generally less coordinated with the broader functions of primary care.

Primary Care in Rural Settings

Observations made during site visits to rural areas are consistent with the extensive literature on rural care in noting what one host called the "fragility" of many programs providing primary care to rural populations. Rural care is often dependent on some form of subsidy, as well as on a distant infrastructure that can provide technical assistance and professional backup. The reasons are several: the higher proportion of the uninsured and underinsured in many rural areas; higher costs of transportation; and lower volume of services. Primary care in the rural setting also includes a stronger emphasis on emergency care and the stabilization and transportation of patients with medical emergencies and trauma. Managed care has not yet penetrated most rural settings. The committee observed successful models of rural care, but none that did not have some form of subsidy or assistance (or both). It also observed impressive examples of the importance of community commitment to the maintenance of a primary care capacity in isolated rural areas.

Care of the Urban Poor

Care for low-income or disadvantaged populations, concentrated in the inner cities, is complicated by the lack of universal insurance coverage, the health care needs of illegal immigrants, and the low payments for providers in many states. These problems have often been alleviated by internal cross-subsidies and federal program formulas that favor institutions and care settings that serve a disproportionate share of the poor. The combination of competitive cost pressures and limits on public financing is likely to become much more acute in the near future and to make existing arrangements unstable. In some areas and states, such as Arizona, evidence suggests that managed care may be able to take on an increased share of these populations, but it is not clear how much such an approach can succeed without some form of subsidy that recognizes the extra costs now being incurred to serve the primary care needs of these populations.

Role of Academic Health Centers

In site visits, the committee heard numerous complaints from community programs about the lack of appropriate involvement of academic health centers (AHCs) in primary care and about the resulting lack of fit between the products of their training programs and the needs of managed care and community-based programs. The problems that AHCs face in surviving in the current health care market have been well documented elsewhere (Blumenthal and Meyer, 1993; Fox and Wasserman, 1993; Epstein, 1995; Josiah Macy, Jr. Foundation, 1995). The extra costs of training, the dependence on patient care income from referrals for tertiary services, the higher proportion of the poor in their service area, and governance processes that make difficult a quick response to market changes are all handicaps for these institutions in a highly competitive health care market. For many of these institutions these factors constitute barriers to greater focus on primary care. Despite these barriers, there are also examples of effective involvement of AHCs in strengthening primary care. In one state, an AHC's mission statement was explicit about its commitment to primary care, and this mission was reflected in the curriculum and in assistance to communities in providing primary care.

MOVING TOWARD DELIVERY OF PRIMARY CARE AS DEFINED

Some aspects of the current health care scene favor further emphasis on primary care as the foundation for the health care system. Despite these favorable forces, many obstacles remain to be overcome in reorienting a large and complex health care system. As a sector of the economy that consumes about one-seventh of this society's resources and that is still growing faster than the rest of the economy, many powerful interest groups have a financial and professional stake in the status quo. Market forces seem to have the strength to require significant alterations in that status quo, but as stated earlier the committee remains skeptical that the market, by itself, will achieve a primary care system that meets its definition and that is widely available to the American public.

Because the benefits of primary care are important for meeting the health care goals of this society, the committee believes that a specific objective for the availability of primary care service should be established, focusing on the central relationship of the clinician and the patient.

Recommendation 5.1 Availability of Primary Care for All Americans

The committee recommends development of primary care delivery systems that will make the services of a primary care clinician available to all Americans.

In order to achieve this goal, steps need to be taken to create conditions favorable to primary care. Some steps involve public policies and the commitment of public resources by federal and state governments (even in a time of stringency for public budgets). Other steps entail voluntary actions to shape existing forces for change so that they more nearly match the committee's definition of primary care. Many of the desired changes will not be achieved rapidly. The results may vary widely in their particulars and still constitute movement in the right directions.

Specific actions in isolation from other needed actions are not likely to be successful. In this sense, bringing about the needed changes in primary care is a systems problem in which many elements interrelate. For example, shifts in the education of primary care clinicians to encourage the function of a primary care team, as described in Chapter 7, are unlikely to have the desired result if the practice environment does not also support those changes. The rest of this chapter identifies some of the specific areas where action is needed to shape the course of the delivery of primary care toward the objectives that were identified in the definition.

Financing of Primary Care Services

The failure of comprehensive health care reform at the national level (which aimed at providing universal health insurance coverage) and the retreat from reforms at the state level (such as in Washington and Oregon) mean that many Americans remain without health insurance coverage. Furthermore, cost-competitive market forces are likely to exacerbate some of the problems of providing care to the uninsured. The proportions of the population that are either underinsured or uninsured are rising (EBRI, 1995; Short and Banthin, 1995). As long as significant financial barriers to access continue to exist for many millions of people, the objectives and implementing reforms recommended in this report, even if instituted fully, will not make the benefits of primary care available to many of those without health insurance. Addressing specific ways that health care coverage could be extended to everyone is beyond the scope of this report, but we note in the strongest terms that the primary care agenda for the nation will remain incomplete until this extension takes place.

Recommendation 5.2 Health Care Coverage for All Americans

To assure that the benefits of primary care are more uniformly available, the committee recommends that the federal government and the states develop strategies to provide health care coverage for all Americans.

The importance of this recommendation is accentuated by the effects of market forces in reducing the internal cross-subsidies and other forms of implicit subsidies that have helped to cover the health care needs of the uninsured. Likely reductions in the growth of public financing of health care in coming years will make these subsidies even harder to sustain. Therefore, the current situation of financial barriers to primary care for some of the population is almost sure to worsen without some form of public action.

The committee is aware of the controversies that may be engendered about who should be included under the rubric of "all Americans." It is beyond the scope of this committee to address these complicated issues in detail, especially the issues of coverage of undocumented aliens. If universal coverage is realized, however, the coverage should at least extend to all those who are legal residents, whether or not they are citizens.

In addition to the lack of universal coverage for medical care, this nation seems nowhere near a policy that addresses the need to cover the costs of long-term care for the elderly and the chronically ill. This gap will continue to make more difficult the appropriate coordination of primary care services with long-term care services.

Delivery systems for primary care services need to assure the actual availability of services to all. Universal coverage may by itself encourage availability for some individuals and populations for whom primary care is currently unavailable or very inconvenient. But removing financial barriers to primary care through universal coverage is unlikely by itself to achieve the goal of availability of primary care services set out in Recommendation 5.1, and specific efforts will be required for some populations.

Later sections of this chapter address the need for special efforts to reach some populations with primary care services. Individuals in otherwise well-served areas may also face problems of availability, and these should also be addressed. Arrangements for the financing and monitoring of care would need to include achievement of this goal.

For the large sector of the population that does have health insurance, some methods of paying for services seem more likely than others to encourage primary care. As implemented in the United States, fee-for-service payments have favored procedural services and specialized care. In contrast, financing methods involving a single payment that covers specified services for an enrolled population over a period of time have provided incentives for primary care. Such global capitation payments have been used for many years by HMOs as various forms of managed care have spread and capitation has become more frequent. One study of the development of integrated delivery systems demonstrated that capitated payment mechanisms covering the continuum of care are most likely to promote clinical integration, preventive care, and treatment of patients in the most appropriate setting. As a result there is an incentive to place primary care rather than acute inpatient services at the center of the health care system (Shortell et al., 1994).

By providing an overall cap on resources, however, capitation may also reward health care plans for not providing services, and services necessary for good care could be neglected. Performance monitoring and public dissemination of quality-of-care information, as well as the opportunity for enrollees to change plans at regular intervals, are intended to motivate plans to provide quality services or risk losing their market share in the competitive environment in which most plans function. If these mechanisms to provide good information about plans work, health plans that provide good care efficiently should succeed. Such monitoring mechanisms, however, are still not fully developed in most markets.

Methods for translating capitation into reimbursement for specific primary care services are numerous and evolving rapidly. For example, some group and staff model HMOs pay salaries to primary care clinicians and may include incentives that are tied to the overall performance of the plan. Many network model HMOs reimburse primary care services through a capitation payment to the primary care clinician, sometimes with specific incentives for desired practice patterns and sometimes placing the primary care clinician at risk for the use of specialty services. Other plans have used a mix of fee-for-service and capitation. Still others pay for primary care on a fee-for-service basis coupled with a financial incentive to discourage high utilization of services.

Capitation payments to the individual clinician may provide incentives not to make referrals that would be in the patient's interests or to skimp on the provision of primary care services by spending too little time with the patient. In particular, deGruy (Appendix D) notes that such incentives may affect the ability of the primary care clinician to deal with the mental health problems presented in the primary care setting, if adequate time for interacting with the patient is not provided. The committee did not have the opportunity to explore in detail the specific methods of paying primary care clinicians that would encourage good primary care. It did note during some site visits that innovations in the patterns of primary care and in the use of teams were associated with salary payment mechanisms. The salary approach also reduces incentives to withhold necessary services. The committee also agrees with the observation by Shortell and his colleagues (1994) that global capitation payments have been associated with an emphasis on primary care services within the overall service mix regardless of the specific method of paying the primary care clinician.

Recommendation 5.3 Payment Methods Favorable to Primary Care

The committee recommends that payment methods favorable to the support of primary care be more widely adopted.

These payment methods should include global capitation that covers all defined services for an enrolled population coupled with methods of paying the primary care clinician and the primary care team that support the characteristics of good primary care as described in this report. Among the methods that seem to be consistent with this objective are (a) salary arrangements and (b) forms of capitation or partial capitation payments (in combination with some form of fee-for-service reimbursement) to the individual provider that are structured to reward good primary care.

As capitation is translated into specific methods of payment for primary care clinicians, clinicians need to be given the flexibility to spend the amount of time with patients that is necessary for good primary care. For example, using rigid productivity guidelines regarding the number of patients to be seen per time period is not consistent with good primary care. The translation of capitation into specific payment mechanisms should also support collaborative practice. This implies that productivity or improvement of health status ought to be measured for the entire primary care unit with such measures adjusted appropriately for the socioeconomic and health-related characteristics of the patient panel.

An aspect of indemnity insurance that discourages primary care is the use of deductibles and coinsurance that raise the marginal costs of the use of primary care services while expensive, specialized services are often provided at no further cost to the patient. Substantial financial disincentives to the use of routine and recurring care tend to encourage episodic, acute care; they work to the disadvantage of continuous care, care of the chronically ill, and advice about and coordination of other services. Such copayments and deductibles are also sometimes used within capitated systems. This disincentive for some primary care services is accentuated when certain areas, such as preventive services, are excluded entirely from benefit packages.

Although the methods for paying primary care clinicians are likely to continue to evolve and to include salary and capitation arrangements, fee-for-service reimbursement is likely to remain a method of payment for primary care for the foreseeable future. Such reimbursement may come as direct payment from a fee-for-service health insurance plan, as with indemnity insurance plans and the regular Medicare Part B program, and it may be used as the method of payment for individual clinicians under a capitated health plan.

Fee-for-service payments in the U.S. have not typically favored primary care services because they provide higher payment levels for specialized diagnostic and treatment procedures. Traditional patterns of fee-for-service payment are even less likely to support many of the aspects of primary care that are emphasized in the committee's definition, such as coordination of primary care with community-based services, which take clinician time and infrastructure support. Substantial efforts have been made to develop fee schedules that are more favorable to the primary care functions; the most notable is the Resource-Based Relative Value Scale (RBRVS) being implemented by the Medicare program and some private plans. Implementation of RBRVS in the Medicare program up to this time, however, has been disappointing in terms of encouraging primary care (PPRC, 1994). Because the various forms of fee-for-service methods are likely to continue to be used for reimbursing many clinicians in the foreseeable future, it is important for this payment method to provide better incentives for primary care, and the committee makes the following recommendation.

Recommendation 5.4 Payment for Primary Care Services

The committee recommends that when fee-for-service is used to reimburse clinicians for patient care, payments for primary care be upgraded to reflect better the value of these services.

The committee believes that greater emphasis on primary care clinicians may be more than offset by the savings that come from decreased use of specialty care. This issue of encouraging financing mechanisms that support primary care may also arise in proposals to establish "medical savings accounts" (MSAs). These individual accounts, which are created through tax-exempt contributions from employers or individuals (or both), can be used to pay for all types of medical expenses; typically the individuals benefit financially from any residual in their account. This proposal is usually coupled with insurance protection against catastrophic acute health care expenditures (American Academy of Actuaries, 1995; Joint Committee on Taxation, 1995). As of spring 1996, 15 states have adopted some form of MSA (Alpha Center, 1996).

A major aim of such proposals is to provide incentives to patients to use medical care efficiently by giving them a greater role in paying directly for services and a direct stake in the level of expenditure for the services. Such an approach offers greater economic incentives to limit the use of primary care relative to the use of expensive specialized services for two reasons: (1) most of the costs of the latter would be covered by the catastrophic insurance component of the plan and (2) the costs for primary care come out of MSAs. Another factor might be patients' tendencies to forgo preventive services with long-range benefits or other aspects of primary care, if the full benefits are not apparent to them or lie well in the future.

The concept of consumer sovereignty that underlies proposals for MSAs implies that consumers or patients have adequate knowledge to guide their own medical care decisions, but this is probably not true for many consumers. Consumers may postpone care until a major acute episode takes place, and this may be especially true for lower-income persons for whom the economic incentive to postpone care may loom large.

The committee is concerned that the values of primary care as discussed in Chapter 3 may be undermined by this approach to financing. If the funds are used for the purchase of comprehensive benefits that include good primary care coverage, such as an HMO plan, the effects may not be negative for primary care; but if the funds are used in a way that downgrades the function of primary care, the long-range effect on health outcomes and on aggregate health expenditures may be negative. This issue illustrates the limitations of the pure insurance model when paying for health care if it does not include appropriate primary care incentives (see the IOM report [1993b] on employment and health benefits for discussion of some aspects of this issue).

Another aspect of current approaches to financing that causes concern to the committee is the disruption of continuity that may occur when employers change health plans or when patients, motivated by small savings in health plan costs, switch plans. During the committee site visits, committee members heard from primary care clinicians and from patients that frequent changes in health plans offered by employers had forced patients to change physicians and that they believe this had adverse effects on continuity and access. The committee notes, however, that in some markets employers are beginning to write contracts with health plans that extend for several years rather than just one year. The committee would like to encourage this trend. Three- or even five-year contracts would reduce the possibility that shifts in health plans would force patients to change primary care clinicians. The problem of patient-initiated changes probably needs to be addressed by better education of patients about the benefits to them of continuity in primary care.

Organizing Primary Care Services

The emergence of large integrated delivery systems has emphasized primary care. These organizational arrangements appear to have some economies of scale for the infrastructure of primary care, such as implementing information systems, disseminating clinical decision criteria, developing and evaluating innovative deployment of health personnel and mechanisms of coordinating services, and developing and using patient education materials. Coupled with enrolled populations, these systems offer other potential benefits: improved continuity of care, reduced barriers to movement between different elements of the care system, and pursuit of population-based approaches to disease prevention and health promotion. Whether these goals are realized depends in the longer term on documenting their advantages for patients and for the purchasers of group health benefits. Criteria for success must move beyond crude measures of cost saving to broader measures of systems performance (see discussion of performance measures below).

The committee also has concerns about this trend toward large integrated systems. Its definition emphasizes the importance of the personal relationship between the patient and the clinician or the team of clinicians. Can a large organization nurture and sustain such relationships in the midst of competitive market forces that are sometimes translated into limits on time spent with the patient? Can triage systems be implemented in a manner that appropriately supports regular contact with a clinician who is knowledgeable about the patient and the patient's history? In concept, and in reality, personal relationships can be fostered if the system makes it a high priority reflected in the organization's leadership, procedures, internal incentives, and patient education program.

Another issue is whether integrated systems address effectively the needs of rural populations, the inner city poor, and culturally diverse populations. The record to date is highly variable, and the inclusion of these special populations in large integrated systems has been limited. The trend toward use by states of managed care approaches for the Medicaid population has provided a possible linkage, and the nature and amount of the public funding for these programs will help to determine if integrated systems can meet the needs of these populations for primary care services.

Variation in successful organizational models is great; the committee does not recommend a specific organizational mode as best for primary care. The committee does believe, however, that the potential of integrated systems to provide primary care is substantial and should be encouraged; it also holds that performance measures used for internal and external evaluation of such systems should encompass the desired characteristics of primary care. The use of these systems to meet the needs of vulnerable and underserved populations also needs to be encouraged and measured, although their success in reaching out to these populations will be limited to the extent that these groups continue to lack health insurance coverage.

Understanding Professional Roles in Primary Care

Background

The roles of the various health professions and how those professions should interrelate are both contentious issues. Discussions of professional roles in primary care are influenced by many past tensions: the sometimes strained relationships between nurses and physicians, the struggle of primary care physicians for appropriate status in a medical environment dominated by specialists and subspecialists, and the arguments between such first-contact health professionals as optometrists and some of the medical profession. The tensions have been exacerbated in recent years by the growth of managed care arrangements that make primary care clinicians the path by which patients gain access to specialized medical services.

This shift in power and responsibility for determining the use of medical resources has significant economic implications for most of the health professions. These implications are magnified when many medical specialties are likely to be in surplus and when the hospital is diminishing as a locus of employment for nurses. (See Chapter 6 for an overview of supply and demand issues for physicians, nurse practitioners, and physician assistants.)

For all of these reasons the debate over the label of primary care clinician is intense. At a public hearing organized by this committee and in written statements received by the committee, a wide range of professional groups have expressed the view that their professions provide primary care. The professional and economic stakes are substantial if the function of primary care receives more emphasis at the same time that efforts to hold down expenditures for health care continue. Subsequent discussion of these issues at a workshop on professional roles convened by the study committee provided opportunity to explore further the many dimensions of the roles issue.

From the beginning of its deliberations, the committee has believed that primary care should *not* be defined solely or primarily by who does it. The definition is a functional definition that provides a basis for determining whether a particular professional is a primary care clinician. That function is the overriding guide to this discussion of roles. Starting with the functional definition makes more problematic an *a priori* determination of who is, or is not, a primary care clinician, as was noted in Chapter 2.

For clinicians whose training is explicitly targeted on primary care, their role as primary care clinician is clear. There is little argument that among physicians (both allopathic and osteopathic), family physicians, general internists, and general pediatricians are primary care clinicians. Many nurse practitioners and physician assistants are also trained for primary care and participate in the primary care function. The issues for these professions are mainly how they can work together in the interest of patients. However, the involvement of other physician specialists in primary care is a growing issue, especially for obstetricians and gynecologists and the medical subspecialties. Also at issue is the role of health professionals who independently provide basic services for some health care needs on a first-contact basis—for example, dentists, optometrists, pharmacists, and some physical therapists. Such services form a significant part of health care, but the relationship to primary care is inadequately defined. Each of these issues is addressed in turn below.

The Primary Care Team

In discussing the definition in Chapter 2, the committee indicated that primary care consists of a set of tasks that can often be best carried out by a team rather than by an individual clinician. The team may be organized to achieve a number of purposes: to increase access, to subdivide tasks so that several different kinds of expertise can be brought to bear on the patient's needs through collaborative activity, and to permit the delegation of some tasks by broadening the range of professionals involved in primary care.

Some of these purposes are quite straightforward—accessibility at any hour or on any day is more easily provided by a team than by a single clinician. The achievement of other benefits of collaboration by the team is more complex. Realizing the benefits to patients of truly collaborative practice that draws on the broader expertise of a team of professionals—for instance, health supervision of the child, treatment of recurring infections, palliative care of seriously ill patients, patient education related to a chronic condition such as diabetes, or coordination of community services—will likely require modification of attitudes and beliefs and changes in training and organization. Maintaining a sense of personal relationship between patients and at least some members of the team calls for an organizational emphasis that is sensitive to patients' preferences and needs.

The specific composition of the team will vary with the care setting and the specific needs of the patients being served. The needs of children for routine regular health maintenance will require different knowledge and skills, such as those provided by a pediatric nurse practitioner, than the care of an elderly person with multiple chronic problems and functional limitations that raise problems for their living environment, which may require the continuing involvement of a social worker. Scheffler (Appendix E) offers a conceptual framework for the variety of team functions in primary care.

The team concept used by the committee means a relatively small group that interacts on a regular basis around the primary care of a defined group of patients. The term "health care team" is sometimes used in a looser way to mean all those who are involved in patient care. In our usage, referrals to specialists or other independent professionals, or the independent involvement of other professionals on a recurring, first-contact basis (such as dentistry), do not make these other professionals part of the primary care team, although they are providing essential health services.

In the committee's view, and in the many examples of teams observed on the site visits, the team nearly always will include a primary care physician. This often is the person on the team who deals with more complex decisions and usually plays some role in coordinating the efforts of the team. The health care organizations visited provided care in a wide variety of circumstances: the open spaces of the rural West, multicultural urban poverty in south-central Los Angeles, middle-class areas of the Twin Cities. For nearly all, the experience is that most patients want to have access to a physician as an important part of their primary care. Nevertheless, a variety of team arrangements can meet the needs of patients and still have another team member carrying out principal contact with patients for important aspects of their care.

To be efficient, larger and more complex teams that interact face-to-face on a regular basis require a substantial panel of patients. When providing services to an isolated rural population, such teams can be geographically dispersed if they take advantage of modern communication technologies as a substitute for face-to-face contact.

All in all, the committee believes that teams offer the best means to bring to bear the wide range of talents and knowledge needed for primary care. Teams provide a way to achieve efficiencies in the delivery of primary care and to improve access to services on a timely basis while maintaining appropriate personal knowledge of the patient.

Recommendation 5.5 *Practice by Interdisciplinary Teams*

The committee believes that the quality, efficiency, and responsiveness of primary care are enhanced by the use of interdisciplinary teams and recommends the adoption of the team concept of primary care, wherever feasible.

Role of Specialists in Primary Care

Physician specialists have long had a role in the delivery of primary care. A major study based on a national sample of physicians during 1973–1976, using a definition of primary care that is more limited than the one adopted by this committee, indicated that approximately 20 percent of Americans received continuing care for the majority of their health problems from specialists (Aiken et al., 1979). Those data are now old, but anecdotal evidence and statements presented to this committee by several specialty groups indicate that some specialists still provide substantial portions of their patients' care, although this care may or may not meet the committee's definition.

Two conflicting trends influence specialist delivery of primary care. First is the continued increase in the number of specialists in the past two decades, both in absolute numbers and relative to the number of primary care physicians. The second trend is the growth of managed care plans, which emphasize primary care and control the use of care provided by specialists. The combined effect of these trends is what many analyses have concluded to be a substantial surplus of physicians in many of the specialties, a surplus that is likely to increase in coming years (COGME, 1994; Weiner, 1994; Pew Health Professions Commission, 1995; IOM, 1996). The lack of opportunities to practice their specialty may provide strong incentives for some specialists to increase their involvement in primary care. This involvement can take several forms.

Mixed practices. One form is a mixed practice in which the physician carries out a specialty referral role for some patients and acts as primary care physician for others. The American Society of Internal Medicine (ASIM) has argued for the acceptability of mixed practices. A recent ASIM survey (ASIM, 1995) found that 55 percent of 53 HMOs that responded allow a physician to designate themselves as both a primary care physician carrying out the "gatekeeper" role and a consulting specialist within the same plan; 43 percent make the physician choose one role or another. One plan allowed the specialist to choose only the consulting role. Most (83 percent) permitted the specialist to act as the primary care physician for any patient and not just for those patients with diseases that fall within the physician's specialty (ASIM, 1995). These results suggest that self-designation as primary care physician could become a popular option for the internal medicine subspecialties.

Mixed practice is also reported to be common in the specialty of obstetrics-gynecology (OB/GYN). Women frequently seek general medical care from their OB-GYNs (Horton et al., 1994). One survey reported that about 20 percent of women would choose to receive their primary care from an OB-GYN if asked to make a choice of primary care physician (ACOG, 1993). Nearly all physicians in this specialty also do surgery and provide other specialized care in addition to obstetrics and gynecological care.

Principal physicians. A second pattern of involvement of specialists in primary care is as principal physician. In this role, specialists care for patients whose principal health problems fall within their specialty, e.g., cancer, pulmonary conditions, and advanced heart disease. While providing care for this problem, which often dominates the patients' involvement with health care, specialists can also provide general care for most of the rest of their patients' health care needs; they can make referrals to other specialists as necessary and in some instances refer the patient to a primary care clinician. For these patients, specialists are acting as the principal physician for both specialized and general care, though the extent of preventive care and screening is unknown.

The committee heard many examples of this role for specialists, but it was not able to quantify the extent of this pattern of practice. The data from the 1970s survey mentioned above (Aiken et al., 1979) suggest that, in those years, this pattern may have been common for selected patients. Today most managed care plans control access to specialty care through a designated primary care clinician, so this pattern of specialist practice is likely to be less common for patients in managed care arrangements.

For the committee, the issue is whether these patterns of specialist provision of primary care—mixed practice and the principal physician role—provide primary care as the committee has defined it. The training, experience, and practice patterns of many specialists are not likely to prepare them to engage in the full range of primary care. Two special cases, however, deserve comment.

The first is the case of the many physicians who received training as generalists before going on to specialty training and practice. Physicians in the specialty areas of internal medicine and pediatrics have typically received three years of training in general internal medicine or general pediatrics. Many of their colleagues in these same training programs have gone on to primary care practice. Whether, however, the first three years of training as provided in past years, with its heavy emphasis on hospital-based care of very ill patients, is appropriate for primary care is addressed in Chapter 7. Many of these specialists, especially in the internal medicine subspecialties, have continued to provide services of a primary care nature along with care in their role as specialist consultants.

The second special case is the specialty of OB/GYN. These physicians provide a considerable amount of general care for women, particularly in the childbearing years. Based on this pattern of practice, the American College of Obstetricians and Gynecologists (ACOG) has advocated that the specialty should be recognized as a primary care specialty and has sought to formalize this recognition in state and federal legislation (ACOG testimony to the IOM Committee on the Future of Primary Care, 1994). Reacting to the concern that obstetricians and gynecologists may not be appropriately trained for primary care, ACOG had also sought to strengthen the training for primary care in the OB-GYN residency.

In both of these special cases, the evidence suggests that considerable numbers of patients receive whatever primary care they receive from these specialists and that many members of the specialties perform primary care in the mixed model described above. In both cases, some basis exists for the claim that residency training will prepare these physicians for the primary care role, at least for more recent and future trainees.

No basis exists at the current time either for the complete exclusion of specialists from the provision of primary care or for their automatic inclusion. Both roles exist now, and the salient issues are: (a) Are the functions of primary care, as defined, being fulfilled? (b) Does the specialist physician have the appropriate knowledge and training to carry out the functions well? The committee believes that primary care requires appropriate training just as specialty care does. Chapter 7 addresses the question of retraining. As indicated in Chapter 4 and in the discussion of education for primary care in Chapter 7, primary care has its own characteristics, knowledge base, and decision criteria. Primary care is more than a junior level of specialty care or a triage function for specialty care. To enable the primary care clinician to carry out the primary care function at a level of excellence that best meets patients' needs requires appropriate training, experience, and support systems. The function of primary care is complex and demanding (see Chapter 4); it involves many activities that extend beyond a reductionist focus on the diagnosis and treatment of a specific disease. The committee questions whether this function can be performed adequately by someone whose orientation and time is substantially committed to the different challenges of the specialist role and whose focus is on a particular disease process or organ system and whether someone can keep abreast of the burgeoning literature in both fields.

The committee does not believe that such questions should be answered by legislative fiat. Nor does it believe that primary care is a residual function to which specialists can return solely through self-designation on the basis of their earlier general training. The current trend is toward a more distinct identification of a group of physicians whose specific role is that of primary care physician, and that trend should be encouraged.

Roles of Other First-Contact Health Professionals

Several health professions provide first-contact care for basic health services that are needed by most or all of the population. Principal among these professions are dentistry, optometry, and pharmacy. Each of these professions has a unique history in the American context, and the evolution of each has been largely independent of the development of the medical profession and the development of the other health professions with closer relationships to medicine, such as nursing and many of the allied health professions. The resulting patterns of basic and continuing services being provided by independent service settings are more a product of history than of logic, but there is no mandate from either health professionals or patients to change these historic patterns.

These services can be considered part of primary care. Representatives from dentistry (American Association of Dental Schools) and optometry (American Optometric Association) have advocated (Appendix B) that these professions be included in any classification of primary care clinicians or that these professions be considered part of the primary care team. The roles of these professions in primary care were also discussed at the committee's workshop on professional roles in primary care.

The committee definition clearly describes functions that extend far beyond the services provided by dentists and optometrists. The independence that characterizes their typical practice does not seem to be consistent with their inclusion in the primary care team as it has been described earlier in this chapter. Yet it would seem logical that good health care for the whole person, certainly a focus of primary care, should include good oral health and vision care.

The historical pattern of separation of these professions and the services that they provide is reflected in such practical matters as the design of health benefit packages, the exclusion of these services from the "gatekeeper" requirements of most managed care plans, and the fact that access to these services is typically through direct contact by the patient. The practical issue would seem to be how to strengthen the relationship to the rest of primary care rather than incorporating these professions into primary care which would involve changes in the historic patterns of professional independence that would probably be resisted by many in these professions. Some have argued that the committee should make explicit that it is not dealing with these professions, but only with primary *medical* care. This approach, however, would seem to neglect the opportunity to build desirable relationships among the professions that could lead to a more integrated approach in the future.

The committee, therefore, would encourage strengthening the two-way relationship between the primary care clinician or team and the provision of dental care, routine eye care, and pharmacy services. For example, the primary care clinician could determine whether patients are receiving preventive and restorative dental services and encourage them to obtain such routine care. Some screening for oral health problems can be carried out in the primary care setting and lead to appropriate referral for dental services (specific screening instructions appear in Greene and Greene, 1995). Conversely, the dentist can screen for medical problems to be brought to the attention of the primary care clinician. Screening for oral cancer is already common; screening for diabetes and hypertension would take advantage of the sometimes routine contact between the dentist and patient. Reference to a common, computer-based patient record would facilitate such interaction.

Similar interaction could take place between primary care clinicians or teams and those providing routine vision care, whether optometrists or ophthalmologists. Pharmacists already serve as a frequent source of medical advice for alleviation of common problems, and they often provide patient information regarding the use of pharmaceuticals. Computer systems in the pharmacy can be used to identify possible drug interactions and dosage problems. Again, this interaction could also be strengthened by access to a common computer-based medical record.

In some sites visited by the committee, the interaction of these professions and the primary care team was encouraged and facilitated by a common site of services, particularly in programs that serve the urban and rural poor, such as services provided in community health centers and Indian Health Service clinics. These settings could provide the basis for more systematic study of the benefits of closer integration between these services and primary care, in terms of patient convenience, access, and health outcomes. The extension of a more integrated model of primary care to include a closer relationship would be a logical development in integrated delivery systems, especially because the desirable infrastructure, such as clinical data systems, is already being put in place.

Another set of health professionals, including physical therapists and podiatrists, may also provide first-contact services. Access to these services is often through regular referral mechanisms, and managed care plans frequently require referral by the primary care clinician. Thus, considering these services as referral services seems to be more sensible. In some primary care practices, however, these professions might be a direct part of the primary care team.

In this study we have not dealt with the role of a large group of other health care personnel who provide services on a first-contact basis that might overlap significantly with services provided in a primary care setting. These include chiropractors, traditional folk healers, and other providers outside the dominant medical model. Some of these services are already included in the primary care offered in some settings or are considered a covered health insurance benefit; others are not. To the extent that such services can be established as effective, the committee would welcome a path of greater convergence between these services and primary care. The National Institutes of Health is implementing a program of research in alternative medicine, which may clarify this issue in future years.

Ensuring Primary Care for Underserved Populations

Background

Earlier in this chapter, the special problems in providing primary care services to underserved populations—particularly rural populations and the urban poor—were underscored. These populations often have special health problems related to low income and social circumstances: for example, trauma related to family and community violence, substance abuse, disease such as diabetes aggravated by poor diet, a higher incidence of infectious diseases such as acquired immunodeficiency syndrome (AIDS) and tuberculosis (TB), and health problems caused by occupational hazards such as injuries and exposure to toxic chemicals among agricultural workers. The primary care clinicians in these areas also face special barriers to making services available. These include lack of health insurance coverage; low reimbursement under many state Medicaid programs; geographic isolation of the population to be served; lack of transportation; problems of recruiting and retaining health care personnel, especially physicians; language and cultural differences that often complicate communication; and special challenges in coordinating primary care with other health and social services.

For many years, federal and state programs and private foundations have directed specific resources toward providing primary care for these populations. These efforts take the form of community health center grants, rural health clinics, the National Health Service Corps, the Maternal and Child Health Block Grant program, the Indian Health Service, direct state and local government provision of services through public health clinics, and many others. These targeted programs have supplemented the large subsidy for medical care for the underserved provided through the federal-state Medicaid program. As valuable as these programs have been in helping to provide these populations with primary care, many gaps remain and the future is uncertain.

Primary care for these special populations is embedded in the social and economic circumstances of the communities and individuals, and primary care, by itself, is not likely to alter these fundamental circumstances. Problems of increasing disparities in incomes, social disintegration, and continued declines in rural populations and the infrastructure of rural communities will make the delivery of primary care more difficult. At the same time, health insurance for the working poor seems likely to continue its decline in the absence of comprehensive health care reform (EBRI, 1995; Short and Banthin, 1995), and the programs and policies that have helped make primary care available for many of these populations are now facing budget cuts and policy changes of historic proportions.

Managed Care and Underserved Populations

Managed care arrangements, integrated health delivery systems, and capitated financing of primary care services—which are likely to be the principal arrangements for organizing and financing primary care in future years—have been slow to include many underserved populations, especially those in rural areas. On site visits to rural areas, for example, the committee saw little evidence that managed care had penetrated these particular rural markets. This situation may change significantly in the near future, however, as states move to implement managed care arrangements for their Medicaid programs. According to a recent study (Lewin-VHI, 1995), as of June 1994 all but eight states had implemented one or more models of managed care for their Medicaid programs and total enrollment in these programs had doubled since June 1993.

Furthermore, the fastest growing form of Medicaid managed care has been full-risk capitation programs. While the growth is rapid, these full-risk capitation programs have been implemented in only a few states, usually states that had substantial market penetration by managed care plans for the population as a whole. Overall, however, many other states are implementing or considering moves to more aggressive managed care arrangements for their Medicaid programs. All of the Medicaid managed care models, including partial capitation and primary care case management, emphasize primary care relative to specialty care.

The trend toward managed care in the Medicaid program does not solve the problems of health insurance coverage for those who are ineligible for Medicaid or who lack private health insurance coverage. State contracts with managed care plans do offer some opportunity to assure the provision of primary care for underserved populations that qualify for Medicaid. This objective could be served both by including the committee's definition of primary care in the criteria by which states select managed care plans and by setting up performance monitoring that includes measures of access, quality, and patient satisfaction that relate to the elements of the definition. Among the factors that ought to be included in managed care contracts are integration of services that makes the process of care more seamless for patients; accessibility; development of sustained partnerships between clinicians and patients; and efforts to relate the health care needs of patients to their families and community. This would help ensure that criteria for awards and subsequent renewals of state contracts would extend well beyond the lowest cost package. Many existing community and rural centers that have sought to provide comprehensive primary care that is responsive to the health care needs of their populations might be considered an asset to managed care plans under these criteria.

A higher proportion of the Medicare population may also be moving into managed care, based on trends in markets that have a high proportion of the under-65 population in managed care. This trend might be advanced further by federal policy changes. As Medicare patients move to managed care settings, the Health Care Financing Administration (HCFA) might (a) include the implementation of the IOM's definition of primary care in its criteria for awarding those contracts; and (b) require improved access for underserved Medicare populations. In sum, conditions for success in acquiring Medicaid and Medicare managed care contracts could constitute a powerful incentive to shape the nature of and access to care provided to underserved populations.

Recommendation 5.6 The Underserved and Those with Special Needs

The committee recommends that public or private programs designed to cover underserved populations and those with special needs include the provision of primary care services as defined in this report. It further recommends that the agencies or organizations funding these pro-

grams carefully monitor them to ensure that such primary care is provided.

Other Approaches for Underserved Populations

Regardless of the method of paying for primary care services for underserved populations, the issues remain about whether meeting their primary care needs requires special services and additional expenses. An additional question is how the costs for patients without any form of health insurance will be met. For hospital care, the disproportionate share provision in the federal financing programs is based on the presumption that a hospital's costs are higher if its patients include a large proportion of Medicare and Medicaid beneficiaries and other low-income patients. For primary care programs supported in part by federal grants, the grant covers costs that are above and beyond reimbursement received through Medicaid, Medicare, private health insurance, and self-pay. One fear of these community clinics—urban or rural, public or private—expressed to the committee during its site visits was that as managed care plans spread to these communities, they would fail to recognize the higher costs associated with meeting the health needs of these populations or that such plans would seek to serve only those patients for whom adequate payment was available. This could well jeopardize current arrangements and leave patients who have no insurance even more vulnerable to a loss of local clinics.

The special problems of serving isolated populations and meeting their primary care needs have been well documented (OTA, 1990). Rural health clinics typically combine the primary care function with some functions of emergency medicine, including ambulance service, and transportation and outreach for patients living in remote locations are other important functions. Support for the professional staff, such as locum tenens programs, is sometimes used to retain staff in isolated areas. Low volume of some services may raise unit costs. The economy of the area being served may be in decline, which raises the incidence of problems such as depression and family violence. Coordination with other needed services, such as social services and home care, may be more difficult because of distance, so the primary care unit may need to be more self-sufficient.

For reasons such as these, the committee believes that some form of subsidy and infrastructure support, in addition to third-party reimbursements, will be needed to make these programs viable. Moreover, if the managed care arrangements extend to these communities, then those groups will need to take these extra costs into consideration.

In some circumstances, integrated health care systems providing managed care may be able to provide the capital, support systems, and personnel to help make rural programs viable. However, specific subsidy of the health system may be required to provide compensation for the extra costs, especially if the system is competing in other markets with managed care plans that do not serve isolated rural populations. Some form of internal cross-subsidy may be required; such subsidies were used in public utility regulation where service to rural communities was required for a license to serve affluent, urban populations.

Serving the urban poor with appropriate primary care services also requires attention to the special problems associated with these populations. Primary care services for these populations have often been concentrated in public clinics, community health centers, or the emergency rooms of public hospitals. The extent to which these populations can be included in the mainstream of primary care services provided through integrated health care systems is complicated by the presence of substantial numbers of those with no source of payment, including the illegal immigrant. Administrators of some integrated systems argue that they can provide primary care for populations with Medicaid eligibility and cover the costs of any needed additional services by their greater efficiency. This is also the general presumption of Medicaid managed care plans. Careful monitoring of the results of managed care plans serving these populations, as recommended, will yield useful information about the extent to which primary care, as defined, can be extended to these populations without compromising care through gaps in needed services, subtle barriers to access, or avoidance of high-risk patients.

Coordinating Primary Care with Other Services

Coordination of services by the primary care clinician is necessary to meet the full range of health needs of the patient and to integrate those services so that the care process can be coherent from the perspective of the patient. Many primary care clinicians and integrated health systems devote considerable attention to coordinating services for the patient within the constraints of current organizational and financial arrangements.

Many of those organizational and financial arrangements, however, are not conducive to coordination of an increasingly complex array of services. For example, the coordination function is often not adequately recognized in the payment for primary care services. Separate administrative structures, funding streams, and organizational and professional cultures may impede coordination. Current knowledge of the wide array of services available for the patient may be difficult for the primary care clinician or team to maintain without some organizational assistance. Specific attention to the means of effective coordination across the array of services needs to be part of the explicit mission of the primary care clinicians and the organizational arrangements within which the primary care function is carried out. The complexities of the coordinating function are another argument for the development of integrated health care systems that can provide appropriate resources for effective coordination.

A familiar aspect of coordination involves the role of the primary care clinician in integrating the diagnostic and treatment services provided by medical specialists. The primary care clinician has an active role in coordinating specialty services on the patient's behalf. This role is much more than serving as a triage point or gateway for those services. As medicine becomes more complex, an active coordinating role for the primary care clinician is essential to assure the effective use of specialized resources. The decision to refer should be accompanied by an exchange of information. In this exchange, ideally, the primary care clinician's knowledge of the patient's history, other health problems, and family and community circumstances is provided to the specialist; the specialist reciprocates with information that is relevant to the comprehensive care of the patient over time, including prevention of disease, maintenance of function, and appropriate treatment of the patient's other health problems.

How to achieve this active interaction should be part of the training of both the primary care clinician and the specialist. Also essential is the organization and financing of services to support the coordination of services. Coordination is also necessary within the primary care team so that the functioning of the team appears to be seamless and coherent to the patient. If the trend is toward larger, integrated health care systems, special attention will need to be given to ensuring that the team approach enhances rather than displaces personal attention to the needs of the patient. The idea of shared responsibility can mean that no one individual feels fully accountable.

Another aspect of coordination—coordination of primary care with other service systems—is the focus of the rest of this section. Primary care teams need to deal with many service systems, including school systems and workplaces. The committee illustrates the importance and nature of this coordinating function by describing desirable interactions with three other health activities where close relationships with primary care are often of great importance to the patient. These are *public health, mental health,* and *long-term care.*

Public Health and Primary Care

Basic linkages. In Chapter 2, the committee acknowledges that population-based public health activities aimed at health promotion and disease prevention have a larger impact on improving health status of populations than personal health services. The committee's definition has focused on primary care as a personal health service and has not incorporated the population-based activities that are the heart of public health; it differs from the World Health Organization (WHO) definition of primary care, which includes the population-based activities of public health under the rubric of primary care. The committee recognizes that effective population-based public health services are essential to the health of the public and acknowledges that rising expenditures for personal health services have often competed in public and private budgets with adequate funding for population-based public health activities (IOM, 1988). The committee holds, however, that the population-based functions of public health and the primary care services delivered to individuals are complementary functions, and strengthening the relationship should be the focus of action in both arenas. Incorporating public health in its totality into primary care would obscure rather than enhance the importance of public health, at least in the American context.

Furthermore, the agenda for primary care is already very challenging without adding responsibility for the full range of population-based public health activities to the primary care function; in particular, the committee would not accept the idea that primary care should include the enforcement responsibilities that are an essential part of the public health function and are legally based on the police power of the state. Rather than competing for attention and funds, the committee believes that both primary care and public health would gain if these functions are viewed as natural allies. The issue then becomes: How can the relationship between primary care and public health be strengthened so that each function will enhance the other?

Public health and managed care. An important dimension of this issue is how the growth of managed care and integrated health care systems with enrolled populations should affect the interaction between primary care and public health. The California Medicaid program (MediCal) illustrates this redefining of the roles and relationships of primary care and public health. As MediCal moves to a managed care model, health plans that are chosen to enroll its beneficiaries will be required to work out agreements with county health departments that will specify responsibilities for various aspects of public health programs (James Haughton, Los Angeles County Health Department, personal communication, 1995). For some functions, the county may contract with the plans to carry out activities such as maternal and child health services and some forms of screening. For other services for which the health department has special expertise and experience, such as TB treatment and control, the health department could be identified as the place to which cases of TB are referred.

For the rest of the population enrolled in managed care plans, there are numerous examples of how these plans can play an important role in health promotion and disease prevention functions that involve services to and interaction with individuals. Plans with capitated funding typically include a wide range of preventive services in their benefit package, in contrast to the exclusion of many or most preventive services in traditional health indemnity plans. These services may include immunizations, periodic screening for disease, health education and behavior change programs, and even discounts at health clubs. The combination of an enrolled population and appropriate data systems makes possible the notification of the patient when a preventive service is due.

Granting that this emphasis on health promotion and disease prevention may be used as a marketing strategy to assure enrollment of healthy persons with a strong interest in maintaining their health, the opportunities to use the plans as instruments of a public health agenda are significant. The primary care team and clinicians can, and often do, fulfill important roles as health educators for individuals and as advocates and activists in community health education programs. There are many examples of this natural alliance between primary care and the public health functions, such as the work of the pediatricians in developing a variety of community-based programs that enhance child safety, ranging from encouraging the use of child car seats to child-proof safety caps on medications.

Enhancing the relationship of primary care and public health. Because of the importance of this relationship to the health of the populations being served by both primary care and public health entities, the committee commissioned a paper by Welton and his colleagues on enhancing the relationship (Appendix F). The authors note the many barriers to effective coordination of the spheres of public health, with its population focus, and primary care, with its focus on clinical preventive services and education and behavior change for the individual patient. Commenting that "we must view both public health and primary care as two interacting and mutually supportive components of an increasingly complex integrated system having the single common goal of improving the health of a community and its diverse population," they outline a systems approach for bringing about this integration. This approach involves developing a means by which to identify the functions of the public health agencies for population-based health activities and those of integrated health systems for personal health services (including preventive and health promotion services for individuals). They also describe the role of the public agency in monitoring the health of the population, including inputs from primary care services, through publicly accountable community health information networks.

Welton and his coauthors also identify the many barriers to accomplishing this degree of integration, including the conceptual, educational, and experiential gaps between public health and primary care professionals. The roles and methods of primary care and public health have often been defined independently of each other. Public health agencies are often organized in a compartmentalized way that makes it more difficult to define the functional relationships to primary care. On the health care side, HMOs and other health care organizations differ substantially in the degree of interest in the long-term health of the population being served and their commitment to provide the professional time and infrastructure necessary to coordinate the primary care and public health functions.

The many barriers and obstacles to relating primary care to the health needs of the community identified by the IOM report on community-oriented primary care (COPC) (IOM, 1984) continue at this time (see Chapter 2), and the COPC model has not expanded its practice base in this country to any great extent, despite some excellent models (see Appendix F).

Welton et al. lay out an ambitious plan for bringing about fuller integration of public health and primary care that would create, on the primary care side, fully developed COPC practices in the context of organized health care systems.

The committee endorses efforts in the organization and financing of primary care services that would move in this direction. The path toward a fully integrated approach that is focused on improving the health of populations will be long and arduous, and the particulars and pace of development will vary from place to place. Moving primary care services toward a more population-based approach will also require changes in the education of primary care clinicians (see Chapter 7) that can build on many activities already under way, such as those supported by private foundations under the "Health of the Public" projects of The Robert Wood Johnson Foundation and The Pew Charitable Trusts and the community-oriented health education programs supported by the W.K. Kellogg Foundation.

The committee encourages the many local efforts that are trying to better integrate primary care and public health activities supported by governments at all levels and by private foundations, many of which are focused on underserved populations. The committee would also like to encourage managed health plans to move toward the "natural alliance" between primary care and public health to which we have referred, based on their mutual interest in improving and maintaining the health of the populations they served. A logical starting place is the ongoing effort to encourage (or require) beneficiaries of federal and state programs (Medicare and Medicaid in whatever form they take in the future) to enroll in capitated managed care plans.

Recommendation 5.7 *Primary Care and Public Health*

The committee recommends that health care plans and public health agencies develop specific written agreements regarding their respective roles and relationships in (a) maintaining and improving the health of the communities they serve and (b) ensuring coordination of preventive services and health promotion activities related to primary care.

Agreements with public program beneficiaries could serve as a model for agreements covering managed care enrollees who are privately insured. Because most managed care plans will enroll both public and private beneficiaries, this extension of the agreements for coordination should be a logical development.

Stimulated by these agreements the committee encourages the development of community- (population-) based information systems that will serve the joint purposes of public health agencies and the managed care plans by providing better data on the health problems of communities. Such agreements should also address joint development of health promotion strategies; these would combine the individualized approaches of the health plan with population-based approaches of the health department and other voluntary health agencies, such as those focused on specific diseases. Although the committee has advocated specific agreements in order to move beyond a rhetorical commitment to a common agenda, such agreements should not replace the dynamics of ongoing and voluntary cooperation. Agreements should be modified frequently to reflect new opportunities and should encourage ongoing dialogue among primary care managers, public health officials, and the communities they jointly serve.

The committee recognizes that managed care plans do not now cover the entire population; as long as health insurance is not universally available to the population, this will be true. This means that public health agencies will continue to be responsible for reaching the entire population with disease prevention and health promotion services. In the short term, the public health sector will also have to continue in many places as the primary care provider of last resort.

Mental Health and Primary Care

Another critical interface that requires attention and coordination is the relationship between primary care and mental health. Part of this relationship is encompassed in the referral of patients with mental health problems to specialized mental health providers; at times this follows the usual pattern of referral to individual specialists and at other times involves referral to separate mental health services delivery systems (sometimes called behavioral health care plans) with their own organization and financing. Describing the evolution of these separate delivery systems in both the public and the private sectors is beyond the scope of this report, but the separateness continues in new forms, the latest of which is the growing use of "carve-outs" for mental health and substance abuse services in private health benefit plans.

The existence of this separate, parallel mental health services system implies that the function of primary care regarding mental illness is initial diagnosis and referral for treatment. Yet the reality is that the primary care clinician not only identifies but treats a large portion of mental disorders. Furthermore, as described by deGruy (Appendix D), many aspects of primary care and mental health are indivisible. To quote deGruy:

> A major portion of mental health care is rendered in the primary care setting and always will be, sometimes despite strong disincentives; . . . a sensible vision of primary health care must have mental health woven into its fabric; . . . the primary setting is well suited to the provision of most mental health services; . . . despite suboptimal recognition and management of mental disorders and attention to mental health, the structure and operation of primary care can be modified so as to greatly augment the provision of these services; and . . . current efforts under way in the U.S. to reform the health care system offer an opportunity to find the most effective of these modifications and to discover fruitful collaborative structures both within the primary care setting and between primary care clinicians and mental health professionals.

The issue of referrals is further complicated by the way that mental health services are financed. Many health plans put limits on the number of visits for mental health services, or they set higher co-payments for such services (or they do both). If a managed care plan capitates its primary care clinicians, it may create an inappropriate incentive for patients to be referred to the "carve out" plan. Referral to mental health providers may compromise the ability of primary care clinicians to maintain continuity of care and to focus on patients' related health problems.

A further issue is the underrecognition and undertreatment of mental disorders in the primary care setting. Most studies of these problems have focused on the diagnosis and treatment of depression, and they indicate that from one-half to two-thirds of patients meeting the criteria for mental disorders are not diagnosed in the primary care setting. For depression, evidence suggests that treatments known to be effective are underutilized by primary care clinicians.

An additional complicating issue is the existence of a "primary" mental health system parallel to the primary care system. Entry to this parallel system— essentially comprising community mental health centers and individual mental health professionals—is at the initiative of patients who identify their problem as primarily mental. For patients who have serious mental disorders or who have mental health problems but no other significant health problems, the diagnosis and treatment by the specialized mental health provider is appropriate. However, for patients with significant overlapping health conditions, this self-referral may raise problems for the adequacy of the treatment of other health conditions.

Given these complexities, the problems of effective coordination of services are not simple to solve. The nature of the relationships between primary care and mental health services, as indicated by deGruy's analysis of the literature and current directions in the health care system, indicate some clear directions for more effective coordination.

First, the important role of primary care in the diagnosis and treatment of mental disorders needs to be recognized and strengthened through appropriate training and organization and financing of primary care services. This role includes dealing with the extensive interrelationships of mental and physical illness.

Second, models of assistance to primary care clinicians by mental health professionals need to be further developed, implemented, and evaluated.

Third, financial and organizational disincentives for a strengthened primary care role need to be reduced so that the primary care clinician can and will provide needed and effective services for those mental health problems that will inevitably present in the primary care setting and that are often imbedded in other health problems. Arrangements such as carve-outs for mental health services and special payment and service limits triggered by a diagnosis of mental problems need to be carefully examined, so that disincentives for appropriate roles of either primary care in mental health or specialized referral services are reduced.

Fourth, collaborative service models that integrate rather than separate specialized mental health services and primary care services need to be encouraged.

This will enable patients in either setting to benefit from coordinated treatment plans dealing with the full range of their health problems, and it will improve diagnosis and treatment of mental health problems, including those requiring specialized services. In many care settings, this means increased consultation and involvement of primary care clinicians and mental health professionals with each other's service domains. Integrated health care systems would seem to be the logical home for such collaborative approaches. *Finally*, the primary care research program discussed in Chapter 8 should include a significant focus on the primary care role in mental health, including study and evaluation of care models and natural experiments.

Recommendation 5.8 Primary Care and Mental Health Services

The committee recommends the reduction of financial and organizational disincentives for the expanded role of primary care in the provision of mental health services. It further recommends the development and evaluation of collaborative care models that integrate primary care and mental health services more effectively. These models should involve both primary care clinicians and mental health professionals.

Long-Term Care and Primary Care

The importance of long-term care is growing as the number of the elderly, especially the very old, increases. These services raise difficult issues for coordinating care. Long-term care extends well beyond the provision of personal health services to encompass issues of housing, nutrition, assistance in the activities of daily living, social services, transportation, and the roles of voluntary caregivers. Looming large over the breadth and content of these services is the lack of a coherent set of social policies concerning funding for long-term care services.

The roles of primary care in the provision of long-term care services are intertwined with these issues. Nearly all persons who receive long-term care services, either formally organized or provided by family and friends, are high users of medical services, including primary care. Because the elderly, or the seriously disabled of any age, typically have multiple medical problems, including a high incidence of mental health problems, the problems of coordination by primary care clinicians or teams are compounded. Furthermore, many of these patients are in declining health, and this calls for a different mind-set than does the provision of acute services with the intent of providing cure or significant alleviation of symptoms. Markers of effective performance by clinicians in terms of desired patient outcomes are different at least in degree if not in kind for this population. Maintenance of function and emotional support, rather than treatment of a physiological condition, become even more important objectives for the primary care clinician.

The aspect of the definition that speaks to the context of family and community becomes especially important in these circumstances, and the need for coordination of services is great. Effective treatment of medical problems requires that primary care clinicians be aware of patients' living circumstances, personal capabilities, and other persons involved in their care. Coordination of treatment plans with others involved in provision of long-term care services is often essential. Simply involving primary clinicians often becomes a problem because of the inability of patients to go to a clinician's office; the resulting special demands on clinicians' time, for which there may be little financial or emotional compensation, pose yet further obstacles. Even today, there are complaints that primary care clinicians do not visit the home- or institution-bound patient and do not take an active role in their care or care plans (IOM, 1986b).

Many aspects of improving long-term care have not been adequately addressed by society as a whole. Among these issues are the preoccupation with holding down acute care costs for the elderly served by Medicare; the reluctance to extend entitlement any further; the possibility of new and strong incentives for states to reduce their exposure to long-term care costs through caps on Medicaid expenditure; and the steady increase in the numbers of the very old. Taken together, these factors almost guarantee that coordination of long-term care and primary care will remain beset with problems and frustrations for both clinicians and patients.

Some avenues for improvement and some care models show promise of better integration of services. Demonstration programs such as the Social Health Maintenance Organization (S/HMO) programs, the Program for the All-Inclusive Care of the Elderly (PACE program), and others pool Medicare, Medicaid, and private funding sources to provide a coordinated approach to care that includes medical services (IOM, 1995). Coordination seems more likely in integrated health care systems that are built on a base of primary care and that have an extended primary care team, because these approaches can include nurse practitioners and social workers who are well informed about the care of the dependent elderly and about community resources that can help. These members of the primary care team can also maintain personal contact with patients in the home or long-term care setting and monitor their medical condition and treatment plans. The primary care team members in turn should participate in the joint planning with those providing long-term care services to develop plans that include attention to the patients' needs for primary care and for the coordination of other medical services. A primary care team member can serve as case manager in coordinating an array of services for the individual with long-term care needs or can work with a case manager from outside the team. Finally, the primary care clinicians and team members can help provide emotional support and counseling for patients whose medical and living circumstances interact to accentuate fear and anxiety.

Recommendation 5.9 Primary Care and Long-Term Care

To improve the continuity and effectiveness of services for those requiring long-term care, the committee recommends that third-party payers (including Medicare and Medicaid), health care organizations, and health professionals promote the integration of primary care and long-term care by coordinating or pooling financing and removing regulatory or other barriers to such coordination.

Performance Monitoring for Primary Care

In an era when resource constraints for health care will be a continuing reality, monitoring the performance of the health care system in terms of quality and patient outcomes will become increasingly important. Costs are quantifiable and a source of intense concern to large payers for health care, so one can safely assume that comparative cost data will become more widely available. The debate over future expenditures for the Medicare and Medicaid programs and the close attention to health plan premiums by employers and, where they bear part of the premium cost, by individuals assure that costs will remain in the forefront as one marker of performance.

Other measures of performance, including technical quality of care, health status, and patient satisfaction, are also increasingly available. Examples include HEDIS (Health Plan Employer Data and Information Set), a system to measure HMO performance pioneered by the National Committee for Quality Assurance, and the requirements set out by such private groups as the employers in the Twin Cities area and CALPERS (the California Public Employees Retirement System), which provide fringe benefits for public employees in that state. A governmental equivalent is the competitive contracting process for state Medicaid programs that selects managed care plans to serve the Medicaid population, as in Arizona, Tennessee, and a number of other states.

Performance monitoring systems should also include measures of access, which would require population-based data on such indicators as those recommended by the IOM in 1993 (IOM, 1993a). Such data cannot be gathered entirely by the health plans themselves, at least as long as a growing number of Americans are excluded from any health plan. Regardless of the prevailing interest among elected officials or the public in questions of access, the committee believes that levels of access should be considered an important indicator of overall performance of the health system, including primary care. This view is consistent with the committee's recommendation that access to primary care for everyone should remain an objective for American society (Recommendation 5.1).

Potential users of information about health care performance include employers, governments on behalf of their beneficiaries and employees, individuals choosing among competing health plans, and health plans themselves.

The developing performance monitoring models are aimed at total health system performance, yet most managed care plans make the operating assumption that increasing primary care as a proportion of the total health care activity will make the totality of care less costly without compromising quality or patient satisfaction. (At a minimum plans may assume that outcomes will be sustained at a level that will not cause the plan to lose enrollees or contracts with employers or government agencies.) Therefore, information on how well the primary care component of the plan is performing is likely to be very important to plan managers, purchasers, regulators, and patients.

Until very recent years most of the resources to develop programs to assess quality have focused on inpatient services. In the current health care environment, however, it is imperative that substantial effort be put into further development of approaches to monitor the performance of primary care, particularly on dimensions of health care outcomes, patient health status, and patient satisfaction. The market in health care, even in those locations that have proceeded quite far down the road of competition among managed care plans, seems too compromised by lack of informed choice for the ultimate consumer, the patient, to be the sole arbiter of health system performance. Whichever mix of regulation—choice by large payers on behalf of consumers or direct choice by patients—emerges as the means of shaping desired performance by the health care providers and plans, better information will be the key. In the area of primary care, where the tradition of measurement is less and where the technical challenges of developing and implementing are formidable, an increased level of effort in developing those systems should have a high priority.

As discussed elsewhere, the objective of accountability in primary care requires performance measurement. Other aspects of the definition make this task more rather than less difficult, because they emphasize characteristics of primary care that extend well beyond the competence with which a specific medical encounter is performed. Both process and outcome data will need to relate to the objectives of integration (continuity, comprehensiveness, and coordination), accessibility of services, sustained partnership with patients, the scope of services and the pattern of referrals (already tracked by most managed care plans), and knowledge of relationships to family and community relevant to the provision of primary care. The technical problems of case mix, instability of enrollments, and the multiple factors affecting outcomes, among others, will complicate the measurement task. The unit of review—health care organization or individual primary care clinician or practice—is yet another issue.

Fortunately, this effort can build on work already done; the need to balance information on utilization and cost with information about the other measures of care that are necessary to measure performance and value should provide the motivation to proceed. The issue is not new, however. According to Kerr White, an important early figure in identifying the need for more emphasis on primary care in the U.S. health care system, "Performance and results are the criteria that society is using with increasing sophistication to assess the medical profession and its efforts; activity and costs are no longer adequate measures" (White, 1967, p. 848).

The issue of who should be responsible for developing the measures and how they should be implemented is also complex, given Americans' general skepticism of the role of government. In recent years, the health professions have also become wary of the motivations of health plans competing in a market that is very sensitive to cost. A governmental model is illustrated by the classic state role in licensure of health professionals and institutions, by the quality assurance and improvement efforts for the Medicare program, and by the regulation of nursing homes under a federal-state relationship related mostly to the Medicaid program. Nongovernmental models are illustrated by the decades-long accreditation programs of the Joint Commission on the Accreditation of Healthcare Organizations and NCQA's accreditation of HMOs and the HEDIS effort cited earlier.

A public-private collaborative model might be appropriate for efforts to develop performance measures, especially if it could continue over time to advance the state of the art of performance monitoring. The users could be both governmental agencies and private sector plans, with the public-private entity assuming a data audit function to certify the quality of the data. The committee has no firm view about which model is best, but history would suggest that a public-private consortium would match the distributed nature of health care responsibility in the United States.

Recommendation 5.10 Quality of Primary Care

The committee recommends the development and adoption of uniform methods and measures to monitor the performance of health care systems and individual clinicians in delivering primary care as defined in this report. Performance measures should include cost, quality, access, and patient and clinician satisfaction. The results should be made available to public and private purchasers of care, provider organizations, clinicians, and the general public.

Infrastructure Development for Primary Care

Primary care practices in the future are likely to require an infrastructure that extends beyond the usual capital requirements of facilities, land, and equipment. This factor in turn will call for investments that are beyond the capabilities of the individual primary care unit (i.e., a small group or team). These infrastructure needs constitute a lengthy and very complex list of systems and information sources, such as:

- systems for
  —recording and maintaining clinical data,
  —providing assists to clinical decisionmaking (e.g., clinical practice guidelines, clinical algorithms),
  —monitoring quality of care, and
  —overall practice management;
- patient education materials relating to healthy behaviors and as background information that patients can use in participating in clinical decisionmaking about their care;
- information on the community and the population being served, including disease and injury patterns, environmental and workplace hazards, social and economic characteristics of the locale;
- information about community services available in the community, including health and social services, transportation services for patients without transport options of their own, and for rural areas, emergency medical services capabilities and transport systems, telecommunication links, and locum tenens support; and
- continuing education support for primary care staff.

Extensive as this inventory of infrastructure needs is, it is not all-inclusive. (For example, not mentioned here is support for professional education and research, which are discussed in Chapters 7 and 8.) Furthermore, although the needs have been recognized for many years, a decade ago an IOM committee identified the lack of appropriate infrastructure support as one factor that inhibited the development of COPC practices in the United States (IOM, 1984).

Some of these activities, such as clinical information systems, are generic to all of medical care; *The Computer-Based Patient Record: An Essential Technology for Health Care* (IOM, 1991) highlights this point. Even generic infrastructure needs, however, have aspects that are particularly related to primary care. For example, the chair of the IOM committee on the computer-based patient record has argued that such systems, although often developed in institutional settings, are even more pertinent to primary care because of the need to deal with patient data covering many problems and to follow the patient over substantial time (Detmer and Finney, 1992).

It is not the intent of this report to deal with infrastructure needs separately but rather to address the questions of how, collectively, they might be met. Several basic approaches to infrastructure development and support might be considered:

- Methods of payment for primary care services should recognize the costs of infrastructure, thereby creating a market for these infrastructure services that will then be purchased by the primary care practices. This market would encourage others to bear development and marketing costs, as, for example, vendors of clinical information systems.

• Aggregation of primary care practices into larger integrated systems results in economies of scale that allow use of internal capital to develop infrastructure.

• Direct subsidy of infrastructure development either by public subsidy or voluntary contributions from organizations.

The first two approaches by themselves have drawbacks. For example, low reimbursement rates or inadequate plan incomes in cost-competitive markets may mean that individual plans cannot finance infrastructure purchases. In addition, concentration of market power in a few large entities may give them competitive advantages (in part through well-capitalized infrastructure) that in turn will inhibit market entry by smaller health organizations. The health care market in many locales is likely to remain a mix of small and large primary care organizations in the near and medium term, yet the large organizations, especially for-profit enterprises, will have significant advantages in raising capital. As long as the health care market is skewed by such factors, the third approach may be desirable, at least for underwriting those infrastructure needs that require extensive initial capital for technical development (such as clinical information and decision systems), especially if those technologies are to focus specifically on the requirements of primary care. The development of infrastructure for primary care and assuring its wide dissemination could be advanced by creation of a new organization devoted to this purpose as well as other related functions, including relevant applied research. These are long-term strategic issues, and the committee returns to some of them in its final chapter on implementation.

Role of Academic Health Centers in Delivery Of Care

The academic health center (AHC) has as its principal missions the education of health professionals, patient care, and the conduct of research to advance health. These institutions have been and remain major providers of health care, primarily through their affiliated teaching hospitals and clinics. The patient care function has historically been seen as supportive of the education and research roles. It has been predominantly hospital based and focused on advanced, tertiary care. While most of the AHCs have provided some primary care, the primary care activities have remained a small part of the institutions' service role.

To carry out the education functions discussed in Chapter 7, however, the service role of AHCs must develop a much stronger base in primary care. This requires creative new strategies that may involve affiliation with other health care organizations and primary care practice sites. These sites for primary care will be the equivalent of the historic role of the teaching hospital; they will need to provide high-quality service while fulfilling the teaching and mentoring responsibilities for new professionals and helping to advance the state of the art of primary care through applied research.

The need to strengthen the primary care role of AHCs comes at a time when the financing of these institutions is under great strain; competing health care organizations draw clinical activities and revenues away from the AHCs and opportunities for internal cross-subsidies are limited. Many of these institutions also care for a larger share of the uninsured than do their competitors. As noted in Chapter 7, therefore, these functions will require some direct subsidy, just as the teaching hospital function has been subsidized for decades. Part of the challenge will be to provide primary care experiences that will prepare students for practice in a health care environment that is concerned about efficient use of resources. Therefore, the subsidy for education should not be used to shield the primary care teaching setting from the need to focus on efficiency and value.

This strengthened role in primary care will call for an explicit modification of the mission of these institutions. As noted throughout the committee's site visits, many other health care organizations are skeptical about the commitment of the AHCs to primary care. Actions will be needed on their part to back up statements about the importance of primary care. It is also reasonable, however, for these institutions to expect that the extra costs of the educational function and of research and demonstrations in primary care will be covered by funding sources.

Recommendation 5.11 Primary Care in Academic Health Centers

The committee recommends that academic health centers explicitly accept primary care as one of their core missions and provide leadership in the development of primary care teaching, research, and service delivery programs.

SUMMARY

This chapter has outlined several features of the U.S. health care scene that will influence the extent to which primary care evolves in this country. These include the spread of managed care, the expansion of integrated delivery systems, the consolidation of health plans and systems, growth in for-profit ownership of health plans and integrated delivery systems, the diversity between and within health care markets, the special challenges of primary care in rural areas and for the urban poor, the need for primary care to coordinate with other types of services, current and evolving roles for health care professionals, and the role of academic health centers in primary care delivery.

Having reviewed these topics, the committee considered what conclusions and recommendations it would make to overcome the barriers, or exploit the advantages, that these factors pose, or offer, to full implementation of the committee's vision of primary care in the future. In all, the committee advances 11 separate recommendations in the several different arenas. First, the committee recommends establishing as a goal the availability of the services of a primary care clinician for all Americans. Second, the committee makes several recommendations to assure that mechanisms for financing primary care services provide appropriate incentives for sustaining a strong primary care function. In this context the committee makes a strong statement about the need to have universal health care coverage to make possible universal access to primary care. Another recommendation concerns the organization of primary care and emphasizes the importance of the primary care team. With respect to underserved populations, the committee returns to its earlier themes to underscore the importance of primary care for populations who have special health care needs or who are traditionally underserved. Another major thesis of this chapter is the need for primary care to develop strong relationships with three other types of health activities—public health, mental health, and long-term care—and the committee offers three specific recommendations intended to reinforce the coordination and collaboration efforts in these areas. A tenth recommendation calls for specific steps to develop tools and approaches for monitoring and improving the quality of primary care and to make performance information available to a wide audience. The final recommendation calls on AHCs to make primary care a core element of their mission and to provide leadership in education, research, and service delivery related to primary care.

REFERENCES

ACOG (American College of Obstetricians and Gynecologists). Findings from a study conducted for ACOG by the Gallup Organization to examine women's attitudes and experiences with OB/GYNs as their primary care physicians. Washington, D.C.: ACOG, 1993.

Aiken, L.H., Lewis, C.E., Craig, J., et al. The Contribution of Specialists to the Delivery of Primary Care: A New Perspective. *New England Journal of Medicine* 300:1363-1370, 1979.

Alpha Center. MSAs: Issues for States. *State Initiatives in Health Care Reform*, 16(Jan./Feb.):7, 1996.

American Academy of Actuaries. *Public Policy Monograph. Medical Savings Accounts: An Analysis of the Family Medical Savings and Investment Act of 1995*. Washington, D.C.: American Academy of Actuaries, 1995.

ASIM (American Society of Internal Medicine). Results of a survey of IPA model HMOs. Conveyed in letter dated May 3, 1995, from J.P. DuMoulin, Director, Managed Care and Regulatory Affairs. *ASIM Survey of HMOs*. Washington, D.C.: ASIM, 1995.

Bailit, H.L. Market Strategies and the Growth of Managed Care. Pp. 3–13 in *Academic Health Centers in the Managed Care Environment*. D. Korn, C.J. McLaughlin, and M. Osterweis, eds. Washington, D.C.: Association of Academic Health Centers, 1995.

Blumenthal, D., and Meyer, G.S. The Future of the Academic Medical Center Under Health Reform. *New England Journal of Medicine* 329:1812–1814, 1993.

COGME (Council on Graduate Medical Education). *Recommendations to Improve Access to Health Care Through Physician Workforce Reform.* Fourth Report to Congress and the Department of Health and Human Services Secretary. Rockville, Md.: Health Resources and Services Administration, Department of Health and Human Services, 1994.

COGME. *COGME 1995 Physician Workforce Funding Recommendations for Department of Health and Human Services' Programs.* Seventh Report to Congress and the Department of Health and Human Services. Rockville, Md.: Health Resources and Services Administration, Department of Health and Human Services, 1995.

Detmer, D.E., and Finney, M.D. The Catalyst of Technology: How Will Advances in Information Technology Change the Role of the Primary Care Practitioner? Pp. 167–182 in *Proceedings of the National Primary Care Conference, Vol. 2.* Washington, D.C.: U.S. Department of Health and Human Services, Public Health Service, Health Resources and Services Administration, 1992.

EBRI (Employee Benefit Research Institute). Sources of Health Insurance and Characteristics of the Uninsured: Analysis of the March 1994 Current Population Survey. *EBRI Special Report SR-28 and Issue Brief Number 158.* Washington, D.C.: EBRI, 1995.

Epstein, A.M. U.S. Teaching Hospitals in the Evolving Health Care System. *Journal of the American Medical Association* 273:1203-1207, 1995.

Fox, P.D., and Wasserman, J. Academic Medical Centers and Managed Care: Uneasy Partners. *Health Affairs* 12(1):85-93, 1993.

GHAA (Group Health Association of America). *Patterns in HMO Enrollment.* 4th ed. Washington, D.C.: GHAA, 1995.

Gray, B.H. *The Profit Motive in Patient Care.* Cambridge, Mass.: Harvard University Press, 1991.

Greene, J.C., and Greene, A.R. Chapter 15: Oral Health. Pp. 315–334 in *Health Promotion and Disease Prevention in Clinical Practice.* S.H. Woolf, S. Jonas, and R.S. Lawrence, eds. Baltimore: Williams and Wilkins, 1995.

Horton, J.A., Murphy, P., and Hale, R.W. Obstetrician-Gynecologists as Primary Care Providers: A National Survey of Women. *Primary Care Update for OB/GYNS* 1:212-215, 1994.

Institute for Clinical Systems Integration. *1993 Annual Report.* Minneapolis, Minn.: Institute for Clinical Systems Integration, no date.

IOM. (Institute of Medicine) *Community-Oriented Primary Care: A Practical Assessment. Volume I. The Committee Report.* Washington, D.C.: National Academy Press, 1984.

IOM. *For-Profit Enterprise in Health Care.* B.H. Gray, ed. Washington, D.C.: National Academy Press, 1986a.

IOM. *Improving the Quality of Care in Nursing Homes.* Washington, D.C.: National Academy Press, 1986b.

IOM. *The Future of Public Health.* Washington, D.C.: National Academy Press, 1988.

IOM. *The Computer-Based Patient Record: An Essential Technology for Health Care.* Richard S. Dick and Elaine B. Steen, eds. Washington, D.C.: National Academy Press, 1991.

IOM. *Access to Health Care in America.* M. Millman, ed. Washington, D.C.: National Academy Press, 1993a.

IOM. *Employment and Health Benefits: A Connection at Risk.* M.J. Field and H.T. Shapiro, eds. Washington, D.C.: National Academy Press, 1993b.

IOM. *Real People, Real Problems: An Evaluation of the Long-term Care Ombudsman Programs of the Older Americans Act.* J. Harris-Wehling, J.C. Feasley, and C.L. Estes, eds. Washington, D.C.: National Academy Press, 1995.

IOM. *The Nation's Physician Workforce: Options for Balancing Supply and Requirements.* K.N. Lohr, N.A. Vanselow, and D.E. Detmer, eds. Washington, D.C.: National Academy Press, 1996.

Joint Committee on Taxation. Description and Analysis of H.R. 1818 (The "Family Medical Savings and Investment Act of 1995"). Doc. No. JCX-28-95. Washington, D.C.: Joint Committee on Taxation, U.S. Congress, 1995.

Josiah Macy, Jr. Foundation. *The Financing of Medical Schools in an Era of Health Care Reform. Proceedings of a Conference Chaired by Eli Ginzberg, M.D.* Conference proceedings edited by R.H. Ebert and case studies edited by M. Ostrow. New York: Josiah Macy, Jr. Foundation, 1995.

Lewin-VHI. *The States and Private Sector: Leading Health Care Reform. States as Payers: Managed Care for Medicaid Populations.* Washington, D.C.: The National Institute for Health Care Management, 1995.

Mitka, M. Higher Pay for Primary Care. *American Medical News* 37:3,7, October 3, 1994a.

Mitka, M. Physician Income up 5.4%. *American Medical News* 37:3,12, December 12, 1994b.

Mitka, M. Academic Pay Slowing, Primary Care Growing. *American Medical News* 38:5, July 24, 1995.

OTA (Office of Technology Assessment). *Health Care in Rural America.* Washington, D.C.: U.S. Government Printing Office, 1990.

Pew Health Professions Commission. *Critical Challenges: Revitalizing the Health Professions for the Twenty-First Century.* San Francisco: Pew Health Professions Commission, 1995.

PPRC (Physician Payment Review Commission). *Annual Report to Congress, 1994.* Washington, D.C.: PPRC, 1994.

PPRC. *Annual Report to Congress. 1995.* Washington, D.C.: PPRC, 1995.

Short, P.F., and Banthin, J.S. Caring for the Uninsured and Underinsured: New Estimates of the Underinsured Younger than 65 Years. *Journal of the American Medical Association* 274:1302–1306, 1995.

Shortell, S.M., Gillies, R.R., and Anderson, D.A. The New World of Managed Care: Creating Organized Delivery Systems. *Health Affairs* 13;(Winter):46–64, 1994.

University Hospital Consortium. *Competing in the Maturing Health Care Marketplace: Strategies for Academic Medical Centers.* Prepared in consultation with APM Management Consultants. Oakbrook, Ill.: University Hospital Consortium, 1993.

Weiner, J.P. Assessing the Impact of Managed Care on the U.S. Physician Workforce. Policy paper commissioned by the Bureau of Health Professions of the U.S. Department of Health and Human Services on behalf of the Council on Graduate Medical Education. November 1993.

Weiner, J.P. Forecasting the Effects of Health Reform on U.S. Physician Workforce Requirement: Evidence from HMO Staffing Patterns. *Journal of the American Medical Association* 272:222–230, 1994.

White, K.L. Primary Medical Care for Families—Organization and Evaluation. *New England Journal of Medicine* 277:847–852, 1967.

6

The Primary Care Workforce

This chapter focuses on the principal types of primary care clinicians—physicians, physician assistants (PAs), and nurse practitioners (NPs). They are the personnel most likely, under state practice acts, hospital or health plan credentialing, or customary practice, to have significant patient care authority. The chapter reviews trends in the supply of these components of the health workforce (noting the extreme difficulties of producing reliable and valid estimates of supply and, especially, requirements for clinicians or clinicians' services); it also briefly comments on the education and training infrastructure for such personnel (a topic taken up in greater detail in Chapter 7). The chapter then advances four recommendations concerning important directions that, in the committee's view, the production and use of primary care clinicians ought to take.

The committee's definition of primary care draws attention to the concept of a primary care clinician, where *clinician* is defined by the committee as "an individual who uses a recognized scientific knowledge base and has the authority to direct the delivery of personal health services to patients" (see Chapter 2). This individual might or might not be a physician;[1] that is, the committee view is that primary care clinicians as likely to include at least physicians, PAs, and NPs;

---

[1]For purposes of this chapter, the term *physician* refers to individuals trained in schools of allopathic medicine (who have received an M.D.) and those trained in schools of osteopathic medicine (who have received a D.O.), and no distinction is made between the two categories of physicians (or schools) unless it is explicitly noted.

that is how the term is used in, for instance, Chapter 5. The committee recognizes that the broader primary care team will include various other health care personnel, such as therapists, nutritionists, social workers, allied health personnel, and office staff. This range of professionals is reflected, for example, in the vignettes used in Chapter 3 to illustrate the scope of primary care. Finally, yet other health professionals, such as dentists, deliver primary care within their own fields and disciplines (IOM, 1995a), but as they are not likely to be responsible for the large majority of health care needs of all people, they are not discussed further here.

WORKFORCE TRENDS AND SUPPLY PROJECTIONS: PHYSICIANS

Overall Levels of Supply

An extremely contentious set of issues in the United States in recent years has involved the numbers of physicians and their distribution by geographic area and specialty. Today, essentially all experts agree that the overall levels of physicians in the country point to a surplus; some in fact would characterize the level as a significant oversupply.

These issues were explored in a recent report by an Institute of Medicine committee on aggregate physician supply (IOM, 1996a, pp. 3–4). The report concluded that

• the nation, at present, clearly has an abundant supply of physicians—which some members of the committee were prepared to label a surplus;
• judgments about the implications of those numbers must be made in the context of the overall U.S. health care system and the components of that system of greatest concern—the quality and costs of health care and access to services;
• the increase in the numbers of physicians in training and entering practice each year is sufficient to cause concern that supply in the future will be excessive, regardless of the assumptions made about the structure of the health care system; and
• the steady growth in numbers of physicians coming into practice is attributable primarily to ever-increasing numbers of IMGs [international medical graduates], about which the committee is very concerned.

Other very recent publications are divided. For example, a minority viewpoint has been laid out by Cooper (1995), who argues that projections of the demand for and supply of physicians using more up-to-date assumptions show "no evidence of a major impending national surplus" (p. 1534). Cooper also draws attention to more than twofold differences across the states in the physician-to-population ratios; to the rapid growth of a wide array of nonphysician clinicians (including NPs and PAs); and to the need to develop policies that take into account the full range of practitioners (not just physicians) who will be delivering services to patients in the next century.

In rebuttal, Tarlov (1995) notes the near unanimity of projections of substantial physician surpluses in analyses since 1980 and draws attention to the considerable uncertainties that surround the Cooper assumptions. Tarlov also calls for more creative actions on the part of many parties to deal not only with workforce supply issues but also to achieve other health goals as well, including reducing the disparities in access for underserved populations and increasing the representation of minorities in the medical profession. The most recent publication of the Pew Health Professions Commission comes down forcefully on the side of surplus, using language such as "a large oversupply" that will result in a "dislocation of crisis proportions" (Pew Health Professions Commission, 1995, p. 42). By and large, the IOM committee reporting here subscribes to the majority view; namely, that the nation does face a meaningful oversupply of physicians, in the aggregate, in coming years.

Figure 6-1 provides some basic data on the growth in physicians in this country over the past nearly 50 years. According to federal statistics, the number of active nonfederal M.D. physicians per 100,000 population in 1950, for example, was 126.6; the figure rose to 127.4 in 1960 and 137.4 in 1970 (DHHS, 1993). In effect, for 35 years or so since the end of World War II, the nation believed it had a considerable shortage of physicians. Steps were taken in the 1960s and 1970s both to expand the production of physicians within the country and to liberalize the rules by which foreign (now international) medical graduates could enter the United States for training and remain to practice.

The change in U.S. physician supply was dramatic.[2] Between 1970–1971 and 1991–1992 the *annual* number of medical school graduates increased from approximately 9,000 to more than 15,000 (for allopathic schools, or M.D.s) and from 500 to more than 1,500 (for osteopathic schools, or D.O.s). As a result of these increases and federal policies that allowed more IMGs to practice in the United States, the number of physicians per 100,000 population increased dramatically between 1970 and 1990.

Active physicians numbered 151.4 per 100,000 population in 1970 and 267.5 per 100,000 in 1992 (IOM, 1996a). Put another way, the nation had 1 active physician for every 584 persons in the country in the mid-1970s (DHEW, 1977) and 1 for every 398 persons by the early 1990s. For active nonfederal M.D.s, the physician-to-population figures were 137.4 M.D.s per 100,000 population in 1970 and 219.5 in 1991, a rise of 60 percent. The percentage increase in the ratio of active nonfederal D.O.s was 104 percent (on a considerably smaller base), from 5.7 D.O.s per 100,000 persons in 1970 to 11.6 in 1991.

---

[2]Reporting of these figures differs somewhat across the period and by sources, depending on who is included in the various categories. Sources include DHEW (1977), NCHS (1983), and DHHS (1993).

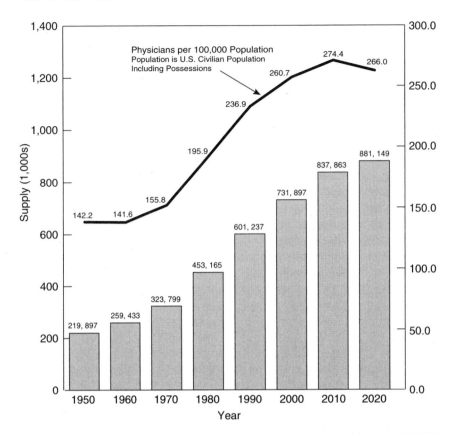

FIGURE 6-1 Numbers of physicians (M.D.s and D.O.s) and physicians per 100,000 population, selected years 1950–2020. SOURCE: IOM, 1996a. Reprinted with permission. Original source: Unpublished data from the Bureau of Health Professions (BHP) provided November 1, 1995. Data for 1950 through 1990 adjusted by BHP from American Medical Association Physician Masterfile and unpublished American Osteopathic Association data. Basic format of figure adapted from Rivo and Satcher (1993, p. 1077).

Table 6-1 provides further information on the U.S. physician supply (both M.D.s and D.O.s) according to various activity categories (e.g., active patient care, research, teaching) for selected years. Of interest is that, in the nearly quarter-century covered by these data, the total numbers of active physicians in patient care and the total numbers in residency training essentially doubled, whereas those in other professional activities rose only a fraction. Table 6-2a shows that, counting all physicians (including those who were inactive or had unknown addresses), the total numbers of federal and nonfederal physicians were 334,028 in 1970; 615,421 in 1990; and 670,336 in 1993.

TABLE 6-1 Supply of Physicians in the United States, 1970, 1980, 1992, by Type of Activity

Type of Activity	Number of Physicians[a]			Number of Physicians per 100,000 population[a]		
	1970	1980	1992	1970	1980	1992
TOTAL	328,020	462,276	685,291	160.9	203.5	267.5
Total Active Physicians[b]	308,487	436,667	627,723	151.4	192.2	245.0
Total active physicians in patient care[c]	222,657	310,533	461,405	109.2	136.7	180.1
Total active physicians in other professional activity	31,582	38,009	39,816	15.5	16.7	15.5
teaching	NA	NA	8,293	NA	NA	3.2
research	NA	NA	16,398	NA	NA	6.4
administration	NA	NA	15,125	NA	NA	5.9
Total physicians in training providing patient care[d]	50,687	61,450	99,138	24.9	27.1	38.7
Not classified[e]	3,561	26,675	27,364	1.7	11.7	10.7
Total Inactive Physicians	19,533	25,609	57,568	9.6	11.3	22.5

NOTE: NA=not available.

[a]Data for 1970 and 1980 are for allopathic physicians (M.D.s) only; data for 1992 include both allopathic and osteopathic physicians.
[b]Includes all physicians and physicians in training except those specifically identified as "inactive."
[c]Although physicians in training clearly provide considerable patient care, they are not included in this total; see their separate line item, below.
[d]"Physicians in training" is defined for 1970 and 1980 as "interns and residents, all years"; for 1992 the term is defined as "residents and fellows."
[e]"Not classified" includes, for 1970 and 1980, those physicians for whom an address is not known.

SOURCES: IOM, 1996a, Table 2-1. Reprinted with permission. Data for 1970 and 1980 adapted from NCHS, 1983, Tables 1 and 55. Data for 1992 adapted from Kindig 1994, Table 1 and text.

TABLE 6-2a Number of Active Federal and Nonfederal Physicians (M.D.s Only) by Specialty, Selected Years

Specialty	1970	1980	1990	1994
Primary Care Specialties				
General practice	57,948	32,519	22,841	18,454
Family practice	NA[a]	27,530	47,639	54,709
General internal medicine	39,924	58,462	76,295	84,951
General pediatrics	17,950	27,582	36,519	41,906
Total primary care specialties	**115,822**	**146,093**	**183,294**	**200,020**
Other Specialties				
Obstetrics-gynecology	18,876	26,305	33,697	36,649
Internal medicine subspecialties[b]	1,948	13,069	22,054	26,476
Pediatrics subspecialties[c]	869	1,880	5,380	7,451
All other specialties	173,414	227,569	302,885	334,752
Total other specialties[d]	**195,107**	**268,823**	**364,016**	**405,328**
Not classified physicians	**NA[e]**	**20,629**	**12,678**	**14,283**
Total active physicians[f]	**310,929**	**435,545**	**559,988**	**619,751**
Total Physicians[g]	**334,028**	**467,679**	**615,421**	**684,414**

NOTE: Data for 1990 and after are as of January 1. Data prior to 1990 are as of December 31.

[a]Data on family practice were not available before 1975.

[b]Internal medicine subspecialties include diabetes; endocrinology, diabetes, and metabolism; hematology; hepatology; cardiac electrophysiology; infectious diseases; clinical and laboratory immunology; geriatric medicine; sports medicine; nephrology; nutrition; medical oncology; and rheumatology.

[c]Pediatric subspecialties include adolescent medicine; pediatric critical care medicine; neonatalperinatal medicine; pediatric allergy; pediatric cardiology; pediatric endocrinology; pediatric pulmonology; pediatric emergency medicine; pediatric gastroenterology; pediatric hematology/oncology; clinical and laboratory immunology; pediatric nephrology; pediatric rheumatology; and sports medicine.

[d]Does not include, for 1994, 120 family practice subspecialty practitioners. Data on family practice subspecialties were not available before 1992.

[e]Data not available before 1972.

[f]Excludes those who are inactive and those for whom the address is unknown.

[g]Includes those who are active, inactive, and those for whom the address is unknown.

SOURCE: AMA, 1996.

Primary Care Physicians

Who Is Included

A major part of the physician workforce debate has centered on whether the supply of *primary care* physicians is sufficient. Although the committee wishes to underscore its view that primary care needs to be considered as a function and that the core of primary care delivery is a team of clinicians (and others), for the purposes of this chapter some denomination of the kinds of physicians typically considered as belonging to the area of primary care is necessary. Thus, to be able to show some numbers relating to supply and to trends over time, the committee focused on the primary care physicians practicing or trained in general practice, family practice, general internal medicine, and general pediatrics.

For purposes of counting practitioners, the committee did not bring obstetricians-gynecologists (OB-GYNs) into its primary care category. It did recognize that many women use OB-GYN specialists as their main, or even sole, health care providers, and the committee agreed that some regular use of this specialty is essential, if only to ensure that women see a physician at least yearly. As discussed in Chapters 2 and 5, however, the committee did not believe that OB-GYNs in general are likely to take on responsibility for "the large majority of health care needs" of their patients (and clearly they are not a source of primary care for men); thus, as a general proposition the practice of OB-GYN does not dovetail with the committee's definition of primary care. Some researchers and others in the workforce policy area, however, do include them in the primary care category, and some elements of the OB-GYN community have successfully argued that they are a part of the primary care workforce.

In general, other specialists and subspecialists are not, for workforce planning purposes, considered primary care physicians. The committee acknowledges that many other types of physicians may render what is recognizably primary care, for at least some of their patients or at least some of the time. No current estimates are available, however, to indicate what proportion of the practices of these other types of specialists is primary care. Thus, for purposes of understanding or influencing workforce policy, the committee is not considering physician specialties beyond those specified above.

Trends in Supply

The supply of primary care clinicians has been studied for many years. The IOM report on primary care in 1978 (IOM, 1978), the report of the Graduate Medical Education National Advisory Committee (GMENAC, 1981), and more recent studies by the Physician Payment Review Commission (PPRC, 1992, 1995) and numerous statements of the Committee on Graduate Medical Education (COGME, especially the fourth and seventh reports [1994, 1995]) have all expressed concern about the adequacy of the supply of primary care physicians. This issue was also addressed in several of the proposals for health care reform, most extensively in the Health Security Act (CCH, 1993). The prevailing view is that the nation has had, and still does, an imbalance between generalists and specialists—too few of the former and too many of the latter.

Specifically, as already noted, the United States has experienced a dramatic change in the composition of its physician workforce. In the early 1930s, 87 percent of private practice physicians were in general practice; 30 years later, only about 50 percent were generalists. Since then, the proportion of primary care physicians has continued to decline—leveling off at about one-third of all active physicians.

Tables 6-2a, 6-2b, and 6-2c provide information on specialty distribution for allopathic physicians for several years beginning with 1970; this information pertains only to M.D.s and takes only active physicians into account. Counting generalist M.D.s to be those in general and family practice, general internal medicine, and general pediatrics, the numbers in primary care increased from about 116,000 (in 1970) to 200,020 (in 1994); the total of all other specialties rose

TABLE 6-2b Physicians (M.D.s only) by Specialty Category as a Percentage of Total Active Physicians, Selected Years

Category	1970	1980	1990	1994
Primary care specialties	37.3	33.5	32.7	32.3
Other specialties	62.8	61.7	65.0	65.4
Not classified	NA	4.7	2.3	2.3
Total active physicians	100.1	99.9	100.0	100.0

NOTE: NA = not available; percentages do not sum to 100.0 because of rounding.

SOURCE: Based on data from AMA, 1996 (see Table 6-2).

TABLE 6-2c Percentage Changes in Numbers of Physicians (M.D.s only) in Primary Care During Selected Periods

Category	1970–1990	1990–1994	1970–1994
All primary care	58.3	8.7	72.7
General/family practice	21.6	3.8	26.3
General internal medicine	91.1	11.4	112.8
General pediatrics	103.4	14.8	133.5

SOURCE: Based on data from AMA, 1996 (see Table 6-2a).

from about 195,000 to more than 405,328 in the same period. In percentage terms (see Table 6-2b), primary care doctors as a percentage of total active physicians went from about 37 percent in 1970 to just over 32 percent in 1994; other specialties were about 63 and 65 percent of all active physicians in those years.

Said another way, in the nearly quarter-century from 1970 to 1994 the total number of M.D.s in the United States more than doubled (from 334,000 to 684,414), and the total of active physicians nearly doubled (about 311,000 to almost 620,000). Most of the growth in the number of allopathic physicians was in specialty medicine—a rise of 108 percent over the period. The primary care workforce (general and family practice, general internal medicine, and general pediatrics) increased by about 73 percent (see Table 6-2c). The percentage increases during 1970–1994 were about 133 percent for general pediatrics, about 113 percent for general internal medicine, and about 26 percent for general and family medicine combined; if just family medicine is considered, the percentage increase from 1980 (the first year of family practice data noted in Table 6-2a) to 1994 was 99 percent. By 1994, of all primary care M.D.s in the United States, 43 percent were in internal medicine, 36 percent in general and family practice (mostly the latter), and 21 percent in pediatrics.

More recently, various expert groups and researchers have concluded that the future demand for physician services including primary care physicians may be attenuated by the rapid growth of managed care plans, which use fewer physicians per enrollee than are used by the rest of the population (Kindig et al., 1993; COGME, 1995; Davis et al., 1995; Gamliel et al., 1995; PPRC, 1995; ProPAC, 1995; Scheffler, Appendix E). Other factors also suggest that the aggregate supply of primary care clinicians may be adequate in the near future. These include the rapid growth in the supply of primary care professionals other than physicians; the provision of primary care by specialist physicians (probably a significant number, although recent data are not available); and a recent turnaround in the numbers of medical students choosing primary care (perhaps a delayed response to market signals that are increasing the incomes of generalists both absolutely and in relationship to specialists incomes). As COGME (1996) notes in its eighth report, however, although projections of the numbers of generalist physicians may suggest that supply will be adequate, there is no guarantee of appropriate geographic distribution of those practitioners.

Education, Training, and Licensure

Today, the United States has a total of 125 schools of allopathic medicine[3] and another 16 schools of osteopathic medicine; up to four new osteopathic

---

[3]Until very recently, the United States had 126 allopathic schools, a number that had remained stable for years. A merger between two schools in Philadelphia changed the figure to 125.

schools are in various stages of planning. Together they currently graduate approximately 17,500 physicians a year—a figure that has been fairly constant for about 15 years. Specifically, the number of M.D. graduates in 1994 was 15,579 (Barzansky et al., 1995), and the number of D.O. graduates that year was 1,775 (Singer, 1994). Graduates from allopathic schools alone are projected to number about 16,400 for the academic years through 1998–1999 (Jonas et al., 1994).

Information on enrollments in allopathic schools is instructive. Total enrollment in 1993–1994 was nearly 66,500; of these, about 40 percent were women. With respect to race and ethnic background, 15.6 percent were Asian and Pacific Islander; nearly 8 percent were Mexican American, Puerto Rican, or of other Hispanic background; 7.2 percent were non-Hispanic African American; 0.6 percent were Native American or Alaskan Native; all other students (white but not of Hispanic origin, and non-U.S. foreign students of any race or ethnicity) made up nearly 70 percent of all students. Of interest is that the ratio of students applying to U.S. medical schools to those accepted is about 2.5 to 1. With respect to the primary care workforce, it is evident from the small proportion of minority students enrolled in medical schools that achieving significant representation of minorities who are trained and practicing in primary care will be difficult, at least in the near term.

Newly graduated physicians take graduate medical education (GME) training in a highly developed graduate training system in this country. Accredited single-specialty and combined-specialty GME programs numbered 7,277 in 1993 (*JAMA,* 1994), with a total of 97,370 resident physicians.[4] Of these programs, 407 are in family practice, 416 in nonsubspecialty internal medicine, and 215 in nonsubspecialty pediatrics; respectively, the total numbers of positions in these programs were on the order of 8,500 (family medicine), 21,300 (internal medicine), and 7,750 (pediatrics).[5] According to Whitcomb (1994), most GME programs (more than 90 percent) are affiliated with a medical school (or a closely related entity).

Groups in both the public and private sectors have sought, over the years, to increase the production of primary care physicians (see also Chapter 7). In the public sector, these steps have included support under Title VII of the Public Health Service Act for the training of primary care physicians. Several state governments have also pressed the medical schools within the state to increase

---

[4]See *JAMA,* 1994. "Straight" residency programs (in generalist or subspecialist disciplines) number just over 7,100 programs; "combined" programs (about 160 in all) are blends such as internal medicine and another specialty (e.g., pediatrics, emergency medicine).

[5]The numbers of programs or positions in "nonsubspecialty" internal medicine or pediatrics may be misleading, however, because historically a majority of those internal medicine residents and a large minority of those in general pediatrics went on to subspecialty training. By contrast, over 90 percent of family practice residents enter family practice.

production of primary care physicians (including Arizona and California). Several private foundations also support programs to increase the training of generalists.

Geographic Distribution of Primary Care Physicians

Of considerable importance is the continuing lack of sufficient primary care clinicians in some geographic areas, particularly rural and some poor urban areas. By and large, problems of geographic maldistribution are set out in terms of aggregate physician presence, not the availability of primary care physicians (or primary care clinicians). For example, in 1993 metropolitan areas had an average ratio of physicians to population of 226 per 100,000 persons, whereas for non-metropolitan areas the ratio was 118 per 100,000 persons (Cooper, 1995). More telling is Cooper's analysis of physician-to-population ratios across the states, which shows a high of 294 in Maryland and the District of Columbia and a low of 118 in Mississippi. Cooper argues that the nation can be characterized as having five regions as follows (physician-to-population ratios are given in parentheses): the Boston-Washington corridor (227 to 294 per 100,000 persons); east and west "arms" including Florida (190 to 212); the central zone (147 to 181); the northern Rockies and Alaska (132 to 143); and Mississippi (118).

Workforce developments in the past 25 years provide ample evidence that increases in aggregate supply, by themselves, are not adequate to correct the problem of shortages in some areas of the country. Although physicians have been moving to smaller or more rural areas since the early 1980s (Schwartz et al., 1980; Williams et al., 1981; Newhouse et al., 1982a, 1982b), the fact that rural areas and inner cities continue to face access problems cannot be gainsaid. Geographic maldistribution in rural areas (e.g., for counties of fewer than 50,000 residents) is worsening, not improving, according to recent data from COGME (1995), a pattern consistent with the data reported by Cooper (1995). The committee returns to the geographic maldistribution issue later in this Chapter 7.

WORKFORCE TRENDS AND SUPPLY PROJECTIONS: NURSE PRACTITIONERS

According to a recent report on nurse staffing in hospitals and nursing homes (IOM, 1996b), the largest group of health care providers in the United States is registered nurses (RNs); in 1992, more than 2.2 million individuals were licensed to practice as RNs, or about 750 RNs per 100,000 population. RNs are prepared in one of three different educational tracks that can take two, three, or four years.[6] In 1993, there were 129 diploma programs, 857 associated degree pro-

---

[6]More information on nursing education can be found in IOM, 1995c.

grams, and 507 baccalaureate programs, which together produced nearly 95,000 graduates; baccalaureate programs alone in 1994 had nearly 113,000 enrollees. Given this diversity of training, RNs differ in terms of both basic and advanced clinical education and skills; consequently, their clinical responsibilities may vary as well, from providing direct patient care at a fairly basic level to managing care for complex cases to directing complex nursing departments in institutions and community sites.

Nurse practitioners are one of a category of advanced practice nurses[7] with significant involvement in primary care. Nurse practitioners have, in general, an average of 580 hours of clinical training (AACN, 1995). NPs "are usually prepared at the master's degree level and also certified in a specialty area of practice, such as pediatrics, family practice, or primary care. Their usual responsibilities include managing clinical care; they conduct physical examinations, track medical histories, make diagnoses, treat minor illnesses and injuries, and perform an array of counseling and educational tasks. [NPs] may also, in some circumstances, order and interpret diagnostic tests and prescribe medications" (IOM, 1996b, 99–100).[8] As for RNs generally, the scope of practice for NPs is governed by state nurse practice acts, which vary considerably across the nation.

Based on a 1992 survey of RNs, approximately 48,200 nurses had formal training as NPs (Moses, 1994). Of this number, roughly three-fifths are certified by a national or state organization, and approximately one-half are practicing as NPs (Moses, 1994).

Table 6-3 shows the growth in number of employed RNs who have nurse practitioner (or nurse midwife) in their title—from nearly 15,500 in 1980 to about 20,600 in 1988 and almost 23,700 in 1992, using data from a national sample survey of nursing that is conducted periodically. In percentage terms, a substantial increase took place between 1984 and 1988 (about 22 percent), with another 14.6 percent rise between 1988 and 1992; the overall percentage change in employed RNs who were either NPs or nurse midwives was more than 53 percent between 1980 and 1992.

The total number of NPs who are practicing is difficult to determine because licensing and educational requirements vary significantly across states (Morgan, 1993; Washington Consulting Group, 1994). For example, some NPs, although graduates of NP programs, do not have and do not need state certification to practice in a health maintenance organization (HMO); thus a count of currently

---

[7]Other types of advanced practice nurses, of which NPs are a part, include certified nurse midwives, certified nurse anesthetists, and clinical nurse specialists. Like their physician counterparts, some of these clinical personnel may well deliver primary care as an element of their practices, but primary care is not their main task or type of training, and for that reason they are not considered further in this report.

[8]Students are RNs who typically take 18 months of training, half of which is in clinical practice (AACN, 1995).

TABLE 6-3 Employed Registered Nurses with Nurse Practitioner or Nurse Midwife in Their Titles, Selected Years, and Percentage Changes between Years

Year	Number of Nurse Practitioners (or Nurse Midwives)	Percentage Change from Previous Year Given
1980	15,443	
1984	16,886	9.3
1988	20,649	22.3
1992	23,658	14.6

SOURCE: National Nursing Sample Survey, 1980, 1984, 1988, 1992 (Bureau of the Health Professions, Health Resources and Services Administration, unpublished).

certified NPs in a given state is likely to result in underestimating those who might be in practice.

Primary Care Nurse Practitioners

The National Nursing Sample Surveys do not specifically break out NPs who are practicing primary care, but the large majority of NPs are thought to be doing so. Table 6-4 shows the number of NP graduates in 1992 by their area of specialization. Most of the categories shown might be considered to have a major primary care focus. Certainly, NPs graduating with a principal area of expertise in family, pediatric, and adult health, and possibly gerontology and women's health, would fall into this category, and together those groups account for about 80 percent of NPs graduating that year.

What is not known, however, is in what areas the nearly 24,000 currently employed NPs are actually practicing. Some NPs who are practicing in what appears to be primary care, for example, consider themselves specialists in a given area, such as diabetes counseling and management of diabetic adolescents. However, the number of such NPs has never been documented, and the extent to which they might also provide large amounts of routine primary care is certainly not known.

Trends in Supply

The number of NPs is expected to grow considerably in the years ahead as a result of the establishment of new education and training programs. A recent survey by the American Association of Colleges of Nursing provides considerable detail on these NP programs. Currently, 644 institutions of higher learning offer at least baccalaureate programs in nursing and, of these, 287 offer master's

TABLE 6-4 U.S. Graduations of Nurse Practitioners by General Area of Practice, 1992

Area of Practice	Number	Percentage[a]
Family	485	29.5
Pediatric	281	17.1
Adult	276	16.8
Gerontology	118	7.2
Midwifery	110	6.7
Psychiatric/mental health	53	3.2
Women's health	142	8.6
School	1	0.1
Other	179	10.9
Total	1,645	100.1

NOTE: American Samoa, Guam, Puerto Rico, and the Virgin Islands are not included.

[a]Total is more than 100 percent because of rounding.

SOURCE: NLN, 1994, Section 2-3, Table 10A.

programs. In all, 206 institutions (32 percent of the baccalaureate-level programs, and 72 percent of those with master's level programs, chiefly in universities) also provide NP education at the level of master's or post-master's training (AACN, 1995, p. 7, Tables 7 and 9);[9] of these, about 30 percent offer a doctoral program as well. In addition, 75 institutions are reported to be planning to add master's degree or post-master's NP education programs to their curricula, a trend that represents rapid growth in NP training programs.

According to the AACN survey (1995), 32,049 individuals were enrolled as of fall 1994 in master's level nursing programs. Of these, 37 percent were in NP areas of study (11,536 in traditional master's programs and 289 in so-called generic programs for persons who had nonnursing college degrees); an additional 3 percent of this entire student body were in combined NP and clinical nurse specialist (CNS) programs (1,023 in traditional and 59 in generic programs). The AACN (1995, p. 3) notes a "dramatic growth in [recent] NP enrollment."

From August 1993 through July 1994, the number of NPs graduating from traditional or generic master's programs totaled 2,153 (AACN, 1995); 183 graduated with combined NP-CNS degrees. Of the 7,999 graduates in that period NPs alone represented about 27 percent and NP-CNSs 2 percent. Comparing these

---

[9]Moses (1994) puts the number of institutions at 507, however, and this may be because of differences in definition.

graduating figures with enrollment data cited just above suggests that the output of nurses with NP (or NP-CNS) training (as a proportion of all nurses being trained at the master's level) will rise in the coming years.

The question of primary care focus within NP training is of interest. Of 125 NP institutions reporting information on this question in the AACN survey (1995), 91 report specialty tracks in family health, 42 tracks in adult health (and an additional 10 in adult acute care), 41 in pediatrics, 27 in gerontology/geriatrics, and 23 in OB-GYN or women's health (other than midwifery). Of the 1,946 full-time and part-time students enrolled in these institutions, nearly 89 percent are enrolled in these specialty areas, suggesting a considerable interest in primary care. The rapid growth in post-master's training may in part reflect the downsizing of hospitals and a shift of hospital-based master's prepared clinical specialists to primary care.

Current Work Environments and Responsibilities

Approximately 29 percent of NPs work in private practices or HMOs, 23 percent in hospital outpatient departments, 23 percent in public or community health centers, and 11 percent in inpatient hospital departments (Washington Consulting Group, 1994). Thus, only about 1 in 10 NPs work in inpatient settings, in contrast to RNs. About two-thirds of RNs work in hospitals, and although available data do not permit a breakdown of inpatient and outpatient settings, it is generally believed that a majority of hospital-based RNs are in inpatient settings (IOM, 1996b; Moses, 1994).

Nearly 70 percent of NPs have primary responsibility for a specific group of patients under either a team or panel approach (PPRC, 1994). NPs in nine states can establish independent practices (Birkholz and Walker, 1994; Henderson and Chovan, 1994; Pearson, 1994). About 1 in 10 NPs have hospital admitting privileges, and 1 in 3 have hospital discharge privileges (Washington Consulting Group, 1994).

WORKFORCE TRENDS AND SUPPLY PROJECTIONS: PHYSICIAN ASSISTANTS

Physician assistants are health personnel who are typically trained in two or more years to render basic health care services that in earlier decades were performed only by physicians (Scheffler and Gillings, 1982; Jones and Cawley, 1994). They represent a "new" category of health personnel that has emerged only since the early 1960s, partly in response to the desire to make good use of experienced hospital corpsmen and combat medics returning from Vietnam. Early models of PA training aimed to produce personnel who would be able to assist doctors in ways that would foster better use of both physicians and nurses. To this day, PAs work under a form of physician supervision (not necessarily direct physical supervision), in which PAs are "agents of their supervising physicians" (Jones and Cawley, 1994, p. 1,269); supervising physicians define the standard to which PA services will be held and are, in effect, vicariously liable for those services (by virtue of being responsible for selecting and supervising PAs).

PA responsibilities have been described by Jones and Cawley (1994) in six areas: evaluation, monitoring, diagnostics, therapeutics, counseling, and referral. Within these categories, the state laws that describe and delimit the scope of PA practice are quite varied. PAs are regulated under states' medical practice acts—a circumstance different from that for nurses, who are regulated under nurse practice acts. This difference means that PAs and nurses may, in some jurisdictions, carry out similar functions, but NPs do so independently and PAs under the supervision (even if distant) of physicians. In any case, the great variation in PA statutes has the effect of not permitting PAs trained in similar ways and exhibiting essentially the same skills to perform the same functions across the nation.

Accurate counts of the number of PAs being graduated in this country date only to about 1967, and figures for the aggregate supply of PAs only to about 1970. The data are collected by the American Academy of Physician Assistants (AAPA), which conducts census surveys of its members; the 1995 mid-year report gives considerable information from a survey of nearly 13,500 PAs (AAPA, 1995). As shown in Table 6-5, in 1967 (the first year that any data were collected) there were 4 new PA graduates; by 1995, the number exceeded 2,100. In the nearly 30 years since any organization began counting, 32,215 PAs have been produced in this country.

Currently, 64 PA programs are operating in the United States. This number includes four new programs begun in the past year (Steven Crane, AAPA, personal communication, November 1995). More than half (55 percent) of entering PA students have baccalaureate degrees, and entering students generally have

TABLE 6-5 New and Cumulative Graduates from Physician Assistant Programs, Selected Years

Year	Number of New Graduates	Cumulative Number of Graduates	Percentage Growth in New Graduates
1967	4	4	NA
1970	195	237	4,775.0
1980	1,489	11,032	663.6
1990	1,195	23,409	−19.7
1995	2,139	32,215	79.0

NOTE: NA = not applicable.

SOURCE: American Academy of Physician Assistants, Masterfile, November 2, 1995.

TABLE 6-6 Number and Percentage of Physician Assistants, by General Area of Practice, Mid-1995

Practice Area	Number	Percentage
Primary Care Specialties	5,922	47.2
Family/general medicine	4,652	37.9
General internal medicine	958	7.8
General pediatrics	312	2.5
Other Specialties	6,612	52.8
Emergency Medicine	1,043	8.3
Obstetrics-gynecology	373	3.0
Industrial and occupational medicine	396	3.2
Geriatrics	115	0.9
Internal medicine subspecialties	925	7.5
Pediatric subspecialties	229	1.9
All surgical specialties	2,767	22.1
All other specialties	764	6.1
Total	12,534	100.0

SOURCE: AAPA, 1995, Table 22a.

had more than four years of health care experience in fields such as nursing and allied health or experience as paramedics and emergency medical technicians (Eugene Jones, personal communication, 1995). PAs in primary care practice with and are supervised by primary care physicians, although in some practices in rural areas the link is electronic and periodic rather than comprising a traditional team practice with shared office space.

Primary Care Physician Assistants

According to a 1995 AAPA report, 5,922 of 12,534 PAs responding to the survey were practicing in federally defined primary care specialties—internal medicine, general pediatrics, and family medicine (Table 6-6). This number represents 47 percent of the respondents (and approximately 34 percent of all PAs surveyed). Although PA practice settings remain diverse, an increasing plurality remain employed in primary care.

Current Work Environments and Settings

According to the AAPA (1995) survey, about 40 percent of PAs work in solo or group practice physician offices, about 10 percent in clinics, nearly 7 percent in health maintenance organizations, and about 25 percent in hospitals. This is a pattern not unlike that for NPs (see above).

TABLE 6-7 Physician Assistants in Practice, by Region, 1994–1995

Region	Number	Percentage
North Central	2,353	19.8
Northeast	3,017	25.4
Southeast	2,867	24.1
South Central	1,631	13.7
West	2,020	17.0
Total	11,888	100.0

SOURCE: AAPA, 1995, Table 6.

Table 6-7 illustrates the geographically uneven distribution of PAs (AAPA, 1995). In 1994–1995, almost one-half (49 percent) were in the East, one-third (34 percent) in the North and South Central regions, and one-sixth (17 percent) in the West.

OTHER FIRST-CONTACT PROVIDERS

First-contact providers such as dentists, optometrists, and pharmacists play an important role in the provision of basic health care services. The committee did not have the resources to track trends in supply of these types of providers, but in general it did not foresee a significant shift in either their numbers or their roles in the near term. With respect, however, to the role of the dental professions in overall health care in this country, a recent IOM report on dental education (IOM, 1995a) calls attention to the following broad health objective (p. 78): "*promoting attention to oral health* (including the oral manifestations of other health problems) not just among dental practitioners but also *among other primary care providers, geriatricians, educators, and public officials*" (emphasis in the original). This committee is generally in agreement with these views.

More broadly, the committee encourages greater coordination between these types of first-contact professionals and primary care clinicians. It believes that a continuation of the typical roles of first-contact providers is not likely to affect the demand for primary care clinicians to any meaningful degree in the near term, and thus it did not explore issues relating to these types of practitioners further.

COMMENT ON WORKFORCE ESTIMATION

The history of workforce projection in health care is not encouraging.[10] The problems lie in the marked difficulties of estimating "need" or "demand" (that is,

---

[10]Reviews of projection methodologies reveal many difficulties inherent in the projection of adequacy of supply and need or demand (i.e., requirements). Feil et al. (1993), for example, present

requirements) for either health care services or health care personnel and the somewhat less troublesome challenges of projecting supply. Tarlov (1995, p. 1,559) notes that some agreement exists about certain factors, such as the state of health of Americans, use of health care, medical training, and growth of nonphysician clinicians; he believes these offer some common ground for making assumptions about supply and requirements that can be used in full-scale workforce models, but he is careful to underscore the uncertainties. Among the trends that complicate forecasting today are the following (Feil et al., 1993): the rate of growth of managed care plans; innovations in the patterns of use of primary care professionals in the future, including the wider use of teams; the rate of spread of those innovations; the acceptance of new patterns of primary care providers by patients as they choose among competing health plans; the degree to which specialists seek to expand their provision of primary care as the pending surplus of specialists cuts back on the opportunities within specialties; the ability of academic health centers and other health organizations to support training of primary care clinicians when the financial viability of the training programs is threatened by the competitive health care market seeking to avoid training costs; and the probable reductions in federal and state budgets for health professional education, including support for GME and nursing training under the Medicare program. In the committee's view, drawing inferences about the expected adequacy of supply relative to requirements must be done with considerable caution, especially for the more distant future, and especially for NPs.

As noted by Scheffler (Appendix E), estimates of the overall impact of NPs and PAs on the size and composition of the future health workforce vary widely because of the different assumptions that forecasters make about patient utilization rates, physician delegation rates, the extent to which HMOs and other managed care organizations are willing to use NPs and PAs, and other variables. The varying assumptions about managed care organizations reflect the fact that so far, researchers have been able to obtain detailed data on physician and nonphysician staffing patterns for only a handful of HMOs, and staffing patterns vary widely among those HMOs that have made data accessible to researchers (Weiner, 1993, 1994).

The case study conducted by Scheffler for the committee compared staffing patterns in two mature HMOs. He found, first, that merely counting physicians and specialist physicians does not provide a useful staffing analysis in a managed care world. Researchers must also examine the use of PAs, NPs, and other

---

a formidable list of factors that introduce uncertainty into projections. Several IOM and National Academy of Sciences reports make the same point about disciplines other than physicians or primary care (IOM, 1995a, 1995b, 1996b; NRC, 1994). The IOM report on the U.S. physician supply has a more detailed review of the major strengths and limitations of standard physician estimation models used for the past 25 years or so, as does the eighth COGME report (1996).

nonphysician clinicians. Second, to make inferences about productivity, researchers cannot merely compare the number of health professionals used by the plan to the total plan enrollment. They need to investigate differences in enrollee and other plan characteristics, including enrollee age and sex distribution, patient severity of illness, patient outcomes, staff productivity, and the organizational structure of the clinical practice. Third, staffing numbers alone cannot reveal some important health workforce parameters, such as complementarity and substitution possibilities within health care teams.

Another salient issue regarding workforce estimates is the lack of current knowledge of the content of clinicians' practices—whether physicians, NPs, or PAs. Regardless of the disciplines in which they receive training, we know little about the proportion of their practice that is, in fact, primary care. Although clearly the numbers of NPs and PAs will increase in the years ahead, their roles in an evolving health care system are uncertain. They may well be used in both specialty care and primary care, for example, making the size of their representation within the primary care clinician category quite problematic at this stage.

CONCLUSIONS AND RECOMMENDATIONS ABOUT THE SUPPLY OF PRIMARY CARE CLINICIANS

Training Programs for Primary Care Clinicians

Basic Goals

Taking all the figures cited above in the admittedly difficult-to-predict context of health care restructuring in this country, the committee concluded that, at the moment, the nation probably has a modest aggregate shortage of primary care clinicians. (Aggregate, in this instance, refers to the combination of physicians, NPs, and PAs in primary care.) In the near term, the aggregate "shortages" may disappear because of several factors. Some relate to demand for health care; others involve current supply and production of various types of primary care professionals.

Market-driven changes will affect the effective economic demand for primary care clinicians. These changes include the growth of managed care, the development by some managed care organizations of innovative models of personnel substitution, and the increased use of primary care teams. All have the potential to affect the demand for primary care clinicians. Because some changes may increase demand and others decrease it, it is difficult to predict the net effect.

Furthermore, the cutbacks in Medicare and Medicaid that can be expected in coming years may attenuate the rate of growth in demand (at least per capita demand) from the elderly population. Certainly the demand for provision of health care services to low-income, disabled, and disadvantaged populations can be expected to drop, if federal entitlements to the Medicaid program are eliminated in favor of state options for health care block grants. The rise in the number of persons underinsured or uninsured in any one year will also affect demand for health care services. So, too, will increases in mandatory out-of-pocket costs, such as higher health care premiums, higher deductibles and copayment requirements, and cutbacks in coverage of certain services such as those for mental health.

Economic demand for health care services is not equivalent to potential need for such services. As Tarlov (1995, p. 1559) notes:

> [A]lso affecting requirements are the emergence of new diseases, sharp changes in demographic composition and the different needs of special populations including the poor, immigrants, some minority groups, children, military personnel, veterans, retirees, elders, and people in underserved rural and urban areas. . . .

The committee is under no illusions: Developing a national consensus about service requirements—i.e., the human need for health care services—is, and will remain, a profound challenge.

Changes on the supply side can be expected to help eliminate shortages in the future. Among these changes are the probable increase in the number of specialists and subspecialists who expand their delivery of primary care services, a rising interest in primary care careers on the part of medical students, and continued rapid growth in training of NPs and PAs.

In general, the committee supports these trends, but it remains unconvinced that the supply of well-prepared primary care clinicians will be sufficient to meet the demand for their services, at least in the short term. In the longer term, of course, these steps may well suffice, but the committee is not persuaded that, collectively, they will produce adequate numbers of appropriately competent personnel able to function in the model of a primary care team and to provide adequate quality of care. To address these concerns, the committee has two points it wishes to emphasize concerning the future of programs that produce primary care physicians, PAs, and NPs.

Recommendation 6.1 Programs Regarding the Primary Care Workforce

The committee recommends (a) that the current level of effort to increase the supply of primary care clinicians be continued and (b) that these primary care training programs and delivery systems focus their efforts on improving the competency of primary care clinicians and on increasing access for populations not now receiving adequate primary care.

General Issues of Access and Quality of Care

In the committee's judgment, the nation does still have an *imbalance* in the supply of primary care clinicians relative to clinicians (chiefly physicians) in specialty and subspecialty disciplines. Recommendation 6.1 is intended to help right that balance, without tipping the scale toward a future excess of primary care clinicians of any type. Its language about the output of current training programs is, therefore, chosen advisedly. That is, the committee believes that the present levels of production of primary care physicians, NPs, and PAs should be maintained—not accelerated, but also not diminished. The committee does not recommend the introduction of major new initiatives aimed at increasing the aggregate supply of primary care clinicians. Rather, as noted just below, the aim is to improve access to primary care for all Americans, taking into account expertise, geographic distribution, ethnic and cultural representation within the primary care workforce, or other factors important to the delivery of high-quality primary care.

The committee's further focus with respect to primary care training programs is on improving primary care competencies. These issues are explored more fully in Chapter 7 on training and education and are touched on in Chapter 8 with respect to accountability for quality of care.

This committee, like others at the IOM, endorses the IOM's stated position about universal access to health care coverage for all Americans (IOM, 1993) and has explicitly offered its own recommendation in this area (Recommendation 5.1). Fulfilling this aim is regarded as especially pertinent for primary care, because of the centrality of primary care to well-rounded, integrated health care, access to appropriate specialists, and better patient outcomes. It is even more important for those populations that do not now receive adequate primary care.

Thus, the committee is especially concerned that training programs be configured so as to prepare students for careers in the full range of settings needed to serve all the American people. These points are also addressed more fully in Chapter 7 in discussions of undergraduate medical education in primary care sites (see Recommendation 7.1) and graduate medical education in nonhospital sites such as HMOs, community clinics, physician offices, and extended care facilities (see Recommendation 7.6).

Minority Participation in Primary Care Training and Practice

The committee also wishes to go on record as supporting special initiatives that will increase the percentage of underrepresented minorities in the health professions, including primary care. This is in keeping with recent recommendations of other IOM committees, especially one on minority representation in the health professions (IOM, 1994) and another on aggregate physician supply (IOM,

1996a); it is also consistent with the "3000 by 2000" goals of the Association of American Medical Colleges.

Specifically, the committee would like to see the ethnic and cultural mix of the present and future supply of primary care clinicians be modified over time by an increase in the proportion of minorities. In this regard, the committee draws attention not only to the problems of underrepresentation among practitioners (i.e., physicians, NPs, or PAs) but also among the health professions faculty and researchers. Consistent with the sentiment of the IOM report *Balancing the Scales of Opportunity: Ensuring Racial and Ethnic Diversity in the Health Professions* (IOM, 1994), the committee is sensitive to the need for health professions schools to develop programs that reflect genuine appreciation and respect for students' various backgrounds, values, and perspectives. It also underscores the need for health professions schools and professional organizations to engage in more outreach to prospective students at the university (indeed, at the high school) level. This view dovetails with the discussion in the next chapter about the need for training programs, professional organizations, and similar groups to emphasize cultural sensitivity and appropriate communication skills (see Recommendation 7.4).

Monitoring Supply And Requirements

Recommendation 6.2 Monitoring the Primary Care Workforce

The committee recommends that state and federal agencies carefully monitor the supply of and requirements for primary care clinicians.

In keeping with the increasingly interdisciplinary nature of primary care, the committee urges that state and federal agencies compile a composite database of primary care clinicians—including physicians, NPs, and PAs providing primary care services. This would help analysts, policymakers, educators, and others understand the changing requirements for primary care clinicians and monitor utilization patterns of employment, geographic distribution, and insurance status of patients served.

Market forces may be able in the future to correct the modest shortage of primary care clinicians. The restructuring presently taking place, however, remains fluid so that the committee cannot be certain that market forces will induce and *maintain* appropriate responses in training and practice choices. Moreover, the committee remains concerned about the rapid changes taking place in the health care sector as a whole. It concludes that ongoing monitoring of supply and requirements is essential to ensure that appropriate public policy and private career decisions can be made.

Currently, the Bureau of the Health Professions (of the Health Resources and Services Administration [BHP/HRSA]), the Council on Graduate Medical Education (COGME), and the National Committee on Nursing Education and Practice have responsibility for monitoring primary care clinician supply and requirements. The committee endorses their efforts and notes the recommendations from a parallel IOM committee (IOM, 1996a) on the same point. Specifically, that panel advocated (p. 90) that

> the Department of Health and Human Services, chiefly through the Health Resources and Services Administration, regularly make information on physician supply and requirements and the status of career opportunities in medicine available to policymakers, educators, professional associations, and the public . . . [and that] the American Medical Association, the Association of American Medical Colleges, the Osteopathic Association, the American Association of Colleges of Osteopathic Medicine, and other professional associations cooperate with the federal government in widely disseminating such information to students indicating an interest in careers in medicine.

Clearly, those recommendations pertain to physicians (and to all physicians, not just those in primary care). This committee would extend that advice to include nurses (especially advanced practice nurses or NPs) and PAs (see IOM, 1996b, for a detailed discussion of the needs for better data on the nurse workforce). Nurses and PAs are health care practitioners of direct interest to BHP/HRSA. The analogous collaboration and cooperation would be sought with a wide array of professional associations, including but not limited to the American Academy of Physician Assistants, American Association of Colleges of Nursing, the American Association of Physician Assistants, American Nurses Association, the National League for Nurses, and the National Organization of Nurse Practitioner Faculties.

Apart from general monitoring of the several professions relevant to primary care (e.g., in terms of current size and composition and future projections of supply and requirements), efforts should also be made to obtain current information on the use of primary care clinicians by managed care plans and integrated health delivery systems. Of particular interest are patterns of substitution across physicians, NPs, and PAs and the impact of the complex interactions of these practitioners on health care costs, access, and quality of care. These points are revisited in Chapter 8 with respect to a primary care research agenda.

Geographic Maldistribution of the Primary Care Workforce

The committee is concerned by the continuing geographic maldistribution of the primary care workforce; there are too few clinicians in inner cities and rural areas. Despite many attempts to address this shortage, the nation simply has not adequately improved access to primary care services in these underserved areas.[11] Although programs such as the National Health Service Corps have filled

---

[11]The history of formally identifying areas that are underserved by health care providers is more

the gap to some extent (especially for rural areas) (Mullan, 1995), significant disparities remain. The latest, dramatic evidence of this for physicians was presented by Cooper (1995), cited earlier; equivalently detailed information for NPs and PAs is not available.

The incompatibility between articulated public policy goals and objectives and the financing mechanisms put in place to support them have created an expansion of the physician supply without actually achieving an adequate workforce supply in underserved areas. Neither "trickle-down" physician workforce policy nor market forces to date have been notably successful in alleviating the problems of inequitable distribution of primary care services and clinicians, across the nation.

The committee has dealt—essentially throughout this report—with the widely recognized issues of maldistribution of physicians by generalist or specialty training and practice. The problem of maldistribution by geographic location is another, and troubling, matter. The committee regards the goal of overcoming imbalances in the geographic distribution of primary care clinicians as an especially significant one. It also believes that, with the rapid changes now taking place in the private sector, managed care organizations and integrated health delivery systems have a significant duty to address this question head-on.

Recommendation 6.3 Addressing Issues of Geographic Maldistribution

The committee recommends that federal and state governments and private foundations fund research projects to explore ways in which managed care and integrated health care systems can be used to alleviate the geographic maldistribution of primary care clinicians.

For purposes of this recommendation, the committee regards rural and inner city jurisdictions as appropriate targets for such projects and for specific attempts to redress the shortage of primary care clinicians in these areas. Clearly, as between rural areas and the core metropolitan areas, the problems, the likely solutions, and the types of personnel and configurations of primary care teams are all likely to differ. In fact, rural areas themselves will vary along these dimensions, as will inner cities.

---

than a quarter-century old, beginning with the development of the Index of Medical Underservice in the early 1970s and continuing with Critical Health Manpower Shortage Areas, Nurse Shortage Areas, Health Manpower Shortage Areas, and now Health Professional Shortage Areas (HPSAs). The last are identified on the basis of several variables, including low physician-to-population ratios, high rates of adverse health events such as infant deaths, and poor access to care. According to the Bureau of Primary Health Care (BPHC, 1995), in 1994 almost 2,740 HPSAs had been designated (of which about two-thirds were rural) covering a population of nearly 48 million individuals. More information on HPSAs and on the entire effort to designate underserved areas and to address their health care professional needs can be found in Lee (1991), Desmarais (1995), and Mullan, (1995).

The committee believes that managed care organizations may be able to deal with some maldistribution problems where earlier efforts have not worked. For instance, integrated delivery systems that wish to expand their businesses into previously uncovered catchment areas, whether rural or inner city, can provide financial incentives, collegial relationships, and telecommunications capabilities that will attract physicians (as well as NPs and PAs) into those areas. Academic health centers may also operate community or school clinics or other types of ambulatory care networks, especially in poor sections of metropolitan areas, that essentially also represent good business and expanded catchment opportunities. The inducements may include acceptable practice sites, competitive salaries, hospital privileges, professional relationships and backup, and appropriate referral networks, but the growing scarcity of practice openings in more affluent areas should not be discounted. The precise combinations of fiscal and professional incentives that might work best for particular types of underserved areas are clearly not known today. Thus, demonstration and evaluation of current efforts would be particularly useful, in the committee's view.

The committee did not call for testing or evaluation of *specific* approaches that managed care and integrated systems might use to address the geographic maldistribution problems of these areas. Consistent with the principles laid out in Chapter 2, however, the committee notes that it would not subscribe to solutions that were based solely on one type of primary care clinician; it believes that innovative programs involving physicians, NPs, and PAs are more desirable, and indeed it would advocate that strategies involving the entire primary care team be investigated.

Finally, this recommendation is couched in terms of research projects and thus should be considered in conjunction with the broad research agenda laid out in Chapter 8. The committee advances it here to underscore the policy issues—specifically, a very uneven presence of primary care clinicians across the states that severely hinders any efforts to bring greater parity in access to health care services to large portions of the U.S. population. Because managed care organizations and integrated systems are gaining such a prominent role in the whole restructuring of the nation's health care system, it was felt that demonstration and evaluation projects conducted by them or under their auspices would shed the most light on how best to address this access issue. In short, the committee believes that as managed care plans and approaches expand, they bring opportunities to improve access to primary care in rural and inner city areas; that efforts to encourage that possibility are called for; and that the successes and failures of such efforts should be thoroughly understood.

Impediments to the Use of Nurse Practitioners and Physician Assistants

"Scope of practice" laws, established by the states, govern what NPs and

PAs are permitted to do. Collectively, these laws constitute a crazy quilt of permitted or disallowed practices and activities. Thus, the legal restrictions on the scope of practice for NPs and PAs in some states seriously impede the involvement of these types of personnel in primary care in some settings and circumstances.

This fact has a number of health care policy and delivery implications. For example, for managed care enterprises that operate in more than one state, the configurations they can use to organize their primary care teams may be different, depending on the state in question. It is not clear to this committee why different structures for the delivery of high-quality primary care ought to turn on what may be quite idiosyncratic or outmoded state practice acts.

Recommendation 6.4 State Practice Acts for Nurse Practitioners and Physician Assistants

The committee recommends that state governments review current restrictions on the scope of practice of primary care nurse practitioners and physician assistants and eliminate or modify those restrictions that impede collaborative practice and reduce access to quality primary care.

The committee is concerned that state statutes presently on the books create obstacles to innovative collaboration among members of primary care teams and that those ordinances by default hinder the provision of effective and efficient health care. These limitations may involve the degree and nature of supervision (such as the requirement in some states for *on-site* supervision of PAs), the ability to prescribe pharmaceuticals, or the ability to order other services needed by the patient without a physician's case-by-case approval.

A recent analysis of the practicing environment in 10 states for NPs and PAs assigned weighted scores regarding scope of practice, requirements for physician supervision, prescriptive and dispensing authority, reimbursement, and so forth. It found total average scores of 63.9 in these 10 states with scores ranging from 0 in Illinois and Ohio where NPs are not recognized at all, to scores over 90 in Maryland, Montana, New Hampshire, and Oregon. Similarly, PAs scores in the same states averaged 60.5 with a range from 0 in Mississippi to over 90 in Iowa, Massachusetts, and Montana (RTI, 1995).

The committee believes that more freedom to structure the divisions of duties and responsibilities should be given to the primary care team. Clearly, reconsideration by the states of these practice acts might also enable some to address their shortage-area problems (discussed earlier) more creatively as well, in part by enabling managed care organizations and integrated delivery systems to develop efficient models of primary care practice that work within their own corporate structures and yet are adaptable to the particular needs of specific frontier, rural, or inner city populations.

SUMMARY

This chapter has reviewed trends in the supply of the principal types of primary care clinicians—physicians, NPs, and PAs—taking care to observe the great difficulties of developing reliable and valid estimates of supply and, especially, requirements for clinicians or clinicians' services. It also briefly comments on the education and training infrastructure for such personnel, which leads into the next chapter. The present chapter then advances four recommendations concerning important directions that, in the committee's view, the production and use of primary care clinicians ought to take. These involve (1) continuing the current level of effort to increase the supply of primary care clinicians but ensuring that primary care training programs and delivery systems focus their efforts on improving the competency of primary care clinicians and on increasing access for populations not now receiving adequate primary care; (2) encouraging state and federal agencies to carefully monitor the supply of and requirements for primary care clinicians; and (3) exploring ways in which managed care and integrated health care systems might be used to alleviate the geographic maldistribution of primary care clinicians; and (4) examining how state practice acts for NPs and PAs might be amended to eliminate outmoded restrictions on practices that currently impede efficient and effective functioning of primary care teams and that reduce access to needed health care.

REFERENCES

AAPA (American Academy of Physician Assistants). 1995 AAPA Membership Census Mid-Year Report, September 1995. Alexandria, Va.: AAPA, 1995.

AACN (American Association of Colleges of Nursing). 1994–1995. *Special Report on: Master's and Post-Master's Nurse Practitioner Programs, Faculty Clinical Practice, Faculty Age Profiles, and Undergraduate Curriculum Expansion In Baccalaureate and Graduate Programs in Nursing.* Publ. No. 94-95-4. Washington, D.C.: AACN, 1995.

AMA (American Medical Association). Physician Characteristics and Distribution in the US. 1995/1996 Edition. Chicago: AMA, 1996.

Barzansky, B., Jonas, H.S., and Etzel, S.I. Educational Programs in U.S. Medical Schools, 1994–95. *Journal of the American Medical Association* 274:716–722, 1995.

Birkholz, G., and Walker, D. Strategies for State Statutory Language Changes Granting Fully Independent Nurse Practitioner Practice. *Nurse Practitioner* 19:54–58, 1994.

BPHC (Bureau of Primary Health Care, Health Resources and Services Administration, Department of Health and Human Services). Health Professional Shortage Area (HPSA) Designations: 1978–1994. Unpublished material from the Division of Shortage Designation, March, 1995.

CCH (Commerce Clearing House). Health Security Act (President Clinton's Health Care Reform Proposal and Health Security Act). Presented to Congress on October 27, 1993. Chicago, Ill.: Commerce Clearing House, 1993.

COGME (Council on Graduate Medical Education). *Recommendations to Improve Access to Health Care Through Physician Workforce Reform.* Fourth report to Congress and the Department of Health and Human Services Secretary. Rockville, Md.: Health Resources and Services Administration, Department of Health and Human Services, January 1994.

COGME. *COGME 1995 Physician Workforce Funding Recommendations for Department of Health and Human Services' Programs.* Seventh report to Congress and the Department of Health and Human Services. Rockville, Md.: Health Resources and Services Administration, Department of Health and Human Services, June 1995.

COGME. *Eighth Report. Patient Care Physician Supply and Requirements: Testing COGME Recommendations.* Rockville, Md.: Health Resources and Services Administration, Department of Health and Human Services, 1996.

Cooper, R.A. Special Communication. Perspectives on the Physician Workforce to the Year 2020. *Journal of the American Medical Association* 274:1534–1543, 1995.

Davis, K., Collins, K.S., Schoen, C., et al. Choice Matters: Enrollees' Views of Their Health Plans. *Health Affairs* 14:99–112, Summer 1995.

Desmarias, H.R. Community Service in U.S. Medical Training and Practice: An Overview. In *Social and Community Service in Medical Training and Professional Practice.* Proceedings of a Conference. G. Herrerra, ed., assisted by G. Carrino and L.G. Herrera. New York: Josiah Macy, Jr. Foundation, 1995.

DHEW (Department of Health, Education and Welfare). *Health United States 1976–1977.* DHEW Publ. No. (HRA) 77-1232. Hyattsville, Md.: Department of Health, Education and Welfare, Health Resources Administration, 1977.

DHHS (Department of Health and Human Services). *Factbook. Health Personnel, United States. March 1993.* DHHS Publ. No. HRSA-P-AM-93-1. Washington, D.C.: Department of Health and Human Services, 1993.

Feil, E.C., Welch, H.G., and Fisher, E.S. Why Estimates of Physician Supply and Requirements Disagree. *Journal of the American Medical Association* 269:2659–2663, 1993.

Gamliel, S., Politzer, R.M., Rivo, M.L., et al. Managed Care on the March: Will Physicians Meet the Challenge? *Health Affairs* 14:131–142, Summer 1995.

GMENAC (Graduate Medical Education National Advisory Committee). *Summary Report to the Secretary, Department of Health and Human Services.* Vol. 1. DHHS Publ. No. (HRA) 81-651. Washington, D.C.: Health Resources Administration, Department of Health and Human Services, April 1981.

Henderson, T., and Chovan, T. *Removing Practice Barriers of Nonphysician Providers: Efforts by States to Improve Access to Primary Care.* Washington, D.C.: Intergovernmental Health Policy Project, The George Washington University, 1994.

IOM (Institute of Medicine). *A Manpower Policy for Primary Health Care: Report of a Study.* Washington, D.C.: National Academy Press, 1978.

IOM. *Assessing Health Care Reform.* M.J. Field, K.N. Lohr, and K.D. Yordy, eds. Washington, D.C.:National Academy Press, 1993.

IOM. *Balancing the Scales of Opportunity: Ensuring Racial and Ethnic Diversity in the Health Professions.* M. E. Lewin and B. Rice, eds. Washington, D.C.: National Academy Press, 1994.

IOM. *Dental Education at the Crossroads: Challenge and Change.* M.J. Field, ed. Washington, D.C.: National Academy Press, 1995a.

IOM. *Health Services Research: Work Force and Educational Issues.* M.J. Field, R.E. Tranquada, and J.C. Feasley, eds. Washington, D.C.: National Academy Press, 1995b.

IOM. *Nursing, Health, and the Environment: Strengthening the Relationship to Improve the Public's Health.* A.M. Pope, M.A. Snyder, and L.H. Mood, eds. Washington, D.C.: National Academy Press, 1995c.

IOM. *The Nation's Physician Workforce: Options for Balancing Supply and Requirements.* K.N. Lohr, N.A. Vanselow, and D.E. Detmer, eds. Washington, D.C.: National Academy Press, 1996a.

IOM. *Nursing Staff in Hospitals and Nursing Homes: Is It Adequate?* G.S. Wunderlich, F. Sloan, and C.K. Davis, eds. Washington, D.C.: National Academy Press, 1996b.

JAMA (*Journal of the American Medical Association*). Appendix II. Graduate Medical Education. Appendix II, Table 1. Resident Physicians on Duty in ACGME-Accredited and in Combined Specialty Graduate Medical Education (GME) Programs in 1993. *Journal of the American Medical Association* 272:725–726, 1994.

Jonas, H.S., Etzel, S.I., and Barzansky, B. Educational Programs in U.S. Medical Schools, 1993–1994. *Journal of the American Medical Association* 272:694–701, 1994.

Jones, P.E., and Cawley, J.F. Physician Assistants and Health System Reform: Clinical Capabilities, Practice Activities and Potential Roles. *Journal of the American Medical Association* 271:1266–1272, 1994.

Kindig, C.A. Counting Generalist Physicians. *Journal of the American Medical Association* 271:1505–1507, 1994.

Kindig, D.A., Cultice, J.M., and Mullan, F. The Elusive Generalist Physician. Can We Reach a 50% Goal? *Journal of the American Medical Association* 270:1069–1073, 1993.

Lee, R.C. Current Approaches to Shortage Area Designation. *Journal of Rural Health* 7(4 Supl.): 437–450, 1991.

Morgan, W.A. Using State Board of Nursing Data to Estimate the Number of Nurse Practitioners in the United States. *Nurse Practitioner* 18:65–66, 69–70, and 73–74, 1993.

Moses, E. *The Registered Nurse Population: Findings from the National Sample Survey of Registered Nurses, 1992.* Division of Nursing, Health Resources and Services Administration, Public Health Service. Washington, D.C.: U.S. Government Printing Office, 1994.

Mullan, F. The National Health Service Corps: Service Conditional Medical Education in the United States. In: *Social and Community Service in Medical Training and Professional Practice.* Proceedings of a Conference. G. Herrera, ed., assisted by G. Carrino and L.G. Herrera. New York: The Josiah Macy, Jr., Foundation, 1995.

NCHS (National Center for Health Statistics). *Health, United States, and Prevention Profile, 1983.* DHHS Publ. No. (PHS) 84-1232. Washington, D.C.: U.S. Government Printing Office, December 1983.

Newhouse, J.P., Williams, A.P., Bennett, B.W., and Schwartz, W.B. Where Have All the Doctors Gone? *Journal of the American Medical Association* 247:2392–2396, 1982a.

Newhouse, J.P., Williams, A.P., Schwartz, W.B., and Bennett, B.W. *The Geographic Distribution of Physicians: Is the Conventional Wisdom Correct?* Publ. No. R-2734-HJK/HHS/RWJ/RC. Santa Monica, Calif.: RAND Corporation, 1982b.

NLN (National League of Nursing). Nursing Datasource 1994. Volume 1, Graduate Education in Nursing. Advanced Practice Nursing Pub. No. 19-2643. New York: NLN Press, 1994.

NRC (National Research Council). *Meeting the Nation's Needs for Biomedical and Behavioral Scientists.* Washington, D.C.: National Academy Press, 1994.

Pearson, L. Annual Update of How Each State Stands on Legislative Issues Affecting Advanced Nursing Practice. *Nurse Practitioner* 19:11–53, 1994.

Pew Health Professions Commission. *Critical Challenges: Revitalizing the Health Professions for the Twenty-First Century.* San Francisco: Pew Health Professions Commission, 1995.

PPRC (Physician Payment Review Commission). *Annual Report to Congress, 1992.* Washington, D.C.: PPRC, 1992.

PPRC. *Annual Report to Congress, 1994.* Washington, D.C.: PPRC, 1994.

PPRC. The Changing Labor Market for Physicians. Chapter 14 in *Annual Report to Congress, 1995.* Washington, D.C.: PPRC, 1995.

ProPAC (Prospective Payment Assessment Commission). *Report and Recommendations to Congress, March 1, 1995.* Washington, D.C.: ProPAC, 1995.

Rivo, M.L., and Satcher, D. Improving Access to Health Care Through Physician Workforce Reform. Directions for the 21st Century. *Journal of the American Medical Assocation* 270:1074–1078, 1993.

RTI (Research Triangle Institute). Characteristics of Practice Environments for Nurse Practitioners and for Physician Assistants. Final Report Deliverable Item 13. Research Triangle Park, N.C.: RTI, July 7, 1995.

Scheffler, R.M., and Gillings, D.B. Survey Approach to Estimating Demand for Physician Assistants. *Social Science and Medicine* 16:1039–1047, 1982.

Schwartz, W.B., Newhouse, J.P., Bennett, B.W., et al. The Changing Geographic Distribution of Board-Certified Physicians. *New England Journal of Medicine* 303:1032–1038, 1980.

Singer, A.M. *1994 Annual Statistical Report.* Rockville, Md.: American Association of Colleges of Osteopathic Medicine, 1994.

Tarlov, A.R. Estimating Physician Workforce Requirements. The Devil Is in the Assumptions. *Journal of the American Medical Association* 274:1558–1559, 1995.

Washington Consulting Group. *Survey of Certified Nurse Practitioners and Clinical Nurse Specialists: December 1992 Final Report to the Bureau of Health Professions.* Washington, D.C.: U.S. Government Printing Office, 1994.

Weiner, J.P. Assessing the Impact of Managed Care on the U.S. Physician Workforce. Policy paper commissioned by the Bureau of Health Professions of the U.S. Department of Health and Human Services on behalf of the Council on Graduate Medical Education. Supported by HRSA P.O. No. 03-339-P. Baltimore, Md.: Weiner, Johns Hopkins University School of Hygiene and Public Health, November, 1993.

Weiner, J.P. Forecasting the Effects of Health Reform on U.S. Physician Workforce Requirement: Evidence from HMO Staffing Patterns. *Journal of the American Medical Association* 272:222–230, 1994.

Whitcomb, M.E. The Role of Medical Schools in Graduate Medical Education. *Journal of the American Medical Association* 272:702–704, 1994.

Williams, A.P., Schwartz, W.B., Newhouse, J.P., and Bennett, B.W. How Many Miles to the Doctor? *New England Journal of Medicine* 309:958–963, 1981.

7

Education and Training for Primary Care

If primary care is to move in the direction advocated by this committee, many aspects of education and training of primary care clinicians must be restructured. The committee has already drawn attention to the wide range of responsibilities that primary care clinicians might have, the equally broad array of settings in which they might practice, and the need for a team approach to the delivery of primary care. Various other issues, more widely examined in the arena of health professions education, also impinge on primary care and have implications for the recommendations this committee is making.

Considerable attention has been focused on these important issues. Christakis (1995) reviewed reform proposals for undergraduate medical education in 19 major reports issued from 1910. He found consistent themes in these reports, including the need to increase generalist training and exposure of students to ambulatory care. In recent years, many statements regarding the content and financing of graduate medical education and primary care education of other health professionals have been issued. Moreover, targeted grants from The Robert Wood Johnson Foundation, The Pew Charitable Trusts, and The W.K. Kellogg Foundation have addressed the changes in academic infrastructure, curricula, and financing that must be implemented to respond successfully to a mandate to increase the availability of well-trained primary care clinicians. Most recently, The Robert Wood Johnson Foundation has funded Generalist Initiative grants to medical schools with a goal of promoting primary care and interesting medical students in generalist training.

To this rich mix the present IOM committee adds its particular perspective, which relates more explicitly to primary care. Specifically, this chapter addresses essential changes that need to be made in undergraduate and graduate health professional training and the need for clinical training to include multidisciplinary team practice; attention is directed to the three types of primary care clinicians—physicians, nurse practitioners, and physician assistants—focused on in Chapter 6. The need to identify common core competencies across these professions is an important ramification of the discussion. The chapter also explores retraining of physicians for primary care. Finally, it offers nine recommendations by which the committee's vision of primary care might be brought closer to reality through appropriate changes in education and training of health care personnel.

APPROPRIATE TRAINING IN PRIMARY CARE

The scope of primary health care services is broad and often complex. Both the content and the challenges of primary care demand a considerable period of education. The committee believes that all newly trained primary care clinicians must have adequate and discipline-appropriate training—that is, specific training in primary care appropriate to their expected roles. For physicians (many of whom will ultimately provide the gamut of primary care services), this means a residency with emphasis on primary care followed by certification by an appropriate specialty board. For the nurse practitioner, it means graduate education and national credentialing. For the physician assistant, it means graduation from an accredited physician assistant program and certification by the National Commission on Certification of Physician Assistants.

THE EDUCATION OF PHYSICIANS

In considering the education of a physician, this committee concluded that attention ought to be directed at both undergraduate and graduate training, because it believes that new efforts to produce a primary care doctor will be far less productive if instituted only at the graduate level. Thus, this section examines issues for both medical students and residents, noting in particular that models of practice to which physicians-to-be and newly graduated physicians are exposed play a critical role in long-term career directions (Stimmel, 1992; GAO, 1994; Martini et al., 1994; Kassebaum and Haynes, 1992).

Undergraduate Medical Education

Experience in Primary Care Settings

The challenges of revamping the undergraduate medical curriculum should not be underestimated, and this committee was not empaneled to explore such issues in depth. One aspect of primary care is especially important in this context, however, and the committee spent considerable time debating it. Specifically, a true appreciation of a patient's family and community context—a tenet of this committee's definition of primary care—requires that students gain experience in practices and sites that are primary care based.

This does not now happen to nearly the extent the committee sees as desirable. The reasons are varied. Financing issues have been a major impediment to undergraduate education in ambulatory settings. Training costs are increased, and the logistics can be complex; finding ways to offset such costs has been difficult. Other objections to ambulatory training have been raised as well (Petersdorf and Turner, 1995). Some faculty, for example, believe that inpatient education with its intense exposure to acute disease provides better education and can be transferred to the ambulatory setting more readily than vice versa. Others are concerned that, during office visits, patients may not be willing to devote the extra time that might be required to accommodate undergraduate teaching and that, similarly, community-based physicians may be unwilling to have their patient schedules disrupted by student involvement.

The committee did not find these arguments about the problems of conducting some undergraduate medical education in outpatient or primary care settings persuasive. Calls for greater emphasis on out-of-hospital primary care training in both undergraduate and graduate medical training are not new; they have been raised with increasing frequency in the last several decades (Alpert and Charney, 1973; IOM, 1983). As discussed below, therefore, the committee concluded that the benefits of such training can and do outweigh the drawbacks and that concrete steps therefore need to be taken to provide all future medical students with such exposure. For this reason, it recommends the following:

Recommendation 7.1 Training in Primary Care Sites

All medical schools should require their undergraduate medical students to experience training in settings that deliver primary care as defined by this committee.

The committee concluded that useful, indeed crucial, educational experiences can take place in doctors' offices, community health centers, and other out-of-hospital community sites. It also judged that such exposure to primary care settings and practices should be relatively intense; that is, an occasional short rotation in several sites is unlikely to provide an adequate experience.

References in this chapter to *ambulatory* in regard to student and resident training should be understood as ambulatory care in primary care settings. The committee strongly cautions against the view that a "rotation in an ambulatory setting" is equivalent to experience with primary care. Substituting ambulatory for inpatient service at either the undergraduate or graduate level will not necessarily yield *primary care* experience to trainees, because much of ambulatory care is not primary care. For example, many procedures that were once performed in an inpatient setting are now done in offices or ambulatory surgery facilities—including subspecialty procedures in ophthalmology, gastroenterology, neurology, and others.

In the committee's view, undergraduate medical education in sites like those in which doctors are expected to practice in the future has several benefits. First, it will expand their knowledge of the goals and processes of primary care, improve the skills required in primary care, and raise students' sensitivity toward core elements of primary care, such as prevention. Second, it may affect the choices that students make about their careers, especially if they encounter, in those sites, role models who are competent and enthusiastic about their work (Osborn, 1993; Martini et al., 1994). Third, past resistance of residents in graduate medical training to off-campus or out-of-hospital clinical rotations is understandable, to some extent, given the absence of any earlier undergraduate experience in community-based, ambulatory settings. Providing such training at the undergraduate level might go far toward reducing such resistance.

Curricular and Other Structural Reforms

Curricula and clerkships. Medical schools of course have a certain degree of latitude to determine what their students must know and be able to do when they graduate, and the committee was heartened by information demonstrating that many schools are responding to the challenge of devising innovative undergraduate programs. In 1992, the Association of American Medical Colleges (AAMC) appointed a Generalist Physician Task Force to develop a policy statement for the association and to recommend actions to help reverse the trend away from generalism. The task force report recommended that, as an overall national goal, a majority of graduating medical students be committed to generalist careers and that appropriate efforts be made by all schools to reach this goal quickly (AAMC, 1992).

The AAMC task force found that medical schools are adding courses with a primary care focus during the first two (preclinical) years and are offering or requiring clerkships in one of the generalist disciplines during the third or fourth years, including clerkships that emphasize experience in primary care settings. At some medical schools, even first-year medical students can apply for primary care clerkships, where they can observe generalist physicians in hospital clinics and doctors' offices. At other medical schools, first-year medical students take required longitudinal primary care clinical care experiences during which they observe generalist physicians in their own office practices. Several schools teach beginning physical diagnosis to their first-year students and supervise patient care interactions such as interviewing and simple clinical examinations.

Many schools now include primary care or ambulatory experiences as part of their basic clerkships.[1] Gradually more of the core clerkships in family practice,

---

[1]A clerkship is a block of educational time that a medical student spends in a particular clinical setting or defined area of medicine.

internal medicine, and pediatrics are being conducted in physicians' offices, community health centers, and group practices. Specialty societies such as the American Academy of Family Practice and the American Society of Internal Medicine (ASIM) actively support such activities with advice, curricula, and evaluation tools. Efforts to encourage states to fund placement of students with practicing preceptors are also under way, with Texas already having passed legislation to fund such programs.

According to a later AAMC report (1994), responses to the 1993 Medical School Graduation Questionnaire found that 36 percent of third-year students and 49 percent of fourth-year students had a primary care clerkship, and 57 percent of these third- and fourth-year respondents had taken the clerkship as a required course.

The AAMC task force also found that curricula are being modified to emphasize the evaluative sciences that are associated with primary care, such as epidemiology and evidence-based medicine. This point is especially relevant with respect to the research agenda issues discussed more fully in Chapter 8. Furthermore, schools are developing programs to provide experience in a number of other fields thought important for a fully rounded primary care education. For example, Dartmouth Medical School requires its students to teach preventive medicine in nearby public schools. Medical students are also matched with needy families whom they advise on health care and social services (*New York Times*, 1992).

These are illustrative examples only, and a broader set of examples of office-based clerkships is provided in a "mentorship kit" developed by the ASIM (ASIM, 1995). This kit encourages local efforts (in part because ASIM is dubious about whether federal funding for such programs will be forthcoming), and it offers practical advice for implementing and evaluating community-based internal medicine teaching for students. Collectively, these examples demonstrate that medical schools across the country can act on, and indeed already are acting on, the above recommendation (Recommendation 7.1) in creative and productive ways. In so doing, schools can also lay the groundwork for acceptance of greater out-of-hospital training during residency years, as discussed more fully below.

Competencies and clerkships. Medical schools and various health policy groups have also begun to consider the competencies that should be required of all graduating medical students. As a case in point, The Pew Health Professions Commission (1994) identified seven capabilities that it believes will be essential for *all* future practitioners, clearly including primary care:

1. Care for the community's health.
2. Provide contemporary clinical care.
3. Participate in the emerging system (including new health care settings and interdisciplinary team arrangements) and accommodate expanded accountability.

4. Ensure cost-effective and appropriate care.
5. Practice prevention and promote healthy lifestyles.
6. Involve patients and families in the decisionmaking process.
7. Manage information and continue to learn.

With increasing interest in the third-year clerkship in primary care, the latest addition to efforts to define appropriate curricula for medical students has been developed by Goroll and Morrison with support from BHP/HRSA (Bureau of the Health Professions of the Health Resources and Services Administration) and approved by the Society of General Internal Medicine (SGIM) and the Clerkship Directors in Internal Medicine (CDIM) (SGIM/CDIM, 1995). This model curriculum for the third-year medicine clerkship is based on a national survey of internal medicine faculty. It emphasizes the importance of training students in basic generalist competencies and shifting a greater portion of their educational experiences from the inpatient to the primary care setting.

As described in their materials, the model curriculum divides the competencies into three categories[2] that should be taught to third-year students:

• Category one competencies (taught in all cases when appropriate): diagnostic decisionmaking; case presentation; history and physical examination; communication and relationships with patients and colleagues; test interpretation; therapeutic decisionmaking; bioethics of care; self-directed learning; and prevention.
• Category two competencies (taught in some but not all cases): coordination of care and teamwork; basic procedures; geriatric care; community health care; and nutrition.
• Category three competencies (taught occasionally): advanced procedures; occupational and environmental health care.

For each competency, a set of corresponding learning objectives, divided into knowledge, skills, and attitudes, has been devised to help guide the learning agenda.

Faculty. Other changes proposed by the AAMC have included raising the prominence of generalist physicians in teaching and medical school administrative positions. Some medical schools have responded by appointing faculty from the generalist disciplines to serve on important administrative committees. For ex-

---

[2]Categories are derived from a survey of faculty to identify and prioritize basic generalist competencies. Respondents used a five-point scale (1 = low, 5 = high) to rank competencies. Category one corresponds to a mean ranking above 3.38; Category two to 2.72—3.38; Category three to 2.09–2.71. Mean rankings below 2.09 were ranked Category four.

ample, in 1990, one medical school had an associate dean for primary care; five years later, eight schools had created such a position, and many more had added special advisers to the dean on primary care (Fein, 1995).

Examinations. The National Board of Medical Examiners (NBME) administers the United States Medical Licensing Examination (USMLE), which was first administered in 1992. Taken by medical students at the end of their undergraduate years, it has also begun to move in a direction that supports greater emphasis on education and training for primary care. In testimony submitted to the committee, the NBME acknowledged that several areas of primary care practice had been underemphasized in its licensure examination—namely, ambulatory care, chronic care, care of the elderly, and preventive care. Acting on its belief that these areas are critically important, it has revamped the examination and placed a priority on generalist knowledge and skills (NBME testimony to the IOM Committee on the Future of Primary Care, 1994).

Remaining issues. Despite these encouraging examples, the dominant model continues to be education in the inpatient services of teaching hospitals, and such training can be expected to have a lasting influence. When medical students begin their third- and fourth-year clinical rotations in the hospital, the role models tend overwhelmingly to be those in the increasingly acute, inpatient setting with high-technology interventions (GAO, 1994). Thus, the committee believes that Recommendation 7.1, above, must be acted on more forcefully at the medical school level as a counter to these long-standing traditional dynamics.

The committee has discussed the system of undergraduate medical education as a whole, perhaps leaving the impression that medical schools are essentially the same institutions across the nation. This is clearly not the case, however. Different medical schools have quite different missions: Some focus more on research and the production of specialists, others focus more on education and the production of primary care clinicians. Moreover, the effect of the structure of universities within which medical schools function and of the history within each institution of its departmental affiliations can be substantial (a point noted in another recent IOM report [IOM, 1995] on dental education). The committee was not ignorant of these factors, but it judged that exploring them would exceed both its charge and its resources. The basic conclusion is that efforts to overcome some of the problems of changing the mission and the curriculum of medical schools will need to take issues of the larger university organization and aim thoroughly into account.

Graduate Medical Education

Graduate medical education (GME) provides the opportunity to train physicians for a field of practice and to prepare them for independent practice and certification. The medical school graduate is an undifferentiated physician who is not capable of independent practice and who must take at least one year of residency training to be eligible for licensure. For practical purposes a physician will require residency training leading to certification to establish his or her place as an appropriately and completely trained physician. Thus, GME becomes as essential for the production of a physician as medical school and is the time when differentiation occurs.

Unlike medical schools, which have relatively broad discretion about teaching curricula, graduate programs in primary care (i.e., residencies) are much more closely defined by the residency review committees (RRCs) of each primary care discipline and by the Accreditation Committee on Graduate Medical Education (ACGME). RRCs approve residency programs, which must comply with their requirements. The specialty boards that examine graduates of residency programs for board certification also influence the curricula by determining what is included—and emphasized—on examinations. In short, regardless of the impact of the above-mentioned changes in medical school curricula, how residency programs are structured will remain a dominant factor in creating a cadre of primary care physicians with the characteristics thought to be significant by this committee.

Residency Programs in Family Practice, Internal Medicine and Pediatrics

Primary care has begun to attract more residents (Fein, 1995). Part of this trend is attributable to external forces, both the growth of managed care (and its greater demand for primary care clinicians) and trends in public policy. For example, several state legislatures have mandated or attempted to mandate that a given proportion, such as 50 percent, of medical school graduates go into primary care residency programs (M. Garg, University of Illinois, Chicago, personal communication, October, 1995). Nevertheless, the main physician specialty areas of primary care—family practice, internal medicine, and pediatrics—have some distance to go in creating training experiences that match the committee's vision of the capabilities that will be needed by primary care clinicians of the future, especially a future dominated by managed care organizations.

Managed care organizations made clear to the committee that the current products of family practice, internal medicine, and pediatric residencies lack key competencies required to function maximally in their systems. Based on its public hearing and site visits, the committee shares with many medical educators and the medical directors of integrated health care delivery systems concerns about traditional GME, especially about the extent to which such training is preparing tomorrow's doctors for the new ways and settings in which they will be expected to function. Graduates of residency programs often lack knowledge of population-based health promotion and disease prevention, evidence-based clinical decisionmaking, and patient interviewing skills (particularly communication and consultation skills). Many are not taught how to function as a member of a team and have little knowledge of information systems or time and resource management.

Internal medicine and pediatrics merit special attention, in the committee's view, because tertiary care and specialty care still constitute too much of the training in their programs; internal medicine residents may lack experience in ambulatory clinical specialty areas such as dermatology, ophthalmology, office gynecology, behavioral health care, behavioral medicine, and preventive medicine (Kantor and Griner, 1981; Kern et al., 1985; Linn et al., 1986; McPhee et al., 1987). Other commonly cited deficiencies are training in clinical nutrition, occupational medicine, working with other primary care clinicians (e.g., nurse practitioners, physician assistants), use of community services, resource management, and setting up an office practice (Barker, 1990).

Primary Care Tracks

Family practice residency programs are unambiguously committed to preparation for primary care practice, whereas internal medicine and pediatric residencies have competing interests in training for referral practice. In the late 1970s, however, residency programs in primary care internal medicine and general pediatrics were established to train more general internists and pediatricians.

Primary care tracks provide more office-based training in gynecology, dermatology, orthopedics, otolaryngology, ophthalmology, psychiatry, and preventive and occupational medicine than traditional programs, and they offer much greater continuity experience. Residents in internal medicine primary care tracks spend considerable time in ambulatory settings, serving as the principal physician for their patients. Less emphasis is placed on hospital-based and subspecialty training; more attention is directed to ambulatory specialties, medical interviewing, and clinical epidemiology (Lipkin et al., 1990). In general these curricula are closer to what the committee is advocating, but they are still small in number and remain the exception rather than the rule.

OTHER CONTENT ISSUES IN TRAINING FOR PRIMARY CARE

Academic health centers educate and train all types of primary care clinicians (physicians, physician assistants, and nurses practitioners) as well as many other health professionals. Their role is evolving, however, as health care restructuring moves rapidly ahead, and their responsibilities with respect to creating innovative education and training programs will likely be more complex in the future than today. One particular challenge will be to identify, in concert with professional and other groups, common core competencies for primary care, so that tomorrow's training efforts will reflect the committee's vision of primary care and primary care teams.

Future Steps for Academic Health Centers

The above-mentioned trends toward reform of undergraduate curricula, changes in graduate training, and more physicians opting for primary care training are encouraging, but they do not tell the entire story. Traditional curricula, training sites, and distinguished role models can all have a powerful reinforcing influence once residents begin their training. Unless primary care faculties are in prestigious administrative and departmental positions (e.g., deans and department chairs), and unless medical students and residents encounter enthusiastic role models, mentors, and teaching methods that support prerequisite skills described in this report, market-driven changes are likely to be short-lived and may eventually give rise to dissatisfied and demoralized physicians who resent not being able to practice medicine as they choose or were trained.

The required changes are complex. Academic health centers must undertake fundamental alterations in their missions, administrative structures, practice environments, and curricula. The logistical difficulties are formidable; for example, emphasizing nonhospital settings is costly under current reimbursement policies. Moreover, they come at a time when academic health centers are struggling to change quickly enough to survive in competitive markets, and these pressures do not foster long-term planning strategies.

The committee believes that the survival of academic health centers depends on their adoption of primary care teaching and service as a central mission, while continuing and maintaining their roles in providing extraordinarily complex patient care and pursuing biomedical research that has justly earned an international reputation. Further, society needs to support these changes by providing funds for primary care just as it has supported the traditional teaching and research missions of the academic health center. In short, academic health centers will have to change to reflect the practice environment in which its graduates will practice; but society, if it is to enjoy the health care system and practitioners it evidently wants, will need to provide the policy and financial support without which academic health centers will not be able to move forward.[3]

Common Core Competencies

Defining core competencies is a requisite for every field in health care. Credentialing of health practitioners—whether by hospitals or managed care organizations—depends on defined competencies. For primary care to prosper, these competencies must be sufficiently well defined for patients, residents, fac-

---

[3]A recent IOM report on aggregate physician supply also drew attention to the potentially precarious state of academic health centers (IOM, 1996), especially if changes in Medicare GME reimbursement bring fewer revenues at the same that their health care service obligations remain steady or increase.

ulty, managed care organizations, other health practitioners, and physicians seeking retraining to understand clearly what is expected of the professional who provides primary care.

Confusion arises over what it means to be a primary care clinician when members of diverse disciplines and specialties (within medicine as well as outside it) declare that they are practicing primary care. Not everyone who declares that he or she is practicing primary care is, in fact, doing so. Despite efforts to define competencies within each discipline and specialty (as illustrated above), no common, cross-discipline competencies have yet been defined and agreed on, either within medicine or across all primary care clinical fields. The remainder of this section reviews efforts by medicine or other health care professions to articulate sets of capabilities or proficiencies for generalist practice.

Defining Core Competencies in Medicine

Medical training programs have remained separate for historical and understandable reasons. Those reasons and the values they represent—clear and justifiable as they may be to those within the medical establishment—are murky to those outside it. The idea of core competencies, however, is reminiscent of the first-year rotating internship that, at one time and in some states, was required for licensure. The committee does not think that GME ought to return to those days. It holds, rather, that in the long term GME programs in primary care would do better to be based on a core set of competencies for all primary care residents and that such core training ought to be augmented by a series of specialty modules (e.g., in the care of the elderly, of children, or of persons in rural areas).

At its most general, training in primary care should equip the clinician to practice competently in a number of areas; for example, for physicians the following competencies would be important:

- periodic assessment of the asymptomatic person,
- screening for early disease detection,
- evaluation and management of acute illness,
- assessment and either management or referral of patients with more complex problems needing the diagnostic and therapeutic tools of the medical specialist and other professionals,
- ongoing management of patients with established chronic diseases,
- coordination of care among specialists, and
- provision of acute hospital care and long-term care.

What specific competencies would enable primary care physicians to fulfill these roles? For half a century or more, the various primary care disciplines have been engaged in defining core competencies within their own fields. For example, in internal medicine, the Federated Council of Internal Medicine Curriculum Task Force (FCIMCTF) has developed a list of learning experiences that would lead to needed competencies in general internal medicine (FCIMCTF, 1996, forthcoming). Another case in point is the American College of Obstetricians and Gynecologists, which has developed program requirements for training residents in obstetrics-gynecology (OB-GYN) (ACOG, 1995). These requirements, which have been approved by the ACGME, include experiences in some areas that reflect a primary care orientation: patient education and counseling, screening appropriate to patients of various ages, management of the health care of patients in a continuous manner, appropriate use of community resources, awareness and knowledge of the behavioral and societal factors that influence health among women, and behavioral medicine and psychosocial problems.

The American Academy of Family Physicians (AAFP) put forward a comprehensive competency-based curriculum for family practice training (Family Health Foundation of America, 1983). The curriculum includes three sets of skills: general skills, systems, and skills needed for care of special problems and populations. General skills include: interaction and involvement with patients and families; the family; health promotion and disease prevention; nutrition; community involvement and public health; patient education; research skills; practice management; medico-legal problems; personal and professional issues; ethical decisions; general laboratory knowledge and medical imaging; and anesthesia. System skills are organized by body system—cardiovascular, musculoskeletal, and so forth. The third set of skills is titled "Special Problems and Special Populations." This set includes pregnancy, childbirth, and the puerperium; the developing child; the elderly; environmental and occupational problems; accidents, poisonings, violence, and emergencies; behavioral and psychological patterns; and recreational and athletic health care. The curriculum was intended to be open-ended and flexible to accommodate changing knowledge and regional differences. Currently a task force of the Society of Teachers of Family Medicine (STFM) is in the process of updating this curriculum (Roger Sherwood, STFM, personal communication, November 1995).

Various joint residencies and activities by specialty boards also reflect concerns about common core competencies, typically involving internal medicine with either pediatrics or family practice (*JAMA*, 1994). A joint statement of the American Board of Internal Medicine and the American Board of Family Practice identified the following essential features of generalist physicians (Kimball and Young, 1994, p. 315):

> Generalist physicians must be highly skilled in using appropriate medical consultation and referral to other specialists and community resources when necessary . . . and must aggressively encourage health promotion and disease prevention and be knowledgeable about the efficient use of resources, behavioral medicine, the information sciences, and the principles of population medicine.

One broad effort reflected a review of residency curricula for family practice, general internal medicine, pediatrics, emergency medicine, and OB-GYN (Rivo et al., 1994). The authors identified 7 categories and 60 key components that primary care clinicians should have. The seven categories were (1) care of the population; (2) care of patients in multiple settings; (3) comprehensive preventive care; (4) treatment of common acute illnesses; (5) ongoing treatment of common chronic conditions; (6) ongoing treatment of common behavioral problems; and (7) other special topics for generalist practice. The authors urged that residency programs require use of these categories and components as the framework for determining resident training.

Barker (1990) offered six "proficiencies" and suggested a residency timetable for achieving the tasks related to each proficiency. Similarly, Lipkin et al. (1984), noting the clinical importance of patient-physician interaction, described a core curriculum for teaching medical interviewing.

Though little collective progress has been made regarding formal approval of a *common* core set of competencies for a generalist curriculum, one thorough analysis of the educational content of curricula developed for pediatrics, family medicine, and general internal medicine residencies identified 15 educational components shared by the three disciplines (Noble et al., 1994):

- Biomedical content: a well-integrated knowledge of biomedical sciences encompassing all the major organ systems and health problems encountered in primary care practice and principles of therapeutics fitted to the requirements of the generalist;
- Special skills: clinical and procedural skills including history taking, physical examination, and office and emergency procedures needed in practice;
- Life cycle: an age-based curriculum taught longitudinally from family planning to care at the end of life;
- Psychosocial and medical interviewing curriculum: specific skill sets that foster the ability to identify and respond appropriately to psychosocial elements within patients and clinicians;
- Multicultural dimensions of health care: understanding international epidemiology, divergent health belief systems, alternative healers, and a range of human behaviors pertinent to health;
- End-of-life care: knowledge of palliation and maintenance of function and quality of life, including, for example, nutrition, pain control, and advance directives;
- Family-oriented care: proficiency in interviewing family members and conducting a family conference; understanding the family life cycle and its influence on health and utilization of medical care, family dynamics in illness, and collaborative care with family therapists;
- Community and population-based practice: training experience in the

community, creating networks of health care workers and services in the community, teaching prevention, and identifying health problems of the community;

• Prevention: prevention of illness, accidents, and health problems;

• Ethics: sensitivity to issues such as those surrounding birth, abortion, emancipated minors, confidentiality and disclosure of information, conflicts of interest, and the obligations of the physician to society;

• Continuous learning: ability to update medical knowledge throughout one's professional life, to appraise literature critically, and to use evidence-based medicine;

• Medical informatics: ability to use computers and information systems and understanding of biostatistics, epidemiology, and health care policy;

• Consultation: the skill set necessary to recognize professional limitations and obtain appropriate consultative assistance, including the rational choice and timing of referrals and effective interaction with colleagues;

• Advocacy: efforts to seek access to care and other needed resources for segments of the population that cannot obtain them; and

• Practice management: some knowledge of the business of practice, financial and legal management, time management, and similar topics.

Although the most comprehensive effort of its sort to date, and although it had the participation of three professional societies, the primary care disciplines have not officially adopted these competencies. These core areas were arrived at despite the differences among the three disciplines (Lipkin et al., 1990). Specifically, pediatrics is distinguished by the young age of patients and by an emphasis on prevention and developmental stages. Family practitioners care for a fuller range of ages of patients and tend to emphasize the family (and sometimes the community) as a unit (as compared to primary care internists), and they may provide obstetrical services; by contrast, internists have more in-depth training in the pathophysiology, diagnosis, and management of complex medical illnesses. Family practitioners tend to see a higher volume of patients in the office setting compared to internists, who focus more on complicated problems and older adult patients in both office and hospital settings. For both internal medicine and family practice, training in geriatrics is becoming essential.

Defining Core Competencies in Nursing

The nursing profession has also recognized the need for core competencies and the desirability of instilling these during training. Nurse training programs for advanced practice, for example, include a primary care track that has separate branches for older adults and for young people.

The National Organization of Nurse Practitioner Faculties (NONPF, 1995) has identified competencies for nurse practitioners, many of which are related to primary care. The competencies are organized into six domains: (1) managing client health or illness status; (2) maintaining the nurse-client relationship; (3) carrying out the teaching-coaching function; (4) developing the professional role; (5) managing and negotiating health care delivery systems; and (6) monitoring and ensuring the quality of health care practice.

Defining Core Competencies Across Primary Care Clinical Fields

Reaching a mutually agreed-upon set of core competencies across all primary care clinical fields—that is, physicians, nurse practitioners, and physician assistants—poses formidable obstacles. The committee supports and encourages the efforts of health professional societies, residency review committees, academic medical centers, and specialty boards to define a set of *common* core competency requirements for primary care.

Recommendation 7.2 Common Core Competencies

The committee recommends that common core competencies for primary care clinicians, regardless of their disciplinary base, be defined by a coalition of appropriate educational and professional organizations and accrediting bodies.

This committee urges the formation of a coalition of appropriate professional organizations, certifying boards, and other groups that provide perspectives about desirable competencies in primary care. Tracking the commonalities of topics and content and mapping them to the definition of primary care is an important task for such a coalition. This is probably a task first for medicine, including schools of medicine; medical residency program directors in family practice, general internal medicine, and general pediatrics; and practicing physicians.

Ideally, however, this effort should eventually include all primary care clinicians, from essentially the same constituencies as for physicians. In addition, important viewpoints will come from representatives with expertise in public health, managed care, the social sciences, and bioethics. The aims are to assist with revamping curricula, promote greater coherence of purpose, and advance understanding and collaboration among primary care clinicians.

The several efforts cited above, such as the 15 components cited by Noble and his coauthors (1994), might form the basis of the work of the coalition proposed in Recommendation 7.2.

Implementing Common Core Competencies

Defining common core competencies will not, in the end, be sufficient. Professional societies and associations, especially those involved with training primary care clinicians and certifying their capabilities at the end of training, have a major role to play as well in implementing the vision of this committee.

Recommendation 7.3 Emphasis on Common Core Competencies by Accrediting and Certifying Bodies

The committee recommends that organizations that accredit primary care training programs and certify individual trainees support curricular reforms that teach the common core competencies and essential elements of primary care.

Apart from the efforts at defining core competencies already mentioned, the committee notes other specific steps being taken by various physician groups. According to the American Board of Internal Medicine, for instance, internal medicine training is in transition to a broader, evidence- and competency-based curriculum; it will place added emphasis on specific ambulatory skills, training in geriatric and behavioral medicine, clinical epidemiology, and medical informatics. It supports generalist training with other primary care (nonphysician) professionals (ABIM testimony to the IOM Committee on the Future of Primary Care, 1994).

The joint statement of the ABIM and the ABFP already cited (Kimball and Young, 1994) praised efforts at designing interdisciplinary generalist clerkships and endorsed the reduction of institutional and interdepartmental barriers to training in coordinated care. Goals for this model include revising curricula and teaching methods and sharing educational resources as a means of conserving educational resources and improving the quality of ambulatory GME programs. These are all worthy steps that other accrediting and certifying bodies, for physicians as well as nurse practitioners and physician assistants, could adopt or adapt.

Special Areas of Curricular Emphasis

Two areas of competency are of particular interest to this committee: communication skills and cultural sensitivity.

Recommendation 7.4 Special Areas of Emphasis in Primary Care Training

The committee recommends that the curricula of all primary care education and training programs emphasize communication skills and cultural sensitivity.

The committee assumes that primary care trainees should and will learn excellent prevention, diagnostic, and management skills and the other types of core competencies described above. It wishes to emphasize, however, the two particular skills mentioned above, communication and cultural sensitivity—one more generally applicable to all patients and the other accommodating the needs of some patients.

Good communication skills are essential for primary care clinicians. These involve interviewing, communicating risks and information, answering questions, addressing the concerns of patients and their families, and helping patients make difficult decisions based on ambiguous or conflicting scientific evidence. Skills in facilitating communication—whether for patients who have hearing impairments, are illiterate, or have language or other barriers to communication—can and should be taught to primary care clinicians. Novack et al. (1992) have described a course for medical students that effectively teaches interview skills using a variety of instructional methods including simulated patients and role-playing.

Apart from straightforward communication skills are issues posed by patients with cultural backgrounds and languages that are different from those of primary care clinicians (or trainees). The ability to accommodate these patients' styles of coping with illness and their values, belief systems, and language is critical. Training could include teaching about the health beliefs, practices, and mores of specific ethnic and cultural groups that are in the patient populations to which trainees or future clinicians are likely to be accountable.

Many examples could be given: African-Americans tend to use eye contact differently from white Americans (Shabazz and Carter, 1992). Asian men may refuse to be examined by a female doctor, and their wives may expect their husbands to be present throughout an examination. Latino patients may speak of *susto*, an illness arising from fright (Allshouse, 1993). Southeast Asians may believe that touching the head is taboo because the head holds the essence of life; consequently, disturbing the head will cause loss of the soul (Sherer, 1993). Other aspects of cross-cultural competence include creating a comfortable atmosphere, encouraging the possibility of disclosure of sexual orientation by using neutral terms, and conveying appropriate trainee and staff behavior toward patients regarding forms of address and rules of propriety (Rigoglioso, 1995).

Emerging links between health professional schools and approximately 600 federally funded health centers are beneficial to both students and health centers because in culturally diverse areas primary care clinicians are expected to be familiar with the cultural context and environmental conditions that affect their patients' health. In many areas of the country, primary care settings are uniquely positioned to fulfill the dual purposes of education—providing students with a very broad set of clinical conditions and offering cultural diversity that helps them gain appropriate cultural competence. Further, given the complexity of presenting problems, especially in underserved communities, students in these settings can learn firsthand about the interdependency of members of a health care team and observe their respect for the complementary skills of individual team members. The W.K. Kellogg Foundation has funded the Community-Based Public Health Initiative to improve the practice and teaching of primary care through collaborative efforts between academic health centers, health professions institutions, and communities. The project involves interdisciplinary education of graduate nurses and medical residents in community clinics.

The shift away from inpatient training permits early access to preventive and primary care. It also reinforces the change that many communities wish to make, namely, away from the prevailing attitude that patients must find their own way to their clinicians, regardless of barriers presented by language, geography, or culture. On their part, communities with significant unmet health problems have begun to welcome involvement with nonhospital-based training programs.

FINANCIAL SUPPORT FOR GRADUATE TRAINING IN PRIMARY CARE

In addition to issues of the content of graduate training in primary care, the committee devoted considerable attention to the question of how such training might be supported in the future. Two topics were paramount: where funding will come from (i.e., what parties in this country ought to be responsible for underwriting graduate training) and how support for primary care training in nontraditional (e.g., nonhospital) settings can best be achieved.

Current Sources of Graduate Medical Education Funding

A considerable array of sources provide GME funding: the Medicare and Medicaid programs, the Department of Defense (DOD) and Department of Veterans Affairs (VA), universities and practice plans, state and local governments, and other third-party payers. The largest single funding source, however, is the federal government, primarily through Medicare. In 1994, Medicare payments for GME totaled $5.8 billion and have been estimated to cost $70,000 per physician resident (COGME, 1994).[4] This program is described in more detail below. The VA and DOD provide 16 percent of total national support of residents' salaries.

Federal funding of a different type comes from the U.S. Public Health Service (Title VII), also described below. This funding is very sparse, however; together with all other sources of support from professional fees, medical school funds, foundation grants, and gifts for GME, it amounts to only 5 percent of total national support (Eisenberg, 1989). Finally, state and local governments provide

---

[4]The actual cost of resident training, which is in part supported by Medicare funds, is unknown because of the complex accounting involved and the well-known difficulty in dissecting the costs of joint products—teaching and patient care, teaching and research, and patient care and research.

an additional 10 percent, and some states also support physician assistant and nursing education.

Medicare Funding

Historically, Medicare funds supporting GME have been divided into two categories: direct (DME) and indirect (IME) payments. DME payments include reimbursements for salaries and fringe benefits of the teaching hospitals' residents, the portion of faculty salaries devoted to teaching, and the overhead allocated by the hospital for teaching. IME payments support teaching hospitals to compensate for higher expenses associated with their teaching mission as well as their patients' greater severity of illness. The payments are based on a set of complex formulas that are intended to recognize the urban location of most teaching institutions, their more complex case mix, the higher costs attributable to inefficiencies as part of the training mission of the teaching hospital (e.g., more testing by residents as part of the teaching process, longer operating room time), and unreimbursed costs of clinical research.

Some readers might wonder why if ambulatory training is so essential for primary care training it has not supplanted hospital-based training. The answer lies to a large extent in how GME is financed. Medicare's system of GME funding makes training in ambulatory care exceedingly difficult to finance. When the Health Care Financing Administration (HCFA) began using the prospective payment system to reimburse hospitals for services to Medicare patients in 1983, it included residents trained in ambulatory settings in its calculations of indirect payments. In 1985, however, a HCFA regulation mandated that training in outpatient settings be excluded from the determination of indirect GME payments. Congress responded by passing the Consolidated Omnibus Budget Reconciliation Act of 1985, which reversed the HCFA regulations and required that Medicare IME payments include training in ambulatory settings. This step did not, however, fully solve the problem.

Before 1986, the time that residents spent in ambulatory settings and the cost of administering outpatient education were recognized by Medicare only if the setting was part of the hospital. In the Omnibus Budget Reconciliation Act of 1986, Congress required that Medicare acknowledge the time that residents spend in ambulatory settings if the hospital incurs "all or substantially all" of the costs of the training. Although this legislation was important in establishing that ambulatory centers do not have to be located in or owned by the hospital, interpreting how much of the cost of education constitutes "substantially all" has made implementation of this law difficult (Eisenberg, 1989).

Furthermore, the rules by which payment is determined for faculty teaching time have also complicated GME financing. Teachers who are not hospital employees cannot be paid through Medicare unless the hospital pays them directly or by written agreement. Even if such an arrangement were made, the hospital would be limited to the costs it showed in 1984, the base year from which Medicare payments are calculated. This has created a financial disincentive to physicians to teach in hospital outpatient training programs and in programs that are separate from the hospital, despite their very real educational advantages (Eisenberg, 1989). Moreover, physical additions to hospitals after 1984 are not recognized in the payment formula, which means that hospitals find it difficult to build new facilities such as outpatient centers to support primary care residency programs.

In addition, resident time spent in outpatient settings other than hospital clinics is not included in the full-time-equivalent calculations for the payment of indirect costs. If a resident's training moves from a hospital-run clinic to a faculty-run clinic—even at the same location—the resident's time no longer counts toward the indirect adjustment (National Governors' Association, 1994). In sum, hospitals have learned that if they want to maximize GME payments for services provided to patients, they should keep trainees as house staff (and thus their site of training) in the hospital.

Another hindrance to the training of primary care physicians is the fact that Medicare GME payments are made to any certified residency program, whether or not such programs further national health care workforce goals and need. In the face of many calls for decreases in the training of specialists and increases in the production of primary care physicians, this aspect of Medicare GME funding in effect encourages the training of more specialists.

Title VII Funds for Primary Care Training

Federal targeted support for residencies in primary care—including general medicine, general pediatrics, and family medicine—was authorized in the 1976 health professions legislation, specifically Title VII, Section 784, of the Public Health Services Act. Title VII also provides support for physician assistant programs and general dentistry. Currently $59.8 million in funds support approximately 405 grants awarded for medical residency training programs, faculty development, and predoctoral training in General Internal Medicine/Pediatric and Family Medicine Programs (Bureau of Health Professions, personal communication, November 1995).

Grant support for physicans assistant (PA) educational programs promotes educational preparation of physicans assistants for roles in primary care settings and utilization in medically under-served areas. Since 1972 these grants have encouraged curricula to focus on primary care and deploying physicans assistants in areas of need. Like the medical training grants, these grants, which totaled $5 million in fiscal year 1993, are administered through the Division of Medicine, Bureau of Health Professions, Health Resources and Services Administration (HRSA) (HRSA, no date). Title VIII provides support for nursing education and is discussed below.

Title VII was not the first federal effort to support primary care graduate medical education. Health professions legislation in the 1960s increased medical school enrollment through capitation and encouraged the establishment of new medical schools. Within a decade medical school enrollments doubled. It was widely believed that by graduating more physicians, the need to produce more generalists would be addressed. Instead, an increasing proportion of the new graduate students pursued subspecialty training.

In 1974, the Bureau of Health Professions in the Health Resources and Services Administration (BHP/HRSA) awarded six contracts to support the development of residencies in general pediatrics and general internal medicine. Shortly thereafter, The Robert Wood Johnson Foundation provided support for some of the original six residency programs as well as others and added a major evaluative component. The documented success of these programs supported continuation of the Title VII effort.

One objective of the 1976 Title VII program was that 50 percent of medical school graduates would choose primary care careers. Consideration was given to requiring 50 percent of graduating students to enter primary care in order for medical schools to receive federal support for GME; however, the legislation did not include such a requirement. Shortly after the legislation was passed, the AAMC reported that 50 percent of GME first-year positions were already in the fields of internal medicine, pediatrics, and family medicine. Of greater concern than the number of the entry-level positions, however, was the number of graduates at the completion of residency training who would be generalists, because many residents who enter general residencies go on to subspecialty training.

The legislation, a product of efforts of the American Academy of Family Practitioners (AAFP) and a small group of academic pediatric and internal medicine generalists, not only supported primary care graduate education but also undergraduate departments of family medicine. Family practice was unquestionably a primary care discipline, and eligibility for grant funding was determined by having an approved residency. The same model did not work for internal medicine and pediatrics because these programs trained large numbers of subspecialists, and no mechanisms were available by which primary care training could be distinguished from the more typical training available to these two specialties.

To help address this problem, BHP/HRSA—with consultation from appropriate medical groups including the AAMC, the AAFP, the American Academy of Pediatrics, and the American College of Physicians—developed eligibility criteria for application to general internal medicine and pediatrics. These criteria included 25 percent "continuity" experience,[5] a psychosocial curriculum, and

---

[5]Generally meaning a block of time spent in outpatient clinics with scheduled patients. The site has to be a single primary care site where patients are assigned on a longitudinal basis (not emergency department or walk-in clinics).

sizeable ambulatory experiences; the last point was especially important for internal medicine, which at that time was 90 percent or more inpatient training. These criteria, although modified in the intervening 20 years, have remained in principle the distinguishing features of primary care training in general internal medicine and pediatrics.

Despite the success of the Title VII program, the period 1980 through 1992 saw funding remain flat (in fact, funding actually decreased because of the failure to keep up with inflation). Funding was especially problematic because various administrations during the period were opposed to reauthorization of the program as a whole. Again, as of this writing, the present climate of budget cutting creates some doubt about whether the Title VII program will be reauthorized.

Funding of Nurse Practitioner Education

Since its original enactment 30 years ago, Title VIII of the Public Health Service Act (P.L. 104-12) has played a significant role in helping to improve health care delivery in our nation by providing federal support to nursing education and students in nursing programs. Specifically, Title VIII programs fund the development of innovative programs to reach underserved areas, the development of educational programs for advanced practice nurses, and the special programs for nursing education for individuals from disadvantaged backgrounds.

Professional Nurse Traineeships for nurse practitioner and other advanced nurse education at the master's and doctoral level are also provided under this authority (Janet Heinrich, American Academy of Nursing, personal communication, January 1996; Bureau of Health Professions, Division of Nursing, 1994). Title VIII support totals roughly $60 million a year and goes directly to educational programs. Of the $60 million, $16.14 is earmarked for nurse practitioner and certified nurse midwife (CNM) programs with $10.9 million for nurse practicition programs and $4.8 million for CNM training. Medicare funds also support nursing, but the $248 million in 1994 Medicare funds support primarily preprofessional (diploma) nursing education (Aiken and Gwyther, 1995).

Graduate Medical Education as a Public Good

A supply of well-trained clinicians is a national resource for all Americans. This benefit, plus the very high cost of graduate training for physicians, justifies the use of public funds to help support such education (Schroeder et al., 1989). Such a resource can be understood, in the classic economic sense, as a public good. "Public goods" are those consumed collectively or those from which everyone can benefit, and where one person's use does not, in theory, prevent any other person from using or benefiting from the goods in question; roads, national defense, and information are cases in point. The contrast is made with "private goods," where consumption or use is exclusive and benefits are internalized; if left to private markets, enough of these goods or services will not be produced to meet public need.

In this context, training (and the costs thereof) should be regarded as a public good; the private market, left to itself, will underproduce GME (or, more specifically, fully trained physicians), whether for primary care or specialty care. Health plans (or health institutions) in the private marketplace will not invest in training clinicians (at least not to the extent necessary). The reason is that the eventual benefits would accrue to all health plans because any physician, having completed his or her training, can work for any plan or institution, but the costs of his or her training are borne by one plan, and those incurred costs might make that plan less competitive.

Furthermore, the costs of training are too great for many medical trainees to pay entirely without incurring very large debts. Indeed, the debt burden incurred by students—which might be repaid sooner if the students enter a highly paid specialty—is often cited as a deterrent to their entering a primary care discipline, where incomes have traditionally been much lower.

To spread GME costs among all sources of payment for medical care, the committee has concluded that the societal benefit of well-trained primary care clinicians is so valuable that it should be supported by all health care payers, including self-insured employers, managed care organizations, and private insurers, as well as federal payers.

Given the importance to our society of a well-trained primary care workforce, this committee recommends that a portion of all health care spending go to supporting primary care training. Because managed care organizations have a clear stake in training primary care clinicians to meet their needs, it is logical that they should play an important role in their education and in the financing of graduate medical education. Medicaid contracts with private sector health plans should, for example, acknowledge the positive role of those organizations that are involved in primary care training. Various legislative, regulatory, professional, or marketplace alternatives might be explored to implement this recommendation (described by Petersdorf, 1985). However such support is structured, the future of primary care depends on explicit support for primary care physicians. Although the committee endorses the support of all primary care clinicians, it emphasizes medical training because that training is long and expensive in comparison to the shorter and less expensive training of nurse practitioners and physician assistants.

Recommendation 7.5 All-Payer Support for Primary Care Training

The committee recommends the development of an all-payer system to support health professions education and training. A portion of this pool of funds should be reserved for education and training in primary care.

In making this recommendation, the committee endorses those of several other groups and commissions, including: COGME (1992, 1994, 1995); PPRC (1993, 1994); the Pew Health Professions Commission (1994, 1995); and previous congressional legislative proposals in both the House of Representatives and the Senate. BHP/HRSA estimates that an allocation of 1 percent of all third-party payments including Medicare would generate approximately $5.5 billion; an allocation of 1.2 percent would provide $6.5 billion (COGME, 1994). Several ways of collecting these funds can be considered; these include a tax on health insurance premiums (or gross revenues) or a tax based on the number of covered lives. The committee is not recommending an increase in funding for GME; rather, it believes that funding should come from all sources, not just Medicare or the much smaller sources cited earlier.

Many health insurance plans now refuse to contract with other health plans, delivery systems, or institutions that have higher costs attributable to teaching. Alternatively, they negotiate rates without regard to these costs and thus avoid paying a share of the cost of education; this is essentially the free-rider problem. If all plans contribute to the financing of GME, however, this problem can be circumvented, and competition among health plans can occur without penalizing a few plans that support primary care training.

Support for Advanced Training in Primary Care Sites

Rather than relying overwhelmingly on public payers such as Medicare, the committee has recommended just above that *all* payers support graduate medical education (indeed, support the education and training of all health professions). It now takes this position one step further and encourages the federal government to implement policies to designate a portion of those funds to support primary care training. This might be done in the context of proposed modifications to federal DME and IME policies now in place in the Medicare program.

Bills before the current Congress have proposed modification of DME and IME Medicare payments, and the financing of GME may be substantially restructured. Whatever the outcome of the current legislation, one thing is certain: if primary care is to achieve the fundamental role in health care that this committee believes it should, continued federal support for training, or at least graduate training, through direct and indirect payments will be necessary. Furthermore, such support will have to be structured to encourage primary care training in ambulatory settings. Finally, financial support should follow the trainee to his or her site of training—whether ambulatory or hospital-based—to produce high-quality primary care clinicians.

Restructuring Medicare GME financing needs to pay specific attention to advanced training for primary care in ambulatory sites. The committee is not alone in this view. For example, in a policy paper for The W.K. Kellogg Foundation, Garg (1995) describes three options for reforming graduate medical educational financing at the federal level. The first option, which is also endorsed by this committee, was that Medicare should extend its direct and indirect reimbursements to ambulatory settings. Thus, to have funds flow to the settings where primary care training for physicians takes place, the committee makes the following recommendation:

Recommendation 7.6 Support for Graduate Medical Education in Primary Care Sites

The committee recommends that a portion of the funds for graduate medical education be reallocated to provide explicit support for the direct and overhead costs of primary care training in nonhospital sites such as health maintenance organizations, community clinics, physician offices, and extended care facilities.

The committee emphasizes that, regardless of the level of training, support from Medicare trust funds should be *reallocated* to ensure that a portion will be used for training in primary care settings. How to ensure through regulation that funds going to plans are used for training at these sites is of concern to the committee, but beyond the scope of its charge.

Regarding support for nurse practitioner (and other advanced nursing) education, many observers have advocated shifting in Medicare monies now spent on diploma education to advanced practice nursing education (Aiken and Gwyther, 1995; Pew Health Professions Commission, 1995).

INTERDISCIPLINARY EDUCATION OF PRIMARY CARE CLINICIANS

Some physicians continue to organize their practices in traditional forms such as single or small, physician-only practices, but multidisciplinary team practice will be an increasingly common mode of practice in the future. Rapid changes of these types are taking place in large managed care organizations. The committee visited many sites that provided team delivery of care and held a three-day conference that explored the roles of health professionals as they practice in teams. In several sites, medical students and other health professional students were incorporated into multidisciplinary teams, and the committee observed the benefits of cross-disciplinary decisionmaking and management that would be useful experiences for students and medical residents during their primary care training. During its site visits, the committee found a remarkable array of organizational uses of health professionals, and it expects that experimentation and evolution will continue. A case study of two mature staff-model health maintenance organizations (HMOs) conducted for the committee illustrated clear diversity and ongoing changes in clinical staffing patterns (Scheffler, Appendix E).

Education must, therefore, equip trainees not only with specific skills but also with the ability to adapt to and create new clinical roles as members of a team.

Surprisingly, however, many students in the health professions are not currently taught in multidisciplinary settings, and they are not exposed at all to working models of team delivery of care in medical and nursing schools or physician assistant programs (MacPherson and Sachs, 1982). The committee urges that this be changed. It is crucial that educational programs recognize the need to prepare their trainees for effective team practice.

Recommendation 7.7 Interdisciplinary Training

The committee recommends that (a) the training of primary care clinicians include experience with the delivery of health care by interdisciplinary teams; and (b) academic health centers work with health maintenance organizations, group practices, community health centers, and other health care delivery organizations using interdisciplinary teams to develop clinical rotations for students and residents.

Educational experiences in interdisciplinary models of practice help trainees to learn the strengths, capabilities, and orientation of other disciplines so that in practice they can more easily appreciate overlapping and complementary skills. The Pew Health Professions Commission recently developed a model curriculum to assist educators in the creation of individualized courses on interdisciplinary collaboration in primary care, and The W.K. Kellogg Foundation has awarded 12 grants for a planning phase to develop interdisciplinary graduate nursing and medical education in community sites. These are important steps.

Such teams need to be truly integrated in how they approach their work and to be organized to provide the kinds of coordinated, comprehensive, and continuous care that primary care trainees are expected to learn. It is difficult to expect such training to take place simply by aggregating medical, nursing, pharmacy, and dental students in the same environment, because of different curricula, scheduling problems, varying levels of preparation, and similar problems.

Rather, students should be incorporated during their training into already functioning teams of practitioners. In this model, students from more than one discipline are assigned to a team that itself reflects an array of health professionals. The committee strongly urges academic health centers to move toward team delivery in their *own* clinics and inpatient settings and that they structure their primary care clinical practices into teams that can be models for teaching students.

Several academic medical centers have taken this approach. For example, since the early 1970s, the George Washington University School of Medicine and Health Sciences has included primary care residents, medical students, nurse practitioner students, and physician assistant students on multidisciplinary teams in its university-affiliated HMO and its geriatric practice. Similarly, in 1994, with support from The Josiah Macy, Jr. Foundation, the Harvard Medical School and then Harvard Community Health Plan began to implement an educational model of this sort that incorporates practicing and learning in a managed care setting (Moore et al., 1994).

The committee is acutely aware of the logistic difficulties of accomplishing this goal in institutions that are organized and funded by program (e.g., physician assistant, nursing, medicine) and by department (e.g., family practice, medicine, pediatrics). Further, these programs and departments may have differing, but deeply held, values that make merging curricula and faculty problematic. It also believes, however, that the commonalities of primary care curriculum content and the realities of the practicing environment make multidisciplinary training both desirable and necessary.

Health professionals must develop a common understanding of each other's roles and feel comfortable working with other health professions; they must have confidence about which clinical areas can be appropriately delegated or referred and to whom, and about whose skills augment their own, especially for the complicated medical and social problems that some patients present. Thus, a considerable amount of innovation, experimentation, study, and evaluation of new approaches is called for, and attention should be directed at the best ways to accomplish such teaching.

Recommendation 7.8 *Experimentation and Evaluation*

The committee recommends that private foundations, health plans, and government agencies support ongoing experimentation and evaluation of interdisciplinary teaching of collaborative primary care to determine how such teaching might best be done.

Although there is no *one* way that teams should be configured, active exploration of different models can improve our understanding of what works best for patient care and, by extension, what works best for teaching primary care. Three questions about teams have been of particular interest: (1) Who should be on the team? (2) How should work be distributed? (3) Who should provide leadership to the primary care team?

Preparing clinicians to practice in a team is a considerable challenge to health professions educators. Long-held distrust between professions, as well as issues of the autonomy of different disciplines, such as nursing and medicine, underlie systems of education. Furthermore, given the differences in length of training and the costs of that training, facilitating the experience of learning together is understandably difficult.

.Despite such financial and political realities, it is nevertheless essential that interdisciplinary education be pursued if there are to be effective primary care teams. Otherwise, it is unrealistic, despite a common commitment to patient care, to expect different health professions magically to come together after the completion of their programs and work effectively and efficiently to provide primary care services.

Students need to be placed on teams that provide good models of primary care in order to appreciate each clinician's role. Cross-professional preceptorships—such as nurse practitioners working with medical or physician assistant students—convey to all concerned the message that all health disciplines have valuable knowledge and skills. Trainees will also learn to manage the conflicts that are bound to arise as the result of different disciplinary approaches, overlapping roles, and competing demands for team resources and time (Doyle et al., 1993).

INTEGRATED DELIVERY SYSTEMS AND PRIMARY CARE TRAINING

Cooperation between academic health centers and integrated delivery systems is currently not occurring to any meaningful degree. Barriers include competition for patients, inflexibility and resistance to change on both sides, and failure of leadership to grasp the long-term potential for community benefit. In the committee's view, however, this should change.

Integrated delivery systems (IDSs) can derive benefits from academic centers, and the converse is also true. Shortages of primary care clinicians can be alleviated by creating or participating in primary care residency programs with IDSs providing training sites. To address an oversupply of specialists, academic health centers and IDSs may cooperate in implementing retraining programs in primary care (discussed below under Physician Retraining).

Other health professional students—in particular physician assistants and nurse practitioners—can and should be included in IDS sites as well. For example, IDSs may develop training programs for physician assistants and nurse practitioners and then employ these clinicians to increase the efficiency of care in their system. They may also develop programs to expand the skill of nurses who are no longer needed in hospitals to enable these nurses to take on roles in homes, skilled nursing facilities, and with medical groups that need personnel for telephone triage and care management.

Such teaching practices can thus be models of multidisciplinary training. If the health plan or system has a primary care residency program, the teaching faculty may be given clinical appointments, and these practices can be the center of physician graduate education. Patients will accept that some clinicians are faculty and that residents and other health professional trainees will participate in their care in these sites. Such partnerships or affiliations between academic health centers and IDSs can include clinical rounds and other linkages with the academic health center as a way to ensure that patients have the benefit of up-to-date clinical knowledge. Teaching practices can also serve as test sites for new models of care and new technologies such as computer-based patient records.

Academic health centers would gain primary care facilities to expand teaching resources in the community. Costs of education and related research could be spread over a broader base. IDSs could provide support for medical, PA education, or advanced practice nursing education in exchange for services and graduates that meet their particular personnel needs. For example, IDS practices that include residents might be able to provide preventive services and continuity of care to a population that otherwise uses an emergency department for its care.

Funding will be a critical issue in considering the role for IDSs in primary care education and training. If funding for teaching in these systems is absent or inadequate, IDSs will refuse to participate or will invest only enough to meet their immediate needs. This may result in short-lived programs and programs of questionable educational quality.

If, however, IDSs are supported by general revenues or other monies for their medical education activities, as recommended above, they are more likely to be longer-term participants. Because IDSs can bring a defined population—even a community—to medical education, they should be understood as indispensable resources for education and training in primary care. Thus, funding to support cooperation between academic medical centers and integrated systems in primary care education is in the public interest and should be encouraged.

CONTINUING MEDICAL EDUCATION

The knowledge base of medicine continues to grow, and clinicians change their practices over time. Attention needs to be paid to how primary care clinicians maintain and improve their skills. Traditional forms of continuing medical education (CME) such as conferences and journals may be augmented increasingly by computer-based methods such as CD-ROM learning materials, telemedicine conferences (both presentations and case conferences), and simulated clinical situations that provide learning experiences tailored to an individual clinician's need and interests. Increasingly powerful search methods are available for locating reference materials, experts, and clinical guidelines through the Internet, and these could be especially useful to those in rural and underserved areas where participation in CME is more difficult. Other promising methods give clinicians feedback about test ordering, prescribing, reminders about needed preventive care, and the like (Davis et al., 1995).

The development of large IDSs may provide especially appropriate settings for relevant CME that can take place in the practice setting itself and bring within reach rural practitioners and those whose care settings are more isolated. This should include training of primary care nurse practitioners, certified nurse midwives, and physician assistants in addition to the training of primary care physicians.

PHYSICIAN RETRAINING

One area of concern to the committee is physicians who are currently practicing in non-primary-care fields and who have not had primary care training. Some of these physicians are now interested in practicing primary care, and some assert that they are already doing so. The basic question is to what extent such physicians, never having had any grounding in primary care, ought now to be regarded as primary care clinicians.

The American Board of Family Practice (ABFP) has taken the position that a full residency is required to qualify one for primary care practice. Nevertheless, the ABFP position may be unrealistic for most subspecialists, because few physicians are able to return to a training program that reduces their incomes by substantial margins for a year or two, and public or private funding is not likely to be available for substantial retraining, especially not for physicians who may already be earning considerable incomes. In any case, it will be necessary (and more practical) to evaluate the results of current shorter programs before concluding that full primary care residencies are needed for retraining purposes.

On the one hand, the committee takes issue with the notion that one can "self-declare" as a primary care physician if one has never received the relevant training or that a weekend or so of continuing medical education will suffice. The committee strongly affirms that primary care requires special training, but it also believes that requiring currently practicing physicians to undertake a full residency equivalent to those of a newly graduated medical student in order to practice primary care is neither desirable nor feasible. "Retraining" is a middle-ground solution.

Experience with retraining of acute-care-based clinical nurse specialists as nurse practitioners has shown that assumptions about the skills that trainees bring to a program based on their educational background are often unwarranted and that more is required than might have been expected. Given discipline-specific demands, nursing should similarly consider that retraining may require significant education.

Although commonly used, the term *"retraining"* in this context is something of a misnomer. Many physicians in medical practice have never been trained in primary care, so retraining in reality refers more to the need to augment the training of clinicians who have been engaged solely or predominantly in subspecialty practice (e.g., a subspecialty of medicine or pediatrics, dermatology, ophthalmology, or anesthesiology) or in specialties that generally involve little or no patient contact (e.g., radiology or pathology). The term does not include training for management positions. A host of issues might be raised about training experienced clinicians to provide primary care.

Reasons for Retraining

Several reasons can be given for retraining. First, from a practical standpoint, some managed care plans now require that physicians be classified as primary care physicians either on the basis of specialty training or by self-declaration; in the latter case, the plans may require evidence of some primary care training. Thus, the most recent impetus for retraining is to enable physicians who are already in practice to participate in managed care plans and to continue to see their patients.

Second, retraining would avoid a waste of human resources and clinical experience in situations where specialists, because of an excess supply in some areas, are unable to practice. Although some might argue that it would be more efficient for specialists to reduce their practice or retire early, 50 percent of all physicians in practice today are 40 years of age or younger with many productive years ahead of them, so early retirement is not an option for many.

Third, there are issues of quality of patient care. On the one hand, if physicians self-identify as primary care clinicians without appropriate training, they may provide poor quality care to their patients. Appropriate training can provide the requisite knowledge and skills. By contrast, newly retrained subspecialists in internal medicine, psychiatry, dermatology, OB-GYN, or other fields could bring needed expertise to a primary care team and thus expand its internal resources.

Fourth, the nation needs some additional primary care clinicians now. Retraining could be an efficient way to produce a well-qualified primary care workforce. By implication, training specialists to practice primary care could help to reduce the specialist-generalist imbalance described in Chapter 6. Because subspecialists may not be needed in many rural areas that would welcome a primary care clinician, it might also assist in recruiting and retaining primary care physicians in rural and urban underserved areas.

Kinds of Retraining

In November 1994 the Pew Health Professions Commission identified 25 different retraining efforts in 13 states (Pew Health Professions Commission, 1994). Of these 25 programs, 10 were in existence, another 6 were under development, 6 task forces or committees were examining research initiatives, and 3 groups were addressing retraining issues. Some of these programs are designed specifically for OB-GYNs; others are directed to internal medicine subspecialists or physicians who have been out of the workforce for a time. One program at the Medical College of Pennsylvania has been in existence for about 20 years, but most are very recent. Length and intensity range widely—from a fully accredited residency program at the University of Tennessee to much briefer programs that might last half a day per week for 6 weeks or more and that are usually described as dependent on the needs of the individual.

A single curriculum is not likely to be either adequate or necessary for all clinicians. Different needs by specialty and type of practice expected (e.g., elderly, large group, urban, rural) are likely to be substantial. Lundberg and Lamm (1993) have made the reasonable suggestion that methods be developed to assess the extent to which practicing specialists possess primary care competencies as a means of determining their retraining needs.

The process of adding competencies will almost surely be different for those who, for example, have had three years of training in internal medicine than for those who were trained in a surgical subspecialty. A different curriculum is required to retrain an internist subspecialist who has had exposure to primary care as a resident and has provided some primary care to his or her patients than to retrain an anesthesiologist who has had no primary care training since medical school and has delivered no primary care as a practitioner. The core set of competencies, when developed (see Recommendations 7.2 and 7.3), could form the basis for a retraining curriculum. The length and intensity of the program needed by an individual would be individually determined, and additional modules could be added as necessary and appropriate. In addition, programs might augment ongoing specialty practice with gradually increasing responsibilities in primary care until "retrainees" can demonstrate adequate capabilities in primary care.

Certification After Retraining

The appropriate certification that should be awarded after retraining is an unresolved question. Many trainees would want a certification that would be more widely transferable than one given by the organization in which they practice or even by a specific state. Without an accreditation policy for retraining or certification examination for individuals based on defined competencies, however, it will not be possible to compare or judge the competence of graduates of widely varying programs. In internal medicine, one section of the recertifying boards is on general internal medicine, and this might be one avenue considered for certification.

Recommendation 7.9 Retraining

The committee recommends that (a) curricula of retraining programs in primary care include instruction in the core competencies proposed for development in Recommendations 7.2 and 7.3 and (b) certifying bodies in the primary care disciplines develop mechanisms for testing and certifying clinicians who have undergone retraining for primary care.

A major oversupply of specialists is perhaps a time-limited problem. In the short term, retraining of specialists may represent an important opportunity to expand the primary physician workforce, but retraining is basically a coping mechanism, not a preferred route to becoming a primary care physician. The committee believes that the specialist oversupply problem may be largely self-correcting in the longer term, as the proportion of newly trained primary care clinicians increases and the supply of specialists decreases. As a start, a study using focus groups to explore issues of specialist retraining has been funded by The Josiah Macy, Jr. Foundation. The committee suggests that foundations and federal agencies such as HRSA and HCFA conduct or support studies on retraining. These studies should include examination of needed competencies and the feasibility and outcomes of various approaches to retraining for various kinds of clinicians. Questions that might be studied include the following:

1. What is the level of interest in retraining and who are the interested clinicians?

2. Which critical primary care competencies are already known and which need to be taught? Can this be viewed as expanding an impressive set of skills rather than starting over?

3. What types of physicians are successfully retrained and enter primary care practice?

4. What sort of retraining is most appropriate and for what kinds of programs? What elements of GME and CME work best for retraining of the sort contemplated here? Are short CME courses, part-time study, tailored mini-residencies, full residencies, or on-the-job training adequate?

5. What are the characteristics of appropriate mentors or preceptors for experienced colleagues, and are these characteristics different for new residents? What are the most appropriate learning methods for mid-career physicians?

6. Who should do the training? Medical schools? Professional associations? HMOs?

7. Who should pay for retraining—the trainee, the organizations that will or have hired them, or state or federal government?

8. Does the incorporation of retrained specialist and subspecialty physicians into a primary care team augment that team's resources, add a new dimension to the team's capabilities, and allow it to function more effectively?

9. What sorts of standards are needed for retraining? Currently the specialty boards such as those for family practice, internal medicine, and pediatrics have taken different positions. What types of standards could be used, or imposed, by the managed care industry?

SUMMARY

If primary care is to move in the directions advocated by this committee, then many aspects of health professions education and training will need to be restructured. This chapter explored the changes likely to be required in undergraduate and graduate training, argued that clinical training ought to involve exposure to multidisciplinary team practice, and examined issues of retraining physicians for primary care.

To reach these goals, the committee put forward several recommendations. With respect to undergraduate medical education, the committee was concerned that students gain experience in primary care settings; with respect to graduate training, the committee explored issues of residency programs in family practice, internal medicine, and pediatrics and the value of primary care tracks. Education in ambulatory sites, community health clinics, and managed care organizations is essential to create a primary care workforce that will serve the needs of men and women, children and adults, rich and poor, individuals in rural and urban locations, and persons of all ethnic backgrounds.

More broadly, the committee examined questions of advanced training for all primary care clinicians and called attention to the need for the development of a set of common core competencies for all primary care clinicians. In addition, the committee highlighted its concerns about two special areas of emphasis—communication skills and cultural sensitivity.

A major consideration for the committee was financial support for primary care training. Consistent with earlier recommendations about universal coverage for health care, the committee called for an all-payer system to support health professions education and training, with some of this support reserved for primary care and directed to training in nonhospital sites such as offices, clinics, and extended care facilities. Adopting the recommendations in this chapter will require a realignment of funding and power to create incentives for different institutional behaviors (for example, in academic health centers and in integrated delivery systems) to focus on primary care and on training in ambulatory as well as hospital-based settings. Similarly, funding mechanisms for graduate medical education will need to be revamped to support training sites other than the traditional hospital base. Because the graduates of these programs will increasingly be needed by integrated delivery systems and the managed care industry generally, the committee believed that all payers should share the burden of establishing and maintaining the required educational infrastructure.

Finally, the committee examined other elements of education and training and called for the development of more innovative and interdisciplinary training programs. It also advocated that better mechanisms be created by which non-primary-care physicians can be formally and adequately retrained for primary care practice.

REFERENCES

AAMC (Association of American Medical Colleges). Task Force on the Generalist Physician, October 8, 1992.

AAMC. *Academic Medicine and Health Care Reform: Roles for Medical Education in Health Care Reform.* Washington, D.C.: AAMC, 1994.

ACOG (American College of Obstetricians and Gynecologists). Primary Care Provisions: Program Requirements for Residency Training in Obstetrics and Gynecology. Accreditation Council for Graduate Medical Education, February 1995 (effective January 1996).

Aiken, L.H. and Gwyther, M.E. Medicare Funding of Nurse Education. The Case for Policy Change. *Journal of the American Medical Association* 273:1528–1532, 1995.

Allshouse, K.D. Treating Patients and Individuals. Pp. 19–27 in *Through the Patient's Eyes: Understanding and Promoting Patient-Centered Care.* M. Gerteis, S. Edgman-Levitan, J. Daley, and T.L. Delbanco, eds. San Francisco: Jossey-Bass, 1993.

Alpert, J.J., and Charney, E. *The Education of Physicians for Primary Care.* DHEW Publ. No. (HRA)74–3113. Rockville, Md.: Bureau of Health Services Research, Health Resources and Services Administration, Department of Health, Education, and Welfare, 1973.

ASIM (American Society of Internal Medicine). *What's So Special About Being an Internist? A Resource Kit for Internists on Internal Medicine Preceptorship Programs.* Washington, D.C.: ASIM, 1995.

Barker, L.R. What and How to Teach. Curriculum for Ambulatory Care Training in Medical Residency: Rationale, Attitudes, and Generic Proficiencies. *Journal of General Internal Medicine* 5 (Jan./Feb. Suppl.):S3–S14, 1990.

Bureau of Health Professions, Division of Nursing. Fact sheets on advanced nurse education; nurse practitioner and nurse midwifery grants; professional nurse traineeships; and nurse anesthetist traineeships. Rockville, Md.: Division of Nursing, Health Resources and Services Administration, Public Health Service, 1994.

Christakis, N.A. The Similarity and Frequency of Proposals to Reform U.S. Medical Education. *Journal of the American Medical Association* 274:706–711, 1995.

COGME (Council on Graduate Medical Education). *Third Report. Improving Access to Health Care Through Physician Workforce Reform: Directions for the 21st Century.* Rockville, Md.: Health Resources and Services Administration, Department of Health and Human Services, 1992.

COGME. *Recommendations to Improve Access to Health Care Through Physician Workforce Reform.* Rockville, Md.: Health Resources and Services Administration, Department of Health and Human Services, 1994.

COGME. *Council on Graduate Medical Education Seventh Report—COGME 1995 Physician Workforce Funding Recommendation for Department of Health and Human Services' Programs.* Rockville, Md.: Health Resources and Services Administration, Department of Health and Human Services, 1995.

Davis, D.A., Thomson, M.A., Oxman, A.D. and Haynes, R.B. Changing Physician Performance. A Systematic Review of the Effect of Continuing Medical Education Strategies. *Journal of the American Medical Association* 274:700–705, 1995.

Doyle, D., Hanks, W.C., and MacDonald, N. The Interdisciplinary Team. Pp. 21–28 in *Oxford Textbook of Palliative Medicine.* New York: Oxford University Press, 1993.

Eisenberg, J.M. Special Article. How Can We Pay for Graduate Medical Education in Ambulatory Care? *New England Journal of Medicine* 320:1525–1531, 1989.

Family Health Foundation of America. MERIT Project. A Compendium of Topics for Curricular Development in Family Practice. Vols. I and II. Kansas City, Mo.: American Academy of Family Physicians Foundation, 1983.

FCIMCTF (Federated Council of Internal Medicine Curriculum Task Force). November 1995 draft, Curriculum report developed by the FCIM Task Force on Curriculum, 1996, forthcoming.

Fein, E.B. More Young Doctors Forsake Specialty for General Practice. *New York Times,* October 16, 1995.

GAO (General Accounting Office). *Medical Education: Curriculum and Financing Strategies Need to Encourage Primary Care Training.* Washington, D.C.: General Accounting Office, 1994.

Garg, M.L.. *Primary-Care Physicians: The Case for Reforming Public Financing of Medical Education.* January, 1995, working paper.

HRSA. Physician Assistants in the Health Workforce 1994. Rockville, Md: U.S. Public Health Service, no date.

IOM (Institute of Medicine). *Medical Education and Societal Needs: A Planning Report for the Health Professions.* Washington, D.C.: National Academy Press, 1983.

IOM. *Dental Education at the Crossroads: Challenge and Change.* M.J. Field, ed. Washington, D.C.: National Academy Press, 1995.

IOM. *The Nation's Physician Workforce: Options for Balancing Supply and Requirements.* K.N. Lohr, N.A. Vanselow, and D.E. Detmer, eds. Washington, D.C.: National Academy Press, 1996.

JAMA (Journal of the American Medical Association). Appendix II. Graduate Medical Education. Table 1. Resident Physicians on Duty in ACGME-Accredited and in Combined Specialty Graduate Medical Education (GME) Programs in 1993. *Journal of the American Medical Association* 272:725–726, 1994.

Kantor, S.M., and Griner, P.F. Educational Needs in General Internal Medicine as Perceived by Prior Residents. *Journal of Medical Education* 56:748–756, 1981.

Kassebaum, D.G., and Haynes, R.A. Relationship Between Third-Year Clerkships in Family Medicine and Graduating Students' Choices of Family Practice Careers. *Academic Medicine* 67:217–219, 1992.

Kern, D.C., Parrino, T.A., and Korst, D.R. The Lasting Value of Clinical Skills. *Journal of the American Medical Association* 254:70–76, 1985.

Kimball, H., and Young, P. Commentary. A Statement on the Generalist Physician From the American Boards of Family Practice and Internal Medicine. *Journal of the American Medical Association* 271:315–316, 1994.

Linn, L.S., Brook, R.H., Clark, V.A., et al. Evaluation of Ambulatory Care Training by Graduates of Internal Medicine Residencies. *Journal of Medical Education* 61:293–302, 1986.

Lipkin, M., Quill, T.E., and Napodano, R.J. The Medical Interview: A Core Curriculum for Residencies in Internal Medicine. *Annals of Internal Medicine* 100:277–284, 1984.

Lipkin, M., Levinson W., Barker, R., et al. Primary Care Internal Medicine: A Challenging Career Choice for the 1990s. *Annals of Internal Medicine* 112: 371–378, 1990.

Lundberg, G.D., and Lamm, R.D. Editorial. Solving Our Primary Care Crisis by Retraining Specialists to Gain Specific Primary Care Competencies. *Journal of the American Medical Association* 270:380–381, 1993.

MacPherson C., and Sachs, L.A. Health Care Team Training in U.S. and Canadian Medical Schools. *Journal of Medical Education* 57:282–287, 1982.

Martini, C.J.M., Veloski, J.J., Barzansky, B., et al. Medical School and Student Characteristics that Influence Choosing a Generalist Career. *Journal of the American Medical Association* 272: 661–668, 1994.

McPhee, S.J., Mitchell, T.F., Schroeder, S.A., et al. Training in a Primary Care Internal Medicine Residency Program: The First Ten Years. *Journal of the American Medical Association* 258:1491–1495, 1987.

Moore, G.T., Inui, T.S., Ludden, J.M., and Schoenbaum, S.C. The "Teaching HMO:" A New Academic Partner. *Academic Medicine* 69:595–600, 1994.

National Governors' Association, Curley, T., Orloff, T., et al. *Health Professions Education Linkages: Community-Based Primary Care Training.* Washington, D.C.: National Governors' Association, 1994.

New York Times. Dartmouth Redesigns Medical Training to Give Future Doctors a Human Touch. *New York Times,* (Education, part 1–3): Sept. 2, 1992.

Noble, J., Bithoney, W., MacDonald, P., et al. The Core Content of a Generalist Curriculum for General Internal Medicine, Family Practice and Pediatrics. *Journal of General Internal Medicine* 9(Supplement 1):S31–S42, 1994.

NONPF (National Organization of Nurse Practitioner Faculties). *Curriculum Guidelines & Program Standards for Nurse Practitioner Education.* Washington, D.C.: NONPF, 1995.

Novack, D.H., Dube, C., and Goldstein, M.G. Teaching Medical Interviewing. A Basic Course in Interviewing and the Physician-Patient Relationship. *Archives of Internal Medicine* 152:1814–1820, 1992.

Osborn, E.H.S. Factors Influencing Students' Choices of Primary Care or Other Specialties. *Academic Medicine* 68:572–574, 1993.

Petersdorf, R.G. A Proposal for Financing Graduate Medical Education. *New England Journal of Medicine* 312:1322–1324, 1985.

Petersdorf, R.G., and Turner, K.S. Medical Education in the 1990s—and Beyond: A View from the United States. *Academic Medicine* 70(Suppl.):S41–47, 1995.

Pew Health Professions Commission. *Primary Care Workforce 2000. Federal Policy Paper.* San Francisco: Pew Health Professions Commission, 1994.

Pew Health Professions Commission. *Shifting the Supply of Our Health Care Workforce. A Guide to Redirecting Federal Subsidy of Medical Education.* San Francisco: Pew Health Professions Commission, 1995.

PPRC (Physician Payment Review Commission). *Annual Report to Congress, 1993.* Washington, D.C.: PPRC, 1993.

PPRC. *Annual Report to Congress, 1994.* Washington, D.C.: PPRC, 1994.

Rigoglioso, R.L. Multiculturalism in Practice. *The Picker Report* 3(2):1,12,13, 1995.

Rivo, M.L., Saultz, J.W., Wartman, S.A., et al. Defining the Generalist Physician's Training. *Journal of the American Medical Association* 271:1499–1504, 1994.

Schroeder, S.A., Zones, J.S., and Showstack, J.A. Academic Medicine as a Public Trust. *Journal of the American Medical Association* 262:803–812, 1989.

SGIM/CDIM (Society of General Internal Medicine and the Clerkship Directors in Internal Medicine). *Core Medicine Clerkship Curriculum Guide: A Manual for Faculty.* A.H. Goroll, and G. Morrison. (project investigators). Rockville, Md.: Division of Medicine, Bureau of Health Professions, Health Resources and Services Administration, 1995.

Shabazz, C.D., and Carter, J.H. Multicultural Diversity in Medicine (editorial). *Journal of the National Medical Association* 84:313–314, 1992.

Sherer, J. New Waves: Hospitals Struggle to Meet the Challenge of Multiculturalism Now—And in the Future. *Hospitals* May 20, pp. 29–31, 1993.

Stimmel, B. The Crises in Primary Care and the Role of Medical Schools: Defining the Issues. *Journal of the American Medical Association* 268:2060–2065, 1992.

8

Research and Evaluation in Primary Care

Primary care can be investigated, and almost certainly improved, using scientific methods. The committee reached this view through testimony at public hearings, its workshop on the science base of primary care (Donaldson and Vanselow, 1996; Green, 1996; Povar, 1996) and a review of published literature. Although primary care research overlaps the field of health services research (IOM, 1995), it has certain special facets and concerns. As conceptualized by this committee, therefore, the primary care research enterprise was thought to be in a fledgling state—long on potential and short on actual accomplishment.

Funding and infrastructure to support primary care research stand in sharp contrast to the organized commitment to advancing knowledge in various subspecialty areas of medicine, typically using the methods of biomedical research and clinical investigation. This has three important ramifications. For one, current clinical research may have little to offer to primary care clinicians,[1] as evidenced by the observation that "[a]lthough primary care practitioners can use some of the knowledge generated by [specialty-oriented] research, in fact, most of it is not relevant to primary care because of its focus on singly developed diseases, carefully selected patients, and the reporting of strictly physiological outcomes" (AHCPR Task Force, 1993, p. iii). For another, lessons from well-done primary care research are not available to inform the larger picture of health

---

[1]By primary care clinician, the committee explicitly means physicians, nurse practitioners, and physician assistants, as discussed in Chapter 2 and the committee's interim report (IOM, 1994a). More generally, in referring to primary care, the committee means to imply primary care as defined in Chapter 2.

care organization and delivery. Finally, this paucity of primary care research and development leaves primary care insufficiently prepared to confront the challenges and opportunities inherent in the committee's definition.

One broad explanation for the mismatch between the bulk of clinical care and the bulk of health-related research is the misperception that primary care is already sufficiently understood (Nutting, 1996). Discussions in the workshop and elsewhere during this study made clear, however, that primary care is a distinct and quite complex field, that it is inadequately described to and poorly understood by the broader health care community and the public generally, *and* that it is apparently an important source of variation leading to different health (or disease) states and clinical management strategies. For all these reasons, the committee determined that setting out a coherent program for research and evaluation in primary care would be an important contribution of its report.

In this regard, the committee took note of Starfield's position (Starfield, 1996) that primary care research is "research *done in* a primary care context." Starfield argues that it is a fallacy to conclude either that primary care research can be done in anything other than primary care settings or that information purportedly about primary care that is drawn from research not done in primary care settings is *a priori* valid for the primary care clinician. With those cautions in mind, one can draw a reasonable inference that the nation has engaged in little primary care research.

To help redress this imbalance, this chapter explores the need for a primary care research infrastructure and identifies key areas of primary care research that warrant high-priority attention. In the first main section, the committee discusses four topics relating to the necessary infrastructure for primary care research and offers four recommendations designed to overcome existing barriers to such work and foster a stronger framework within which a broad range of studies might be conducted. In the second main section, the committee identifies high-priority areas of research. Although these topics are often in the health services research arena, they are highlighted here for two reasons: (1) to draw attention to the core elements of the committee's definition of primary care, and (2) to underscore the importance of conducting much of this work in settings that deliver primary care as conceived by this committee. The chapter ends with some commentary about the long-term impact of primary care research on the quality and costs of health care in this nation.

The committee's views on primary care research and an appropriate infrastructure in which to pursue it do not imply that the committee believes this part of the research enterprise should be separated from the rest of the research effort in this nation. Primary care research cannot be done in a vacuum. Rather, this work should be done in the context of developing data and insights for the entire approach to health care in this country—the realm of health services research (IOM, 1995)—so that a responsive, cost-effective, and high-quality system can be built in the ensuing years.

SUPPORT FOR THE INFRASTRUCTURE FOR
PRIMARY CARE RESEARCH

The committee found challenging declarations of research agendas for primary care (e.g., Williams and Brook, 1978; Mayfield and Grady, 1990; AHCPR Task Force, 1993; Starfield, 1996); there is no lack of questions to be asked and answered. What does seem to be missing is a widely held commitment to the exploration and explication of primary care using all the methods of science and the array of settings in which primary care is delivered. At present, no adequate infrastructure exists that is designed to undergird an enduring primary care research enterprise. In this committee's view, it is unlikely that primary care can be grounded in an adequate science base unless such infrastructures are created.

The untapped opportunities in primary care research leave us ignorant about why some people get sick while others stay well and why some people recover from their illnesses and others do not. Primary care research can determine the transition of signs and symptoms and vague concerns into clinically more significant diseases and diagnoses so that prognostication can be improved and the needs of newly forming integrated delivery systems and the patients that they serve can be met. The most urgent need, however, is not for a particular investigation but the building of the nation's capacity to investigate multiple primary care questions. In other words, the overriding goal must be to establish a viable primary care research infrastructure.

Key elements of such an infrastructure have been defined. Among them are

• a designated lead agency at the federal level that would be held accountable for advancing primary care research;
• national health and health care utilization surveys and databases that capture the relevant aspects of and data on primary care;
• primary care research laboratories, such as practice-based research networks that link primary care practitioners with those who carry out scientific investigations;
• appropriate data standards and classification systems for primary care;
• training programs for primary care clinician-scientists; and
• stable career ladders for primary care researchers.

The committee found exemplary efforts in each of these areas. Some are well known, such as the large population surveys of the National Center for Health Statistics (NCHS) or the Agency for Health Care Policy and Research (AHCPR) in the Department of Health and Human Services (DHHS). Similarly, the international classification system for primary care (the International Classification of Primary Care, or ICPC) is widely known in certain circles (especially abroad) and clearly opens the door to the episode-oriented epidemiology critical to capturing the phenomena of primary care.[2] Other advances are not widely recognized or are too new to be broadly known; the idea of primary care laboratories or primary care practice-based networks for research (discussed below) is a case in point. Yet others are in a developmental stage; the lead agency for primary care research falls into this category.

In many ways, apart from long-standing federal surveys, what has been achieved so far has been largely through a patchwork of research efforts and the successes of occasional champions, relying on budgets that seem trivial when compared to the nation's other research commitments relevant to health, such as the biomedical research institutes. The future of primary care will be strengthened if genuine capacity for conducting primary care research is clearly established. The following subsections discuss in more detail specific needs that must be met to set a primary care research infrastructure solidly in place; where relevant, the committee's recommendations are given.

Federal Leadership and Support for Primary Care Research

The nation might be said to have either a surfeit of agencies conducting or supporting what they regard as primary care research or essentially no such capacity. The stand one might take on this depends in part on the breadth and content of one's concept of primary care research. Certainly if the focus is on research that is carried out in primary care settings to answer epidemiological, clinical, organizational, or other questions about primary care needs and health care delivery, then capacity and output to date have been low. That is essentially the conclusion of this committee. To address this gap, the committee reached consensus on the proposition that substantially greater emphasis, focus, and support for primary care research is needed at the federal level.

Recommendation 8.1 Federal Support for Primary Care Research

The committee recommends that (a) the Department of Health and Human Services identify a lead agency for primary care research and (b) the Congress of the United States appropriate funds for this agency in an amount adequate both to build the infrastructure required to conduct primary care research and fund high-priority research projects.

A lead agency is necessary for two main reasons. First, primary care research should not be a crazy quilt of independent research efforts, none working with another, none building on previous or ongoing work. Thus, the coordinating

---

[2]See, for example, Lamberts et al., 1993, for a more complete explication of the ICPC and its use among members of the European community; these points are also explored in Lamberts and Hofmans-Okkes, 1996a. An illustrative presentation of data on episodes of care using this classification system appears in Appendix 4A of this report.

and "bully pulpit" functions of a lead agency will be very important in developing synergistic programs of research and in raising the visibility of primary care research. Second, this is a period of unprecedented belt tightening at the federal level, and the nation cannot afford to squander any resources devoted to primary care research. A lead agency is thought to be a useful vehicle for shepherding the nation's scarce research dollars in this area and for making the most efficient use possible of the resources that are available.

Placement and Role of a Lead Agency

The committee did not take a stand on precisely what unit within the Department of Health and Human Services (DHHS) might be assigned the lead, as it judged that the best decision could be made by the Secretary of DHHS in light of evolving organizational change within the department. The committee recognizes, however, the importance of AHCPR as the only federal agency explicitly authorized to investigate primary care as it is conceived of by this committee, and the agency has mounted an important effort to do just that in the past two years or so. Furthermore, in mid-1995 the reorganization plan for the agency (*Federal Register*, 1995) included a "Center for Primary Care Research." It was assigned the responsibility of conducting and supporting projects in the following five areas: (1) primary care settings and systems; (2) rural health care services and systems; (3) care for special populations; (4) effectiveness of education, supply, and distribution of the health care workforce; and (5) international activities. To the committee's knowledge, no other element of DHHS has this charge or responsibility.

As this report was being prepared, the Institute of Medicine issued a report on the health services research workforce, and it noted that the leading sponsor of broad-based health services research in this country is AHCPR (IOM, 1995). The primary care committee observed that many of the issues addressed by health services researchers for the past quarter-century, many of the settings in which it is conducted, and many of the methodological and statistical approaches employed by health services researchers are relevant to primary care research as envisioned here.

The responsibilities of such a lead agency could be to conduct, oversee, and coordinate activities relating to a broad agenda of primary care research (see below). In addition, it could assist or advise other agencies on matters relating to the supply of primary care clinicians or of appropriately trained researchers; for example, a lead agency for primary care research could work with the Bureau of Health Professions (BHP) in the Health Resources and Services Administration (HRSA) in that agency's efforts to monitor the supply of physicians, nurses, and other health professionals. Furthermore, a lead agency could support research training programs as well as offer technical and methodologic assistance to other federal, state, or local agencies wishing to pursue primary care research on their own. A lead agency would be in a strategic position to synthesize and dissemi-nate information from the full array of primary care research projects being carried on in the nation (whether it is actively funding them or not). A final, important responsibility of such an agency would be to build an understanding of the need for such research and a constituency that will demand, use, and act on the results of such projects.

Collaborative Responsibilities of a Lead Agency

A lead federal agency for primary care research should interact and collabo-rate with both other elements of DHHS and other federal departments. An agency within the Public Health Service (PHS), such as AHCPR, could develop cooperative arrangements and communication avenues with other PHS agencies. These include the Centers for Disease Control and Prevention (CDC), offices and bureaus in HRSA (such as BHP and the Maternal and Child Health Bureau), and the National Institutes of Health (especially those institutes that carry out clinical investigations about primary care concerns or support clinical trials in ambula-tory settings). Collaboration with the CDC might be especially important, given that agency's responsibilities in the area of prevention.

In addition, a lead agency for primary care research (if placed in the PHS) would need to develop collaborative relationships with several other DHHS agen-cies. Primary among these is the Health Care Financing Administration (HCFA), given its responsibilities for the Medicare and Medicaid programs and its own health services and policy research agenda. Other elements of the department also have interests that intersect with primary care research because of their focus on ensuring high-quality services to specific populations; among these are the Administration on Aging and the Administration on Children and Families.

A formally designated lead agency could also forge links with two other departments with significant primary care concerns and responsibilities for large numbers of individuals across the age span—namely, the Department of Veterans Affairs (VA) and the Department of Defense (DOD). Research efforts sponsored, for example, by the VA's Health Services Research and Development program or by DOD/Health Affairs (which cuts across all the armed services) could present important opportunities for joint research efforts and interaction, especially to the extent to which VA and DOD efforts are carried out in primary care settings.

Many entities in the private sector underwrite various types of primary care research or programs to build capacity for such work. For example, the Robert Wood Johnson (RWJ) Clinical Scholars program has produced, through its more than 20-year history, a cadre of primary care clinicians capable of independent health services and policy research. Other RWJ programs have involved Gener-alist Academic Fellows in pediatrics and medicine. The Pew Charitable Trusts have for 10 years also supported training in health services research, and many of its Fellows come from or conduct research in primary care disciplines. The community development orientation of The W. K. Kellogg Foundation has also provided a context for innovative demonstration projects that relate to the delivery of primary care services. In addition, the committee learned of both medical and nursing schools that support primary care faculty to some extent to carry out research in this field.

Finally, as discussed more fully below, more than 30 practice-based research networks are either operating or serving as laboratories for various kinds of primary care research (see Recommendation 8.3). The committee judged that collaborative public-private partnerships are the wave of the future (see also Recommendation 9.1 in the following chapter). Thus, it believed that, in all these cases, a lead agency could better foster mutually productive relationships than could multiple agencies operating independently.

Data Sources and Needs

Need for a Primary Care Database

Research often demands complex primary data collection, particularly when specific hypotheses are to be tested using experimental or quasi-experimental designs. By and large, the details of such data sources and methods for collecting or analyzing such information must be specific to the research project at hand. Although the committee did not explore the issue of primary data collection directly, it was cognizant of the fact that much useful work can be done with analyses of secondary, survey, or administrative data, providing that the data are reliable, valid, accessible, and current. Such information offers a means by which the relevant phenomena of primary care can be captured to answer such questions as "What is the great majority of health care needs to which primary care responds?" "Who is delivering that care today?" "In what settings?" and "At what cost?" Thus, the committee looked into the characteristics of major surveys and databases that might be seen as part of the infrastructure for primary care research, giving particular attention to whether they collect and array data in ways that would permit analyses to be done on episodes of care.

Existing Data Sources Relevant to Primary Care Research

The federal government conducts a great variety of surveys and oversees an array of databases that have relevance for primary care and primary care research.[3] These are the responsibility of several departments in the executive

---

[3]For more detail on the nature and breadth of federal health data sources, see CBASSE/IOM, 1992, especially Appendix C, and the sources cited there. As this report was being prepared, DHHS was designing a major restructuring and consolidation of core DHHS surveys, as a means of reduc-

branch. The great majority of these activities reside, of course, in DHHS. A selected few, briefly described below, are of special importance for primary care research; these include the programs of NCHS (which is the lead agency for the "production, analysis, and dissemination of general-purpose health statistics" [CBASSE/IOM, 1992, p. 129] and is a part of the CDC), those of AHCPR (the lead agency for health services research), and those of HCFA (which administers the Medicare program and the federal portion of the Medicaid program).

NCHS conducts many general and special purpose surveys. The best known are the National Health Interview Survey (NHIS) and the National Health and Nutrition Examination Survey (NHANES). The NHIS is a cross-sectional household interview sample survey providing information on the general health status of the civilian, noninstitutionalized population; it yields national estimates of the incidence of acute illnesses and injuries, the prevalence of chronic conditions and impairments, the use of health care services, and various other health-related topics. This annual survey comprises both a core set of questions (on measurement of illness and injuries, days of disability, limitations of activities, use of health care, perceived health status, and socioeconomic characteristics) and a variety of items (in supplements) that change from year to year depending on the health issues of the day.

The NHANES evolved from the Health Examination Survey first launched in 1959. It involves direct standardized physical examinations, clinical (e.g., visual acuity) and laboratory (e.g., biochemical and hematologic) tests, measurements of nutritional status, and interviews. The aim is to obtain information on "undiagnosed" and "nonmanifest" diseases and the prevalence of defined diseases or conditions as well as to gather normative health-related data.

Since 1973, the National Ambulatory Medical Care Survey (NAMCS), a national sample survey, has gathered and disseminated information on patient visits to physicians' offices. It excludes services provided by nonphysician personnel and telephone contacts. NAMCS collects information on characteristics of patients, diagnoses and symptoms, diagnostic and therapeutic interventions, and characteristics of the physician and payment source. Only since the establishment of the National Hospital Ambulatory Medical Care (NHAMC) survey in 1991 has similar information been collected on health care provided by hospital emergency and outpatient departments.

AHCPR administers the National Medical Expenditures Survey (NMES), which is intended to provide national estimates of the use of and expenditures on

---

ing duplication and increasing survey efficiency, meeting a broad set of user needs, filling existing data gaps, and improving the efficiency of the survey enterprise. As the details of these proposals were not available to the committee, it was not able to take them further into account for this report. It is clear, however, that the committee's ideas about a primary care survey and database (discussed in Recommendation 8.2) are consistent with the general thrust of the DHHS plans.

health care services and the extent of health insurance coverage in the nation. The three major components of this survey (a household survey, an institutional population component, and a survey of American Indians and Alaska Natives) yield population-based estimates of health and functional status, insurance coverage and health care utilization, outlays, sources of payment, and various other socioeconomic data on respondents. A long-term care supplement provides information on persons with functional disabilities and impairments and their use of formal home and community-based services. This survey, although comprehensive with respect to these topics, is conducted only infrequently, and data are not readily accessible; it was undergoing considerable revision in terms of sampling design and similar matters as this report was being prepared.

A final survey of great potential for primary care focuses on the Medicare beneficiary population. Administered by HCFA, the Medicare Current Beneficiary Survey (MCBS) is intended to be an ongoing multipurpose interview survey focused on health care use and expenditures; it also includes health and functional status and various socioeconomic and demographic characteristics, including family support. This survey, because it is of a representative panel of Medicare beneficiaries over time, can provide data sets appropriate for either longitudinal or cross-sectional studies.

Although all the above are critical elements of the nation's infrastructure for health statistics, and although all yield some information pertinent to primary care research, they are not (either individually or collectively) completely satisfactory as a base for analyzing the range of issues that this committee believes ought to be included in the primary care research agenda. For instance, with the exception of the MCBS, they are not person-specific and do not yield longitudinal data on particular individuals; this means that episodes of care for specific people and their particular conditions cannot be created or analyzed from these files. In addition, they do not include information on nonphysician primary care clinicians at the level of detail necessary to understand who is providing what kinds of services to which patients for which problems; thus, they cannot illuminate the concept of the primary care team.

The committee spent some time discussing the strengths and limitations of various large-scale data sources of this type, with specific attention to the national surveys conducted by DHHS agencies. In general, none of these surveys was considered wholly adequate for the purpose of providing information to answer a broad set of primary care research questions, and indeed even collectively they would not suffice. To address this need, therefore, the committee agreed on a recommendation concerning a primary-care-specific database that would be created from a periodic national sample survey.

Recommendation 8.2 National Database and Primary Care Data Set

The committee recommends that the Department of Health and Hu-

man Services support the development of and provide ongoing support for a national database (based on a sample survey) that reflects the majority of health care needs in the United States and includes a uniform primary care data set based on episodes of care. This national survey should capture data on the entire U.S. population, regardless of insurance status.

Episodes of Care

Defining episodes of care. Key elements of the committee's definition of primary care involve continuity and coordination of care. Research in this area must, therefore, be able to track the care for specific conditions through time and across clinicians and settings. This condition in turn requires the ability to create what analysts term "episodes of care." An episode of care has been defined as "all care for a given spell of illness, for a specific injury, or for a particular chronic illness" (Lohr et al., 1986, p. S9); this is similar in concept to the definition advanced in Chapter 4 and its appendix that an episode refers to a problem or illness during the time from its first presentation to a clinician until completion of the last encounter for that problem.

Ideally, one would prefer to study episodes of *illness* and of *disease*; for economic analyses at least, an episode of illness has been characterized as the "natural unit of decisionmaking" (Newhouse and the Insurance Experiment Group, 1993, p. 80). An entire episode of disease is not by and large a measurable concept, because the beginning date of an acute or (especially) a chronic problem can rarely if ever be known, especially for conditions with insidious onset or lack of symptoms until the disease is well advanced. The exceptions may be episodes starting with an acute traumatic injury and well-child care starting with the birth (although the latter is not typically regarded as illness). In addition, long-term chronic disorders that have periods of remission and flare-up add to the conceptual complexity of an episode of disease.

For these reasons, most episode-based research focuses on episodes of *care*. These typically date to an office visit, emergency room visit, hospitalization, or the like that appears to be the first identifiable service for a symptom or condition; they end, depending on the analysis in question, at death, at the end of traceable services for that problem, or at the end of a year.[4]

---

[4]This brief commentary about episodes of care masks the true complexity of defining, creating, and analyzing episodes of care. Among the issues that researchers must take into account are episodes with no obvious start; episodes that apparently involve services that are not recorded anywhere (e.g., not in patient records, not in insurance claim databases) but that can be presumed to have occurred; overlapping episodes (e.g., when a person with a serious chronic condition suffers an accidental injury); and situations in which services apparently relating to two different episodes

The content of an episode of care can be extremely complex; even for ambulatory care, it can include visits to various clinicians (or visits by various clinicians to a home or other setting), laboratory tests (and ideally their results), diagnostic procedures (and results), and both inpatient and outpatient treatments of all sorts, including prescription (and, ideally, nonprescription) medications. This characterization of episodes of care is not easy to realize on a routine basis, however, and in many circumstances an "episode" may relate only to visits linked over time.

Reasons for using episodes of care. The analytic rationale for using episodes involves the ability (a) to describe better the full set of services directed at a particular clinical problem or provided to a specific individual for preventive or for diagnostic and therapeutic reasons and (b) to capture more fully the cost and quality consequences of the patterns of care. In addition, using episodes of care permits better modeling of care decisions by both patients (or family members) and clinicians than would be possible simply with counts of physician or clinic visits.

Barriers to creating and using episodes of care. By and large, current databases (such as the survey files described earlier) cannot provide the types and levels of information required to create, let alone analyze, episodes of care. The ability to examine complete episodes of care that may extend over time and space is a critical feature of a "primary-care-informative" data set that most existing databases do not have.

None of the current data sets adequately overcome the limits of their cross-sectional design. For example, even though some surveys (such as the NHIS) ask respondents to give their answers about events in terms of a recent time frame, the files are not (and cannot be) constructed in a way that would permit care to be viewed as a longitudinal series of visits and activities that occur over time and in different parts of the health care system. To give another illustration, past NMES databases link events for individual patients over time and thus in theory might have been very useful in primary care research, but the 1987 NMES was not designed for this purpose and may not contain the necessary level of detailed data

---

occur simultaneously (e.g., a follow-up visit for precancerous uterine fibroids that also involves counseling for possible alcohol abuse). In addition, some investigators distinguish between an "episode of disease," which they characterize as "a health problem from its onset through its resolution or until the patient's death," and an "episode of illness," or "the period during which a person suffers from symptoms or complaints experienced as an illness" (Hornbrook et al., 1985; Lamberts and Hofmans-Okkes, 1996a, p. 161). For practical purposes, the distinction may not matter much, because the researchable concept is far more likely to be an episode of care, although the idea of "health maintenance episodes" can perhaps be usefully considered a special form of episodes of care (but not disease or illness) (Lamberts and Hofmans-Okkes, 1996a).

on physicians seen and services provided (as contrasted with economic information on charges and reimbursements or out-of-pocket expenditures). Finally, the likely requirement to maintain the confidentiality of respondents' identity in survey data amassed with public funds can clearly hamper any linkage of information over time.

Somewhat the same problems plague administrative insurance claim files (such as the Medicare databases). Medicare files—which many regard as the best source of condition-specific utilization information that the nation has today—do not, for example, cover prescription medications and do not code laboratory tests or other services at a sufficient level of detail. (Obviously, these files yield no information on the general population of nonelderly individuals.)

Good insurance files for private sector plans that cover a generous benefit package (explicitly, those that cover preventive services and prescription medications in addition to traditional outpatient and inpatient services) can be used to create episodes of care, but doing so requires considerable clinical, analytic, and computer expertise to develop the "rules" by which various different kinds of services are linked correctly into diagnosis- or problem-specific episodes over time. Furthermore, such files may or may not be available for research purposes, depending on who owns them, although clearly such organizations can carry out internal research related to primary care. By and large, patient records and data files maintained by health maintenance organizations, physician networks, or integrated delivery systems today cannot provide, in any routine way, the episode-based information that would be needed to measure primary care. In any case, it would be unusual for specialized episode-of-care information to be made available to outside investigators; but as with insurance files, these managed care organizations can and do conduct their own studies on primary care issues (which might be episode based).

It is quite possible to create episodes of care using algorithms that are based on diagnoses; indeed, this is the preferred approach. This was done in early work in the Indian Health Service (Paul Nutting, University of Colorado Health Sciences Center, personal communication, September 30, 1995), for example, and much of the analyses done in the RAND Health Insurance Experiment were based on complex diagnosis-specific episodes created from the research-oriented insurance claim files of that study (see, for example, Keeler et al., 1982; Lohr et al., 1986). Today, unfortunately, coding of diagnoses may often be related less to the reality of patient illness than to the complexities of reimbursement rules established by third-party payers (IOM, 1994b) or to the desire to circumvent stringent physician profiling programs of managed care or accreditation organizations.

Incompatibility of concepts. Apart from the conceptual and practical issues about episodes of care discussed above, the committee acknowledges the likely difficulty of operationalizing several parts of its definition for survey or database purposes. To illustrate the point: In the data exercise conducted for the committee, the notion of "practicing in a family and community context" proved especially problematic. Although, clearly, reliable survey questions can be devised to tap this domain, a nontrivial amount of methodologic work might need to be done to capture the concept adequately in terms that lay respondents would understand.

Getting at these concepts through present-day administrative databases or existing surveys is almost certainly not possible. One might try to use diagnostic or reason-for-visit codes of "family problems" or similar nomenclature as an indicator measure of family context. In the data exercise conducted for the committee, however, this diagnostic cluster appeared too infrequently to be useful. Another alternative might be to examine patterns of diagnosis-specific services that are rendered to several members of one family. An example might be the constellations of (ostensibly related) services for one parent who is terminally ill with cancer, counseling for that individual's young children who have behavioral problems at school or are visibly depressed, and respite services for the spouse. The methodologic challenges of creating such analytic units are extreme, however. Moreover, in general the committee believed that practicing in a family and community context implies a great deal more than simply providing related (or unrelated) care to more than one family member. In addition, the above analytic tactics obviously do not adequately address the idea of "community."

Finally, none of the current data sets adequately addresses the problem of properly labeling the events of primary care. This requires attention to both the patient's multiple reasons for visits and the physician's appraisal of the problem(s) as it (or they) evolve over multiple visits. Classification systems now mainly used outside the United States (such as the ICPC) may, however, help overcome this problem if they become more widely used here (Lamberts et al., 1993). The point is taken up again in the discussion of data collection standards below.

Structure of a Primary-Care-Oriented Survey

The committee did not discuss in any depth the details of a new or modified survey that would satisfy the goals set out in Recommendation 8.2, nor did it come to consensus on what federal entity within DHHS might conduct such a survey on a routine basis. It did, however, believe that such a survey should follow a probability sample of individuals of all ages over time and that it should focus on core elements of the primary care definition.

One possibility might be for such a survey to be fielded independently of any of the current NCHS surveys but to use the same or a variant of the person-specific (rather than provider-specific) sampling frames used in, for instance, the NHIS or NHANES. Yet another option might be for the next NMES (now referred to as the Medical Expenditures Panel Survey, or MEPS) to be expanded or for a supplement to be fielded that would target significant primary care questions.

Toward A National Health Care Survey (CBASSE/IOM, 1992) had recommended that NCHS develop a new survey that would address current limitations of certain NCHS surveys and improve their ability to measure the longitudinal dimensions of care. The aim was to overcome one major drawback, namely, that the starting point is a sampling of events rather than a sampling of patients. That committee recommended that person-level data be collected "on health care received by individuals over time and over the entire progression of an episode of illness" (p. 4). Moving in this direction would clearly go a long way toward reaching the goal of the present committee with respect to a primary-care-oriented national database.

Regardless of the mechanics,[5] the committee wishes to go on record as favoring large-scale, episode-oriented morbidity studies in the population that can provide the databases needed to enable the nation to assess how well the concepts in the IOM definition are being achieved. In the research arena the committee has emphasized surveys or other types of data collection strategies that would feed into databases that could be tapped for various types of primary care studies. In addition, the committee calls attention to the opportunities offered by practice-based research networks to be an important source of such survey information (see the discussion for Recommendation 8.3 below). Because such information would come from the front lines of primary care practice, the resulting database would comprise clinically important information for research, policy, and practice applications.

The committee also holds that the development of computer-based patient records ought to be a high priority as well, consistent with the recommendations of two earlier IOM committees (IOM, 1991a, 1994b). In this way, it may be possible in the future to have a data collection structure that permits data to be organized into episodes of care in sufficient clinical and demographic detail to measure the components of primary care far more appropriately than is true today. In particular, the committee would urge managed care organizations to adapt their information systems in such a way that they can measure episodes of care for their enrollees within the conceptual framework of the definition of primary care given in Chapter 2.

---

[5]As indicated in note No. 3 (above), the considerable changes to DHHS surveys now being designed may make these ideas less relevant for future years than they were in 1995. The advantages to the person-specific (i.e., population-based) orientation are clear, however. In addition, Kerr White (Charlottesville, Va., personal communication, December 21, 1995) notes: "Linkages at the individual level among the several national surveys conducted by NCHS, AHCPR, and HCFA could be especially useful for further testing hypotheses that bear on the origins of diseases and their natural history, in addition to their importance in tracking the use of services. Until these surveys are linked at the individual level, they will continue to be plagued by the 'ecological fallacy' in which changes of an attribute in one population may or may not be causally related to changes observed in a second population."

Primary Care Research in Practice-Based Research Networks

Several barriers to primary care research need to be overcome. Among them are "a lack of a critical mass of researchers, competing demands faced by investigators, lack of a research culture, and difficulties in operationalizing practice-based wisdom into researchable theories, measures, and appropriate study designs" (Stange, 1996). The shortage of funding for research in primary care, which Stange attributes in part to the typical "categorical" nature of much research support and which is not in keeping with the generalist underpinnings of primary care, is a major obstacle.

Another major unmet need lies in the area of simultaneously providing sophisticated methodologic training for a relatively small cadre of primary care researchers while also opening up opportunities for large numbers of clinicians to participate in such research (Stange, 1996). Nerenz (1996) also discusses the strengths and limitations of primary care research within integrated health systems. Multidisciplinary collaboration and support for such work must be increased,[6] through mechanisms such as primary care research centers and practice-based research networks.

According to Nutting (1996), studying the relevant phenomena of primary care presents a logistical challenge that might be satisfactorily addressed through the use of practice-based research networks. Analogous to the networks of major tertiary care centers that conduct the great bulk of the nation's basic biomedical research, primary care networks serve as laboratories by which health care events and the health status of many patients might be studied in "real world" settings.

Although less well known in this country than elsewhere, practice-based research networks have operated in other countries for years, often with considerable support from central governments. Niebauer and Nutting (1994) reported that at least 28 such networks now operate in North America. Among them are networks associated chiefly with family medicine that date to the mid-1970s, including the Dartmouth Primary Care Cooperative Information Project (or Dartmouth COOP), the Ambulatory Sentinel Practice Network (ASPN), the Michigan Research Network, the Minnesota Academy of Family Practice Research Panel and the Wisconsin Research Network (WREN). The American Academy of Pediatrics practice network has also been in operation since the 1980s.

Nutting (1996) describes practice-based research networks as having the following four characteristics:

---

[6]A similar argument about the need for and value of multidisciplinary research was made by a recent IOM committee examining issues related to the health services research workforce (IOM, 1995).

1. Capturing health and health care events relating to community-based patient populations;

2. Providing access to the full range of practice experiences of all primary care clinicians;

3. Focusing activities on research questions that are relevant to actual practice, using sophisticated research designs and statistical methods; and

4. Involving in a systematic way the networks' own clinicians in defining the research issues, designing the project, and interpreting the study results.

The committee sees practice-based research networks as a significant underpinning for studies in primary care, noting not only their attractiveness conceptually but the growing recognition of their value as reflected in the rise in the number of such entities in recent years. For this reason, the committee reached consensus on a recommendation that these enterprises should receive high-priority attention and funding to carry out the variety of studies that will contribute to the science base of the future for primary care.

Recommendation 8.3 Research in Practice-Based Primary Care Research Networks

The committee recommends that the Department of Health and Human Services provide adequate and stable financial support to practice-based primary care research networks.

Using Practice-Based Research Networks

Some commentators raise the question of directing such support to primary care research networks, believing that such groups can compete satisfactorily in the traditional investigator-initiated research mode. In the committee's view, however, these types of research networks have been successful in the past and today offer the most promising infrastructural development it could find to support better science in primary care.

Primary care research is not being defined as research solely about problems that exist in primary care; as noted earlier, it is not to be conducted in a vacuum. Rather, the committee is acting on its understanding of the ingredients of an effective scientific enterprise: Scientists have to get the questions straight and observe the relevant phenomena, so that their investigations can be done with reliable estimates of error and bias. Primary care practices, and the research networks that link them, are the sources of the right questions, and they offer an efficient mechanism of relating those questions to the appropriate events that need to be studied.

According to Kerr White (Charlottesville, Va., personal communication, December 21, 1995):

Asking the "right" questions is at the heart of all research. Asking "important" and "researchable" questions is also an essential element of every investigator's basic preparation. Describing the distributions of diseases, conditions, services, interventions, and costs is of great importance. Equally if not more important, however, should be deep concern on the part of the primary care establishment, especially its academic components, with adding to the essential fund of knowledge bearing on the origins of diseases and ultimately their prevention or amelioration. The enormous strengths of biomedical research during the past half century have been its outstanding contributions to our understanding of disease mechanisms and processes and the development of a cornucopia of efficacious interventions. The primary care fraternity in recent decades has contributed precious little to medical science. . . . If primary care is to take its rightful place in medicine and the healing sciences, then it must contribute to fundamental medical knowledge, not just to knowledge about services, education, and training, and about epiphenomena bearing on its own ministrations.

Funding for Research Through Practice-Based Networks

A major concern about these research networks—which in reality generalize to the entire primary care research enterprise—is predictable funding. Stable financial support is necessary for two principal reasons. First, it enables investigators with ambitious and innovative projects to begin and complete them and to disseminate their results. Second, it sends a message to researchers and clinicians (i.e., potential investigators or participants in research projects) that they can have reasonable expectations of a career in primary care research.

The committee did not, in the end, establish a target figure for research funding in primary care. After protracted debate on the point, it did agree on the following propositions. First, the level of funding ought to be proportionate to the nation's outlays on primary health care. The bulk of the medical enterprise in this country lies in primary care, but the bulk of the research enterprise lies elsewhere. The disproportion between that investment (i.e., in basic biomedical research and clinical investigation) and the resources directed at primary care research is extreme, and the committee believed that some redress of this imbalance is in order.

Second, the committee estimated that federal investments in primary care research today total between $15 million and $20 million annually, depending on what is included. This level is one that the committee regards as absurdly inadequate to the task. Although arriving at a realistic figure for federal funding of primary care research was not possible, the committee generally believes that levels of support four to five times the present investment were not unreasonable. An amount of this magnitude, the committee judged, would enable the nation to support useful research projects and, at the same time, begin to build the infrastructure required to carry the primary care research enterprise forward into the next century.

As noted in Chapter 7, the committee recommends an all-payer approach to support education and training in primary care (see Recommendation 7.5). The committee believes that this strategy can and ought to be used to lend some long-term stability to the funding for primary care research as well. One tactic might be to direct a small, specified percentage of whatever sums are raised through an all-payer program for education and training to the "lead agency" specified in Recommendation 8.1 above, for the explicit purpose of broad-scale support of research or more targeted funding of primary care research networks or other centers that may combine training and research.

Finally, although Recommendation 8.1 is directed at DHHS, the committee wishes to go on record as urging the nation's premier health care foundations to promote an even greater level of research activity in primary care. The general cutbacks in federal research dollars are coming just at the time that the need for increased investment in primary care research is becoming acute. Thus, although foundations have played a role in this arena for some years, in the committee's view it is even more important for them to do so now. The committee would encourage foundations that have not been deeply involved with primary care issues to enter the field, and it sees this as a major area in which foundations now being created from former health care provider and payer organizations might have a considerable interest.

Standards for Data Collection

The committee was very aware of the significant problems that occur in using existing data for primary care research purposes. These include consistency of definitions of clinical, health services, epidemiologic, and demographic variables; coding of diagnoses and procedures; and similar data standards problems. These matters extend well beyond primary care; for example, a similar plea for improved coding and definition of minimum data sets was put forward by the IOM committee on emergency medical services for children (IOM, 1993b) and by a different committee concerned with the use, disclosure, and privacy of health data (IOM, 1994b). In discussing the necessary "upgrades" in the primary care research infrastructure, however, the committee concluded that specific attention to standards for data collection that could be promulgated by appropriate authorities in both the public and the private sectors is necessary.

Recommendation 8.4 Data Standards

The committee recommends that the federal government foster the development of standards for data collection that will ensure the consistency of data elements and definitions of terms, improve coding, permit analysis of episodes of care, and reflect the content of primary care.

The issues represented by this recommendation are broad indeed. The committee has commented elsewhere in Chapter 4 and earlier in this chapter about the desirability of conducting research in terms of episodes of care. Doing so, however, calls for better classification systems for reasons for visit (or encounter), diagnoses, and services. This in turn requires that all those responsible for developing databases or recording and reporting health data work from a consistent understanding of desirable (or at least necessary) data elements and of how those data elements are to be defined and described. The difficulties that this set of requirements presents should not be underestimated. As just noted, at least two other IOM committees in recent years have directed a considerable amount of attention to data and data systems (IOM, 1993b; IOM, 1994b), and readers are directed to those reports for more detailed discussion of these issues.

Coding of clinical conditions, diagnoses, symptoms, and complaints as well as services rendered is especially problematic, particularly if the full range of primary care as envisioned by this committee is to be adequately taken into account and reflected appropriately in research data sets. Also likely to be questionable is the information typically recorded on what types of practitioners (e.g., physicians, nurse practitioners, or physician assistants) may have actually provided the services in question. Lacking reliable approaches for defining and coding such information, certain types of primary care research may face considerable methodologic challenges.

A final comment is that the recommendation calls for the federal government to develop standards for data collection. Among the issues that such an effort might address are formal, quantitative or qualitative standards involving reliability, validity, and practicality of data collection instruments and methods. One background guide for such effort might be the recently published criteria from the Medical Outcomes Trust, by which it evaluates standardized measurement instruments in the area of health outcomes (Perrin, 1995). These criteria include specific elements related to: the conceptual and measurement model; reliability (both internal consistency and reproducibility [test-retest and inter-observer or inter-interviewer reproducibility]); validity (content, construct, and criterion); responsiveness (ability of the instrument to detect change); interpretability (the degree to which one can assign qualitative meaning to quantitative scores); respondent and administrative burden; alternative forms of an index measurement instrument; and cultural and language adaptations of an index instrument (Scientific Advisory Committee, 1995). This listing alone makes clear the challenges of adequately meeting the committee's aspirations in this area.

PRIORITY AREAS FOR PRIMARY CARE RESEARCH

As noted above, many issues confronting investigators in primary care are similar to those addressed by health services researchers. The committee wished to highlight certain topics, however, as they relate to the committee's conceptualization of primary care (in Chapter 2) and its view of the settings within which primary care research ought to be conducted. Thus, this section briefly discusses the links that must be forged with elements of the infrastructure discussed above and with other types of research. It then offers a selected set of topics that the committee judged, drawing on the outcomes of its research workshop and its own expertise, warranted early or high-priority attention.

Links to Infrastructure Capabilities

As should be clear by this point, the committee concluded that the scientific underpinnings for primary care are of uneven quality. The mismatch between the scope of, expectations for, and potential of primary care (on the one hand) and the research base that documents those characteristics of primary care (on the other) is considerable. The recommendations offered above for strengthening the infrastructure, visibility, priority, and funding for primary care research are means by which the committee hopes that this situation will be ameliorated. Nonetheless, the committee recognized that resources for primary care research are always likely to be scarce (at least relative to desirable levels) and that priorities need to be set on researchable questions that warrant near-term attention. One way of organizing the myriad suggestions and opportunities for primary care research is to focus on the infrastructure elements discussed already in this chapter.

Having a lead agency is critical to operationalizing the research agenda from the perspective of federal funding. A lead agency might also be especially well placed to foster cross-cutting research projects that link "basic" primary care research with other research areas, such as methodologic investigations of outcomes or patient satisfaction measures or studies of the impact of family support systems or cultural competency on the need for long-term care services.

A national, survey-based data set that captures episodes of care contributes to understanding the epidemiology of health care needs (e.g., incidence and prevalence of disease; utilization of services). Such data files also provide critical information about the access to care that all members of the population (however defined) actually have and about the integration (i.e., continuity and coordination) of health care services. Improved data collection and coding standards, especially if linked to primary care research supported by a lead agency, will reinforce efforts to explore issues relating to the large majority of health care needs. Finally, practice-based research networks are intended to provide the venues in which all of the core elements might be studied, but they would be in a particularly good position to investigate issues of access to care, coordination and continuity, sustained partnerships, accountability, and family and community context; a special point about practice-based networks may be their ability to investigate how various parts of the nation differ in these respects.

Other Linkages

An underlying issue for this committee is the recognition that research in this area requires that health be understood not just in relation to traditional biomedical models, but also in terms of physical and cognitive functioning, emotional well-being, and changing states of health. The concepts of functioning and well-being are multidimensional (Inui, 1996), and this very "messiness" makes primary care research both challenging and rewarding in terms of what can be learned about effective health care. It also calls attention to other important linkages, particularly with health services and clinical research and between physical and mental health.

Links to Health Services Research

The scope of primary care research includes or interacts with other major areas of health services research (IOM, 1995). Among these are outcomes and effectiveness research; quality assessment and improvement; development and dissemination of clinical practice guidelines; a wide array of methodologic questions, including refinement of instruments to measure health-related quality of life, patient utilities and preference weights, and improved methods for severity and risk adjustment; organization and financing of health care delivery and the general area of health economics; health professions workforce (e.g., effective education and training programs, supply and demand modeling); sociological issues (e.g., the role of social support and self-efficacy); and information systems (e.g., uses of computer-based patient records and clinical applications of telemedicine and telecommunications technologies).

Put another way, the above-mentioned topics are not unique to primary care. Rather, they are applicable in many instances to primary care; conversely, research in the primary care arena is likely to contribute to advances in the knowledge base on these issues. For example, the involvement of ambulatory patients is likely to provide insights about patient or practitioner satisfaction or outcomes of care quite different from those emanating from research in the inpatient or long-term care setting.

Links Between Primary Care Research and Clinical Trials

Almost all research and teaching in the United States today are conducted in tertiary care centers. The knowledge derived there, especially from classic randomized clinical trials (RCTs), does not easily apply to primary care. Generalization to the patients seen in primary care practices is difficult because of exclusion criteria commonly set for study populations. For example, RCTs often exclude patients with comorbidities and indistinct conditions, individuals of certain ages (especially the elderly and healthy children) or gender (until recently, especially women of childbearing age), and hard-to-reach or non-English-speaking groups. Furthermore, because of cost and time constraints RCTs must use intermediate (often anatomic or physiologic) end points rather than broad measures of health status, functioning, and health-related quality of life.

These limitations do not fit the model of primary care practice and thus are drawbacks from the point of view of primary care research. Patients seen in primary care settings can present with multiple diagnoses, puzzling complaints, and unacknowledged disorders (e.g., mental and emotional trauma). This comorbidity is part and parcel of the primary care enterprise, and it may or may not be well reflected in classic RCT investigations.[7]

Links between Physical and Mental Health

A particularly important element of primary care involves the fact that emotional and physical problems tend to be intertwined, such that one can only be understood in its relationship to the other and to the context of a patient's life. In a paper prepared for this committee (see Appendix D of this report), deGruy makes the following point:

> Systems of care that force the separation of "mental" from "physical" problems consign the clinicians in each arm of this dichotomy to a misconceived and incomplete clinical reality that produces duplication of effort, undermines comprehensiveness of care, hamstrings clinicians with incomplete data, and ensures that the patient cannot be completely understood.

This committee agrees: Those who can and do take responsibility for the quality of patient care in a primary care setting (indeed, in any setting) must never lose sight of this inextricable, inevitable relationship between the physical and mental domains of health. The lesson for researchers is that they must themselves undertake to examine these domains of health in tandem, especially in projects that relate to continuity and coordination, accountability for quality of care, and family and community contexts.

---

[7]In commenting on this topic, Kerr White (Charlottesville, Va., personal communication, December 21, 1995) observed: "Opportunities to study the origins and natural history of disease through collaborative efforts between primary care investigators and colleagues in various specialties and the basic sciences are abundant. Such collaborative work may be a good way to enhance the research skills of all parties, broaden the portfolio of problems and questions that deserve study by all those parties, and enhance respect for primary care. An added advantage of such work may also be that research into the origins of disease, in addition to research into disease processes and mechanisms, may attract more generous funding from a variety of federal or private sources."

Primary Care and Specialist Physicians

The committee has not, to this point in this chapter, singled out the concept of "primary care clinician" as an appropriate target of research (recalling that the term *clinician* in this context refers to physicians, nurse practitioners, and physician assistants [see Chapter 2]). On numerous occasions throughout the study, however, two questions arose: Who today actually delivers primary care, and to what effect on patient outcomes? Of particular concern was the notion that in the future even more physicians (than is true at present) who are trained and practicing in various specialties and subspecialties will be providing primary care services. In the committee's view, this phenomenon deserves explicit attention as part of a broad primary care research agenda. For that reason, it states the fifth recommendation of this chapter.

Recommendation 8.5 Study of Specialist Provision of Primary Care

The committee recommends that the appropriate federal agencies and private foundations commission studies of (a) the extent to which primary care, as defined by the IOM, is delivered by physician specialists and subspecialists, (b) the impact of such care delivery on primary care workforce requirements, and (c) the effects of these patterns of health care delivery or such care on the costs and quality of and access to health care.

The committee reached this recommendation after reflecting on several trends in health care today, especially the accelerating growth of various types of managed care organizations. First, it has become clear that a good deal of primary care is delivered today by specialists and subspecialists, particularly those in internal medicine and pediatrics. Second, many of these practitioners will likely try to raise the proportion of primary care in their practices, as a result of specialist oversupply (see Chapter 6) and the increasing difficulty of making a career solely in specialty practice. Third, no one can say with certainty what net effects these overlaps in primary and specialty care have on costs and quality (IOM, 1996a).

These issues intersect with some already alluded to, including those relating to access to care, the idea of a sustained partnership between patients and clinicians, and accountability for high-quality health care. The committee judged, however, that the basic phenomenon was sufficiently troublesome to warrant a very high ranking in any primary care research agenda. The reasons are several: problems of quality of care if physicians practice outside their usual areas of competence; questions of the adequacy of "retraining" programs for subspecialists (see Chapter 7); and ramifications for overall physician workforce supply and demand modeling and projections. Also of concern is the appropriateness, from either a cost or a quality standpoint, of managed care systems requiring specialists to (a) choose to be either wholly a specialist or wholly a primary care physician or (b) elect to do both. Finally, the last study of primary care delivered by specialists and subspecialists was the Mendenhall study in the 1970s (Mendenhall et al., 1978a, 1978b; Aiken et al., 1979), when physician supply, health care organization and financing, and other aspects of the U.S. health care system were quite different from those that obtain today. On the grounds of timeliness alone, revisiting these important questions can be justified.

Priority Areas Based on the IOM Definition

If the capacity to investigate primary care were to exist, what would it do? This was a major focus of the workshop organized by this committee in January 1995. To some extent, workshop results echoed earlier AHCPR findings (Mayfield and Grady, 1990; AHCPR Task Force, 1993). The remainder of this chapter identifies high-priority research topics tied to core elements of the IOM definition of primary care in Chapter 2.[8]

Large Majority of Health Care Needs

Documenting and getting consensus on what constitutes the "large majority of personal health care needs" in this country are formidable tasks. The questions (and the answers) differ by population and individual patient—for instance, families without children in contrast to those with children; patients with a chronic disease who do, or do not, have significant comorbid conditions; and rural, suburban, and inner city populations. Different ethnic groups, communities, and individuals may have quite different perceptions of illness and care-seeking behaviors, meaning that uniform definitions of this concept may be difficult to arrive at. Finally, within the full range of health care needs, what rightly belongs in the primary care ambit and what can properly be regarded as specialty care deserves explication.

Health and health services should be broadly defined. Prevention is a principal element, so risk assessment and health risk appraisal are important. Both physical and mental health must be considered. Patients whose basic needs are

---

[8]The points made in this section are deliberately selective and illustrative. Interested readers are also directed to the materials cited at the outset of the chapter as well as to research agendas in related areas, such as aging (IOM, 1991b); quality of care (IOM, 1990; 1994b); and pediatric emergency medical services (IOM, 1993b). The committee draws specific attention to the plans for the AHCPR Center for Primary Care Research (*Federal Register,* 1995). Finally, the February 1996 issue of the *Journal of Family Practice* contains articles about the science base of primary care, some of which pertain to the barriers to and opportunities in primary care research.

palliative or comfort-related (e.g., those with terminal illness), together with family members and other significant persons in their lives, are also an important population, even if the assistance lies more in social services, sophisticated pain management, or respite care than in traditional primary care.

Accessible and Integrated Health Care Services

Access to care. The IOM is on record as supporting universal access to insurance and health care (IOM, 1993a, p. 7): "All or virtually all persons—whether employed or not, whether ill or well, whether old or young—must participate in a health benefits plan." This committee, in identifying accessibility as a core element of primary care, subscribes to this same goal (see Chapter 5). The nation is moving in the opposite direction, however; for instance, Short and Banthin (1995) report that, of persons under 65 years of age who are insured, more than 22 percent are now underinsured for all or part of a year; overall, more than 35 percent of the nonelderly (between 75 million and 79 million persons) have inadequate health insurance today.

Primary care research must continue to examine patterns of use of services by all members of a given population (e.g., a community, a managed care plan, or special groups such as the homeless), with particular emphasis on the care provided to the uninsured and the underserved. The national survey-based data set on primary care recommended earlier would help provide information on (a sample of) all individuals, not simply on users of services. Several special aspects of the access issue warrant early attention:

• To what extent are physical health and mental health concerns and services treated in a parallel manner? More specifically, are services for mental disorders and substance abuse given reasonable parity with those for physical ailments?

• To what degree can certain populations gain access to services in "nontraditional" settings? For example, how available in school-based settings are counseling or preventive services for sexually active teenagers?

Integration of health care services—coordination and continuity. Methodologically, questions in this area lend themselves best to analyses of episodes of care, and practice-based networks may have a comparative advantage for such work. Among the key issues:

• What are the most efficient and highest quality ways to coordinate and combine health care services, taking time, type of provider, type of setting, and patient disease and sociodemographic characteristics into account? For example, what works best for major chronic conditions (e.g., diabetes, multiple sclerosis)?

elective or emergency surgical procedures (e.g., hip replacement)? mental or cognitive problems (e.g., dementia)?

• What impact on coordination and continuity does comorbidity have? For instance, how best might integration of services be accomplished for acute problems among patients with long-standing chronic illness? Would the answers differ for the major causes of morbidity and mortality in this country, such as cancer, cardiovascular disease, acquired immunodeficiency syndrome (AIDS), or violence-related problems among the young?

• What distinguishes an effective primary care team from an ineffective one? What impact does team delivery have on costs, quality, and access?

• What patterns of "substitution" of clinicians are emerging in managed care plans? in inpatient settings such as hospitals and nursing homes (IOM, 1996b)? What effect does such "substitution" have on patient outcomes and satisfaction with care? on provider and clinician satisfaction with performance?

Sustained Partnership

A core element of primary care is the notion that individuals and families will have a "usual clinician" (i.e., physician, nurse practitioner, or physician assistant) with whom they will have a long-standing relationship based on mutual trust and respect. For today's health care market, however, several issues emerge:

• Do most people today have a usual clinician or source of personal health care? Does the answer to this still depend heavily on insurance status and, if so, how?

• What types of usual clinician do various people prefer? What types of clinician do they actually have?

• What responsibilities do patients expect such clinicians to have? What do clinicians themselves see as their responsibilities as a usual source of care?

Part of the appeal of a sustained partnership is the belief that clinicians will come to a deep understanding of their patients' preferences (or, in the research vernacular, utilities) for different health outcomes. Among the topics of interest:

• Does understanding patient preferences derive from, and contribute to, better communication between practitioners and patients? Does it need to involve communication between members of a primary care team? between team members (on the one hand) and families (on the other)?

• Does a better understanding of patient utilities make any difference in the types or intensity of services offered? in the kinds of services demanded or accepted by patients and families? in the health outcomes achieved? For instance, what is the effect of trust (manifested through sustained partnerships) in improving the decisionmaking and outcomes in "difficult" diseases or circumstances, such as schizophrenia or at the end of life?

Accountability for Quality of Care

Traditionally, among the most difficult and contentious areas to conceptualize and measure is quality of care. This becomes especially true as the managed care revolution begins to shift incentives away from the utilization- and cost-inducing ones of the country's traditional fee-for-service system of health care and toward the utilization- and cost-constraining incentives of managed care, and as the language turns more toward informed purchasing and accountability and away from quality improvement. These shifts pose numerous questions, including simply defining accountability, performance monitoring, informed purchasing and clarifying how they are similar to, and how different from, quality assessment and quality improvement.

Measuring and improving quality of care and evaluating quality assurance and quality management programs in health care are crucial to primary care. In 1990, an IOM committee concerned with the Medicare program's quality assurance strategy laid out a research agenda for quality of care that categorized research priorities into one of three stages: basic research, applied research, and diffusion. It called for

> basic research [in] the following topics: (1) variations, effectiveness, and appropriateness of medical care interventions; (2) process-of-care measures for both the technical aspects of care and the art of care; (3) outcomes, health status, and quality of life; and (4) continuous improvement models. Priorities in applied research included: (1) linking process and outcomes; (2) practice guidelines; (3) effectiveness of quality assurance interventions; (4) various setting-specific issues (relating to hospitals, ambulatory care, home health care, and HMOs); (5) rural health care; and (6) the effects of organizational and financing arrangements on quality of care and quality assurance. Finally, with respect to diffusion, . . . the following areas [warrant] continued work and investigation: (1) data systems and hardware; (2) data sharing; (3) data feedback and disclosure; and (4) program evaluation [IOM, 1990, p. 364].

To this broad agenda can be added:

- How best should patient (consumer, purchaser) satisfaction be measured? clinician satisfaction?
- Do patient and clinician satisfaction interact and, if so, how?
- In today's rapidly changing market, who has final responsibility for decisions about adopting new technologies? for abandoning obsolete technologies?
- As more and more tasks are delegated across members of the primary care team, what are necessary skills for use of various technologies and procedures? How can appropriate levels and modes of training help to ensure those skills?

Finding the answers to ethical dilemmas is among the greatest challenges in health care today. It may prove especially demanding for those in the front lines—that is, primary care. Even posing the questions about the mission of primary care, research priorities, and criteria for quality assessment can be difficult when different value systems and models of health care delivery intersect (Lamberts and Hofmans-Okkes, 1996b). Among the questions are:

• Who exactly is accountable to whom in the health plan-clinician-patient triad?
• Are physicians or other clinicians now employed by managed care plans and integrated delivery systems finding themselves in a "dual agent" position, ostensibly accountable not just to their patients but also to the plans and systems within which they practice? How are they to reconcile their duties to systems and to individual patients? How should primary care clinicians harmonize either of those sets of obligations to those posed by society at large?

Family and Community Context

In this committee's view, primary care must be practiced in the context of family and community. In research terms, numerous issues arise:

• How should a "family" be defined or characterized today? a "community"?
• How can proper account be taken of cultural and ethnic differences in a society as diverse as that of the United States?
• What constitutes "dysfunctional" families and communities, and how might these factors affect the way primary care is practiced and the health outcomes expected?
• What role do families and external social support systems play in episodes of care for a particular individual? For instance, what is the impact of social support networks on family functioning and patient outcomes? What role should primary care clinicians play in mobilizing family (or outside) support and involvement in the ongoing care for individuals? What role do they play?

The committee gave special attention to the bond between primary care and public health (see Chapter 5). For research purposes, three sets of topics warrant focused attention:

• What, in today's fiscal and political environment, does the link between primary health care and public health functions actually mean in practical terms? Does this differ by geographic area? political jurisdiction?
• How permeable are the boundaries between health care and public health?

• What "clusters" of problems (e.g., infectious disease, violence, or trauma) can be identified within families? within communities?

SUMMARY

Primary care in the United States represents a largely uncharted frontier, awaiting discovery and exploration. Expanded research in this area is timely because of the accelerating movement toward a variety of managed care and integrated delivery systems, most of which will rely increasingly on primary care models and clinicians. To the degree that this is so, improved primary care that can bring about a better balance between patients' and populations' needs and the health care services they receive is critical.

The science base for primary care is modest, and the infrastructure underlying the knowledge base is skeletal at best. Thus, the committee in this chapter has advanced four recommendations intended to strengthen the underpinnings of a primary care research enterprise. Those relate to (1) federal support for primary care research, including the designation of a lead agency in this effort; (2) development of a national database on primary care, ideally through some form of ongoing survey mechanism; (3) support of research through primary care practice-based research networks; and (4) development of standards for data collection, including attention to data element definition and improved coding. The committee also identified several subjects that it believes warrant high priority in any primary care research agenda. Prominent among these was the committee's recommended study of specialist provision of primary care. Other areas involve major elements of the committee's conceptualization of primary care, such as the large majority of personal health care needs, accountability, and practicing in a family and community context.

This chapter has pulled together the threads of the committee's views about the value, nature, and delivery of primary care into a formidable research agenda and a call for infrastructure development. The final chapter of this report takes those themes, together with the issues raised about the primary care workforce and education and training, to offer the committee's views about how its vision of the future of primary care might be implemented in coming years.

REFERENCES

AHCPR Task Force. *Putting Research into Practice. Report of the Task Force on Building Capacity for Research in Primary Care.* AHCPR Publication No. 94–0062. Rockville, Md.: Agency for Health Care Policy and Research, Department of Health and Human Services, August 1993.

Aiken, L.H., Lewis, C.E., Craig, J., et al. The Contribution of Specialists to the Delivery of Primary Care. *New England Journal of Medicine* 300:1363–1370, 1979.

CBASSE/IOM (Commission on Behavioral and Social Sciences and Education and Institute of Medicine). *Toward A National Health Care Survey: A Data System for the 21st Century.* G.S. Wunderlich, ed. Washington, D.C.: National Academy Press, 1992.

Donaldson, M.S., and Vanselow, N.A. The Nature of Primary Care. *Journal of Family Practice* 42:113–116, 1996.

Federal Register. Department of Health and Human Services, Office of the Secretary. Agency for Health Care Policy and Research; General Reorganization; Statement of Organization, Functions, and Delegations of Authority. *Federal Register* 60:37898–37900, July 24, 1995.

Green, L.A. Science and the Future of Primary Care. *Journal of Family Practice* 42:119–122, 1996.

Hornbrook, M.C., Hurtado, R.V., and Johnson, R.E. Health Care Episodes. Definition, Measurement, and Use. *Medical Care Review* 42:163–218, 1985.

Inui, T.S. What Are the Sciences of Relationship-Centered Primary Care? *Journal of Family Practice* 42:171–177, 1996.

Journal of Family Practice 42:113–203, 1996.

IOM (Institute of Medicine). *Medicare: A Strategy for Quality Assurance.* K.N. Lohr, ed. Washington, D.C.: National Academy Press, 1990.

IOM. *The Computer-Based Patient Record: An Essential Technology for Health Care.* R. Dick and E. Steen, eds. Washington, D.C.: National Academy Press, 1991a.

IOM. *Extending Life, Enhancing Life: A National Research Agenda on Aging.* E.T. Lonergan, ed. Washington, DC: National Academy Press, 1991b.

IOM. *Assessing Health Care Reform.* M.J. Field, K.N. Lohr, and K.D. Yordy, eds. Washington, D.C.: National Academy Press, 1993a.

IOM. *Emergency Medical Services for Children.* J.S. Durch and K.N Lohr, eds. Washington, D.C.: National Academy Press, 1993b.

IOM. *Defining Primary Care: An Interim Report.* M. Donaldson, K. Yordy, and N. Vanselow, eds. Washington, D.C.: National Academy Press, 1994a.

IOM. *Health Data in the Information Age: Use, Disclosure, and Privacy.* M.S. Donaldson and K.N. Lohr, eds. Washington, D.C.: National Academy Press, 1994b.

IOM. *Health Services Research: Work Force and Educational Issues.* M.J. Field, R.E. Tranquada, and J.C. Feasley, eds. Washington, D.C.: National Academy Press, 1995.

IOM. *The Nation's Physician Workforce: Options for Balancing Supply and Requirements.* K.N. Lohr, N.A. Vanselow, and D.E. Detmer, eds. Washington, D.C.: National Academy Press, 1996a.

IOM. *Nursing Staff in Hospitals and Nursing Homes: Is It Adequate?* G.S. Wunderlich, F. Sloan, and C. Davis, eds. Washington, D.C.: National Academy Press, 1996b.

Keeler, E.B., Rolph, J.E., et al. *The Demand for Episodes of Medical Treatment: Interim Results from the Health Insurance Experiment.* R-2829-HHS. Santa Monica, Calif.: RAND Corporation, 1982.

Lamberts, H., and Hofmans-Okkes, I. Episode of Care: A Core Concept in Family Practice. *Journal of Family Practice* 42:161–167, 1996a.

Lamberts, H., and Hofmans-Okkes, I. Values and Roles in Primary Care. *Journal of Family Practice* 42:178–180, 1996b.

Lamberts, H., Wood, M., and Hofmans-Okkes, I., eds. *The International Classification of Primary Care in the European Community with a Multi-Language Layer.* New York: Oxford University Press, 1993.

Lohr, K.N., Brook, R.H., Kamberg, C.J., et al. Use of Medical Care in the Rand Health Insurance Experiment: Diagnosis- and Service-Specific Analyses in a Randomized Controlled Trial. *Medical Care* 24(9 Suppl.):S1–S87, 1986.

Mayfield, J., and Grady, M.L., eds. *Primary Care Research: An Agenda for the 90s.* DHHS Publication No. (PHS) 90–3460. Rockville, Md.: Agency for Health Care Policy and Research, September 1990.

Mendenhall, R.C., Girard, R.A., and Abrahamson, S. A National Study of Medical and Surgical Specialties. I. Background, Purpose, and Methodology. *Journal of the American Medical Association* 240:848–852, 1978a.

Mendenhall, R.C., Lloyd, J.S., Repicky, P.A., et al. A National Study of Medical and Surgical Specialties. II. Description of the Survey Instrument. *Journal of the American Medical Association* 240:1160–1168, 1978b.

Nerenz, D.R. Primary Care Research from a Health Systems Perspective. *Journal of Family Practice* 42:186–191, 1996.

Newhouse, J.P., and the Insurance Experiment Group. *Free for All? Lessons from the RAND Health Insurance Experiment.* Cambridge, Mass.: Harvard University Press, 1993.

Niebauer, L.J., and Nutting, P.A. Primary Care Practice-Based Research Networks Active in North America. *Journal of Family Practice* 38:425–426, 1994.

Nutting, P.A. Practice-Based Research Networks: Building the Infrastructure of Primary Care Research. *Journal of Family Practice* 42:199–203, 1996.

Perrin, E.B. SAC Instrument Review Process. *Medical Outcomes Trust Bulletin* 3(4):1, September 1995.

Povar, G.J. Primary Care: Questions Raised by a Definition. *Journal of Family Practice* 42:124–128, 1996.

Scientific Advisory Committee. Instrument Review Criteria. *Medical Outcomes Trust Bulletin* 3(4):I–IV, September 1995.

Short, P.F., and Banthin, J.S. Caring for the Uninsured and Underinsured: New Estimates of the Underinsured Younger Than 65 Years. *Journal of the American Medical Association* 274:1302–1306, 1995.

Stange, K.C. Primary Care Research: Barriers and Opportunities. *Journal of Family Practice* 42:192–198, 1996.

Starfield, B. A Framework for Primary Care Research. *Journal of Family Practice* 42:181–185, 1996.

Williams, K.N., and Brook, R.H. Research Opportunities in Primary Care. *The Mount Sinai Journal of Medicine* 45:663–672, 1978.

9

Implementation Strategy

GUIDING PERSPECTIVES

The committee believes that the recommendations presented in this report are essential steps toward strengthening primary care as the firm foundation for health care in this country. Chapter 1 presented underlying principles to guide these steps, but only through effective implementation will the benefits of these steps be achieved. Successful implementation will demand understanding of the importance of primary care as a foundation for effective, responsive, and efficient health care. That understanding must be shared by the public, in its capacity both as patients and as those who will ultimately determine the directions for health care in this free society. It will also require a commitment to action by public and private health policymakers and funders, the health professions, health care organizations, and those responsible for health professions education.

To provide focus for the implementation effort, this chapter presents specific means for implementing the committee's recommendations and identifies the many parties whose commitment will be necessary. This plan for implementation is guided by several perspectives that, in the view of the committee, are essential for success.

Mounting a Coordinated Strategy

If primary care is to be strengthened in the directions indicated by this report, simultaneous actions will be required of many parties. The breadth of these actions reflects the breadth of primary care itself, for primary care is multidimensional and inclusive. A comprehensive strategy that deals with these many inter-related dimensions seems more likely to succeed. Focusing on needed changes one at a time is unlikely to be as successful, as indicated by the failure of many prior efforts to advance primary care to have the hoped-for impact. Actions must be focused toward a common objective, and they must be mutually reinforcing. For example, changes in education for primary care are unlikely to bring about desired changes in the practice of primary care unless the changes are reinforced by the organization and financing of services.

The common objective is provided by the committee's definition. The many elements that together can advance primary care toward that objective can be viewed as a system—that is, "a set or arrangement of things so related or con-nected as to form a unity or organic whole" (*Webster's New World Dictionary*, Second College Edition).

Taking a Long-Range Perspective

In addition to this systems view of the challenges of implementation, the committee believes that the strategy for implementation must have a long-range perspective, with action steps that can be taken in the shorter term to advance the strategy. Making intended changes in an enterprise as complex and fluid as health care is neither simple nor quick; continued learning from experience and from the development of new knowledge will be mandatory. The research and data recommendations outlined in Chapter 8 should help provide the means for this continuous learning process over the long term, but in the meantime we believe that we know the direction to take and enough about the needed action steps so that progress can begin immediately.

Taking Advantage of Factors Favoring Primary Care

Many of the actions recommended in this report are intended to shape changes already under way, rather than to mark the start of new efforts. The forces for change at work today can be important potential allies of the imple-mentation strategy. Those forces were described in some detail in Chapter 5.

For example, the growth of managed care and integrated health care systems that emphasize the role of primary care has raised the demand for primary care clinicians thus reducing the differential between the incomes of primary care clinicians and the incomes of medical specialists. Federal and state policymakers have also shown growing interest in the availability of primary care, particularly in rural areas, in the training of adequate numbers of primary care clinicians, and in the removal of legal barriers to the wider involvement of nurses and other types of health professionals in primary care. The rapid development of Medicaid managed care programs, and the likely continued growth of the enrollment of Medicare beneficiaries in managed care arrangements, will continue to merge the interests of government health care programs with the trend toward managed care in the private sector. Primary care seems to be on the rise in the career choices of physicians and nurses, as those entering the health professions read market signals. Educational programs for the health professions are focusing more attention on the preparation of clinicians for primary care.

Although these forces for change can be allies in implementing the recommendations of this report, they tend still to be focused on achieving cost containment and, to a lesser extent, on improving access to basic services for hard-to-serve populations. Demonstrating the value of primary care to patients and to the broader society, over and above its cost savings alone, will require concerted efforts and time to implement the changes described in this report.

Involving Interested Parties in the Implementation Effort

The intended audiences for this report are very broad, and all must play some role in the implementation of the recommendations. They include:

- the health professions whose principal activity is the provision of comprehensive primary care and the organizations that represent them. These include physicians in family practice, general internal medicine, general pediatrics, and some obstetrician-gynecologists; nurse practitioners; and physician assistants;
- the many health professions that have a role in primary care as first-contact professionals for specific functions, such as dentists, optometrists, pharmacists, and others;
- medical specialists who have some primary care responsibilities or whose referral specialty functions require a relationship to and understanding of the appropriate scope of primary care clinicians;
- managed care plans, other health care insurers, integrated health care systems, community and rural health centers, and other organizations providing or arranging for the provision of primary care;
- academic health centers (AHCs) and other educational institutions providing education and training for primary care;
- federal, state, and local governments, which finance care, provide care, support training programs, license health professionals, regulate health care quality and cost, and carry out public health functions;
- employers and employer groups with health care interests;
- specialty boards and other professional organizations that set standards for training and that help define competencies and scope of practice for the professions;
- health services researchers and organizers of health data systems;
- foundations with interests in health care and education, including primary care;
- consumer health advocates (e.g., the American Association of Retired

Persons, unions, rural health groups, and advocates for the poor and populations with special health care needs); and
- the news media.

Reaching such a broad array of audiences with the contents of this report will require more than the publication and distribution of the report. To involve these groups in implementation of the report's recommendations will call for continuing discussions and dialogue about the issues raised by the report and the development of common agendas of action for at least a critical core of interested parties.

A PRIMARY CARE CONSORTIUM

Mission of a Public-Private Consortium

Coordinated implementation by many participants over time is unlikely to take place unless there is in place an entity whose purpose is to monitor and facilitate implementation, including building appropriate coalitions of the parties necessary for action. The committee regarded the creation of such an organization as central to the accomplishment of much of the primary care agenda laid out in the earlier chapter of this report.

Recommendation 9.1 Establishment of a Primary Care Consortium

The committee recommends the formation of a public-private, non-profit primary care consortium consisting of professional societies, private foundations, government agencies, health care organizations, and representatives of the public.

The mission of a primary care consortium would be to facilitate implementation of the recommendations in this report and to coordinate efforts to promote and enhance primary care. The consortium would also conduct research and development, provide technical assistance, and disseminate information on issues such as primary care infrastructure, innovative models of primary care, and methods to monitor primary care performance. These tasks are briefly discussed below. In addition, later in this chapter the committee comments on implementation of all the other recommendations it has made, noting in some instances where the consortium might be a critical factor in success.

Organization of a Primary Care Consortium

The consortium would take the form of a nonprofit corporation, with a board of directors, a full-time executive director, and other staff sufficient to carry out the functions described below. Because both the public and private sectors need to be involved in implementation, the board should include representatives of both public agencies and the principal nongovernmental organizations with interests in primary care.

In addition, the consortium would clearly have an organizational structure, corporate or legal existence, and physical location. It would also be expected to conduct business, articulate a mission statement, promulgate policies, implement procedures, and carry out data analyses.

The organization would seek grant support from government as well as foundations, health care organizations, professional societies, and business and consumer organizations with a stake in health care. Financing from a wide array of sources is desirable to symbolize the consortium nature of the entity. Some of this support should have a relatively long duration, such as five years, to provide needed stability for the long-term tasks.

Functions of a Primary Care Consortium

In addition to its functions of coalition building and of monitoring progress in implementing steps for the enhancement of primary care, the consortium should also have the capacity to conduct research and development. These activities could be supported by targeted grant funding. Among the activities to foster the primary care agenda that might be supported are (a) development of data systems and other infrastructure needs for primary care, (b) development and validation of primary care competencies, and (c) the evaluation of innovative approaches to primary care. Other functions, as described throughout this report, that would benefit from large-scale coordination could also be pursued or sponsored by the consortium. The full range of functions by this consortium could develop over time as needs are identified by the consortium membership and as funding is made available.

The organization would also provide technical assistance to organizations and professional groups to enhance their primary care activities. This technical assistance could help assure that patients in all types of settings and locations would benefit from advances in primary care, not just those being served by large organizations with the internal infrastructure and capacities to take advantage of improved methods. This technical assistance function would include wide dissemination of information about improved methods and approaches for primary care, including but not limited to the improvements developed through the consortium's own activities. This information dissemination function could be a source of information about "best practices" in primary care, an action that might help to overcome the tendency of health care organizations to limit dissemination of improved methods that are providing the organization with advantages in a highly competitive market.

The consortium could organize national meetings on primary care on a regular basis, perhaps annually, that would provide an opportunity to report on progress in implementing the primary care agenda and to share information about new approaches to improved primary care. An example of this approach to developing a field and monitoring progress are regular meetings held to advance the agenda of prevention and to monitor progress toward the health objectives for the nation.

Although such convening and information-sharing activities are sometimes carried out by the federal government, we believe that the mixed sponsorship and governance outlined here is more in keeping with the wide array of interests in primary care that need to be involved. Government is one of those interests, but many aspects of the agenda proposed in this report require action and commitment by many entities in the private sector and at the state and local levels. The federal government is likely to remain an important force through its funding and direct delivery of health care, its support for data and research, its backing for the development and evaluation of service innovations, and its support for education and training of health professionals. The consortium should be useful to the government in carrying out these functions, but its status as an independent, nonprofit entity, with broad participation of the array of interested parties, should help assure that the consortium is not caught up in the specific federal policy agendas of the moment.

IMPLEMENTATION OF SPECIFIC RECOMMENDATIONS

This section offers a brief commentary about implementation of the specific recommendations presented in Chapters 2 and 5 through 8. The comments identify some of the key parties that need to be involved in implementing each recommendation, make suggestions about next steps, and offer observations about the general time frame for implementation. More complete discussion of each recommendation can be found in the chapter in which it was first introduced.

Recommendation 2.1
To Adopt the Committee's Definition

Primary care is the provision of integrated, accessible health care services by clinicians who are accountable for addressing a large majority of personal health care needs, developing a sustained partnership with patients, and practicing in the context of family and community.

The recommendation that health policymakers, professional groups, and AHCs adopt the committee's definition of primary care is crucial, because building coalitions for action on other recommendations will be facilitated if all parties have agreed on a uniform definition of the primary care function. Even disagreements should have more focus if the beginning point of the discussion is the definition as provided in this report. Uniformity in the particulars of implementation by various parties should not be necessary or desirable if all are moving toward a common set of objectives for primary care.

This recommendation should be implemented immediately, although refinements in interpretation will emerge as the definition is used in real primary care situations. The definition should be revisited at some interval, such as five years, perhaps at one of the national conferences convened by the consortium proposed in this chapter.

Recommendation 5.1
Availability of Primary Care for All Americans

The responsible parties for the full implementation of Recommendation 5.1 are funders of health care, both public and private. Specifically, adequate federal and state support needs to continue for primary care delivery systems for those underserved populations that are not yet being served by managed care plans and integrated delivery systems, including rural populations. Implementation of the recommendation falls as well on managed care plans and integrated delivery systems that are serving fully insured populations. Finally, those institutions with training responsibilities need to assure a supply of primary care clinicians that is adequate to achieving the goal of this recommendation.

Full implementation is not likely in the near term. However, progress toward this objective can be made for those populations that have some form of health care coverage or are served by a delivery system targeted to the underserved (such as community health centers and rural health centers), whether funded by the federal government or by community resources such as free clinics.

Recommendation 5.2
Health Care Coverage for All Americans

Recommendation 5.2 bears on most of the other recommendations in that implementation of the full agenda for the strengthening of primary care will be incomplete in its coverage of the population without progress in making some form of health care coverage available for all Americans. At this writing, health care coverage is shrinking rather than expanding, and proposed changes in the Medicaid program may further shrink coverage, particularly for the working poor. Reversal of this trend is unlikely to occur through purely voluntary activity in the private sector as employers, especially small employers, seek to limit their exposure to the costs of health care coverage for their employees. Therefore, as indicated in the wording of the recommendation (see Chapter 5), the federal and state governments bear the principal responsibility for implementing this recommendation. Some of the foundations have served a useful function in exploring approaches to the wider availability of health care coverage, but those experiences indicate that government support is a necessary element of any approach achieving full coverage. Unfortunately, the failure of comprehensive health care reform at the federal and state levels in recent years would suggest that any implementation of this recommendation will be in the long run.

Recommendation 5.3
Payment Methods Favorable to Primary Care

The principal implementers of Recommendation 5.3 are the managed care plans, integrated health delivery systems, health insurance companies, and federal, state, and local governments that pay for health care services. Most of these payers are already using or developing ways of paying for care that are more favorable to primary care than past payment methods. Many of these plans already use comprehensive capitation for at least part of the population covered by the plan. The continued spread of managed care in the private sector and in public financing programs will probably continue the trend toward the development of a variety of ways of paying for primary care under an overall framework of capitation. While some of the aims of this recommendation are already achieved, full implementation is still in the future.

Recommendation 5.4
Payment for Primary Care Services

The action on Recommendation 5.4, which calls for fee-for-service payments to reflect better the value of primary care, falls to the private and public third-party payers. The work in developing the Resource-Based Relative Value Scale (RBRVS), appropriately modified to address its current deficiencies, provides the basis for a payment methodology that reflects more closely the value of primary care services. The Physician Payment Review Commission and the Health Care Financing Administration are likely to remain key participants in the further refinement and application of the RBRVS, but payment innovations in the private sector can also advance this recommendation. Building on work already done, implementation can proceed without delay.

Recommendation 5.5
Practice by Interdisciplinary Teams

Recommendation 5.5 will be realized chiefly through the actions of clinicians and health care plans, health centers, and integrated delivery systems. Payers can use their influence to encourage the use of teams. The role of foundations and the federal government in supporting and evaluating team delivery models has already been important and should continue. The role of the training programs in encouraging team delivery is covered by Recommendation 7.7. Research on primary care teams is included in the research agenda set out in Chapter 8. Implementation is already under way in many settings. Full implementation will require some time and simultaneous changes in the care and the training environments.

Recommendation 5.6
The Underserved and Those With Special Needs

The implementers of Recommendation 5.6 include public and private payers and care programs directed at these populations. Development of methodologies for monitoring access to appropriate care requires actions by the research community and the supporters of research, both the federal government and the foundations. The consortium described above may be able to play a useful role in stimulating the development and testing of methodologies for tracking access. Implementation can begin immediately. Full implementation, however, would require that tracking methodologies be developed and applied, an accomplishment that could take several years.

Recommendation 5.7
Primary Care and Public Health

The main implementers of Recommendation 5.7 are the public health agencies and the managed care plans. Foundations and government could support models of cooperation. The proposed consortium could play a role in encouraging an ongoing dialogue between the public health and the primary care communities so that issues of population-based health can be adequately addressed.

Implementation can begin now. Because of the many organizational and attitudinal barriers to be overcome, and because of the resource constraints that face parties in both primary care and public health, full implementation in many communities probably lies 5 to 10 years in the future.

Recommendation 5.8
Primary Care and Mental Health Services

Primary care clinicians and mental health professionals are the main implementers of Recommendation 5.8, but payment policies and managed care arrangements must be changed. Mental health "carve-outs" are bringing this issue to the fore. The teaching and research communities involved with both primary care and mental health care need also to emphasize the importance of this interface and develop the needed knowledge base.

While approaches to building this important linkage are under way in some environments, historic patterns of practice push full implementation into future years. The work on bringing these systems together requires effort and tenacity that begins in the near term and deals with the major changes in the way that health care is organized and financed.

Recommendation 5.9
Primary Care and Long-Term Care

Recommendation 5.9 identifies the principal parties at interest as third-party payers, health care organizations, and the health professions. Nurse practitioners and geriatricians are a key resource for accomplishing the goals set forth in this arena. Experimentation with funding methods that are a better match for the needs of long-term care patients should continue, as should the development and evaluation of care models. The foundations and the federal government need to continue their support of innovation and analysis for this issue. Given their heavy role in long-term care, the states should become more uniformly active in supporting this innovation and analysis. A barrier to full implementation is the lack of a coherent national policy about payment for long-term-care services, which leaves serious gaps in coverage and pushes much of the cost burden onto the Medicaid program.

The time for full implementation is probably off in the distance. However, further analysis of this issue can begin now, taking the probable revamping of the Medicaid program into account. The substantial role of private foundations in these issues needs to continue, especially because the public sector is frightened by the future expenditure levels and the possibility of movement toward a new entitlement program.

Recommendation 5.10
Quality of Primary Care

The research community, the existing programs for monitoring quality for public and private programs, primary care clinicians in practice, and representatives of the public all need to be involved in developing improved means for monitoring and improving quality (Recommendation 5.10). Support from private foundations, federal and state governments, and health care plans will continue to be necessary. The proposed consortium may be able to play a role in bringing these parties together around a common agenda, backed by the capacity to evaluate current approaches.

Full implementation will be long term. Useful steps by both private organizations and the federal government have already taken place and provide a basis for further progress.

Recommendation 5.11
Primary Care in Academic Health Centers (AHCs)

The major implementers of Recommendation 5.11 are the AHCs and their faculties. Funders of clinical services and training programs in these centers, including state and federal governments, also need to be supportive of these changes.

Many AHCs are addressing these issues today. However, the magnitude of the changes required, the uncertainty of funding for new approaches, and the normal slowness of decisions in a highly decentralized environment (accentuated by a faculty the majority of whom are not interested in primary care) make a longer time frame for implementation more likely, even when commitment by the leadership is present.

Recommendation 6.1
Programs Regarding the Primary Care Workforce

The current funders of primary care training at the federal and state levels, and to a lesser extent the foundations, are the principal parties for maintaining the current level of support (Recommendation 6.1, first part). The training programs and the health care plans are the implementers of the second part of Recommendation 6.1, which concerns improved competencies and access (see Chapter 6), although some continued subsidy of the services to underserved populations is likely to be needed. The actions called for can be immediate, since maintenance of effort rather than new programs is needed.

Recommendation 6.2
Monitoring the Primary Care Workforce

State and federal agencies, and particularly the Bureau of Health Professions in the Public Health Service, are important implementers of Recommendation 6.2. This conclusion derives from their responsibilities as funders of much of the training of health professionals and their traditional role of providing information and analysis about the health workforce. The cooperation and involvement of the professional societies will also be important for this function. Action can be immediate.

Recommendation 6.3
Addressing Issues of Geographic Maldistribution

Federal and state governments and the foundations are the funding sources for Recommendation 6.3, with health care plans and community health centers being necessary collaborators. Action can be immediate.

Recommendation 6.4
State Practice Acts for Nurse Practitioners and Physician Assistants

State governments are the implementers of Recommendation 6.4. The support and assistance of professional groups will also be necessary. Action can be immediate.

Recommendation 7.1
Training in Primary Care Sites

The medical schools are the implementers of Recommendation 7.1. The controlling factor of the speed of implementation is the availability and adequate funding of primary care sites for training.

Recommendation 7.2 and Recommendation 7.3
Common Core Competencies
Emphasis on Common Core Competencies
by Accrediting and Certifying Bodies

Implementation of Recommendations 7.2 and 7.3 will involve primary care clinicians from all of the groups involved in comprehensive primary care, the relevant specialty boards and equivalent professional bodies, accrediting bodies, certifying organizations for primary care training programs, state licensure officials, and educators. The proposed consortium may play a useful role by serving as a neutral site and convener for this function. Support to facilitate this work could come from foundations.

Implementation could begin immediately. The final product, however, is likely to take several years to develop and several more years to implement; therefore, the final result can be looked for only in the long term.

Recommendation 7.4
Special Areas of Emphasis in Primary Care Training

For addressing questions of communication skills and cultural sensitivity, (Recommendation 7.4), the committee believes that the principal implementers are the training programs. Implementation can begin immediately, especially since curriculum development has already taken place to meet these needs in some programs.

Recommendation 7.5
All-Payer Support for Primary Care Training

All-payer support (Recommendation 7.5) would require federal legislative action. Some of the necessary policy analysis has already been done in the context of developing health care reform proposals. Some states might initiate such action themselves through state legislation that provides some form of tax on health insurance premiums.

The full implementation of such a sweeping change will require a supportive legislative environment, absent a major health care reform proposal. Some progress at the margin might be made by negotiation at the state or local level aimed at achieving voluntary cooperation by the major health care plans. Such a voluntary approach to implementation is unlikely to pick up the small insurers, but their share of the market is likely to decline.

Recommendation 7.6
Support for Graduate Medical Education in Primary Care Sites

Federal legislation will be needed to add a requirement for all-payer support of graduate medical education (Recommendation 7.6) to the Medicare legislation. If an all-payer system is devised, the requirement would need to be included in that proposal. Passage of such legislation could be made part of any changes in the Medicare program. Implementation would need to await legislative action, but it could move ahead soon after the legislation passes and necessary regulations are promulgated. This could take several years even if the legislative change is made in the near future.

Recommendation 7.7
Interdisciplinary Training

The implementers of Recommendation 7.7 are the training programs and the various health care organizations that need to provide the training sites in which service by interdisciplinary teams is ongoing. The limiting factor in implementation for some training programs may be the availability of appropriate training sites. The training programs may need to work with primary care providers to create and fund sites where they do not exist. This could delay implementation by several years.

Recommendation 7.8
Experimentation and Evaluation

As listed in Recommendation 7.8, the funding sources for implementation of this recommendation are foundations, health plans, and government agencies. The training programs and the training sites must also be principal collaborators in the implementation. Because interdisciplinary team models already exist in many locales, design and implementation of these experiments could begin immediately.

Recommendation 7.9
Retraining

The participants in implementation of Recommendation 7.9 would need to include the training programs and the certifying bodies for the primary care disciplines. Full implementation would depend on the development of the common core competencies called for in Recommendation 7.2.

Recommendation 8.1
Federal Support for Primary Care Research

The implementers of Recommendation 8.1 would be the Department of Health and Human Services (DHHS), the Office of Management and Budget, and the appropriations and budget committees in the U.S. Senate and House of Representatives. In the current budgetary climate, implementation in the near term will be difficult, but the case is strong for some action now that would not require large funds in the context of the federal budget.

Recommendation 8.2
National Database and Primary Care Data Set

The principal implementer of Recommendation 8.2 would be DHHS, but the committee believes consultation with the health services research community, potential users in the health care system, state governments, and the primary care professional groups will be crucial. Other important actors will be practice-based primary care research networks (mentioned below).

Implementation of the consultation and planning phase could begin within the year. Full development and implementation of the survey is probably at least five years away, assuming that funding is found. This might be an area for collaboration between private foundations and the government.

Recommendation 8.3
Research in Practice-Based Primary Care Research Networks

The agency designated by the Secretary of DHHS as the lead agency for primary care research would be the principal implementer of Recommendation 8.3. Assuming available funding, support could be provided within the year.

Recommendation 8.4
Data Standards

The federal government would have the implementing responsibility for Recommendation 8.4, and the committee expects that a collaborative effort involving the agency designated for primary care research, the Health Care Financing Administration, and the National Center for Health Statistics will probably be needed. Extensive consultation with data experts, health care plans, professional groups, the states, and the primary care research community would be in order in developing these standards. Implementation of the planning and design phase could begin immediately.

Recommendation 8.5
Study of Specialist Provision of Primary Care

The federal agency supporting primary care research and the foundations would need to take responsibility for the design and implementation of the study proposed in Recommendation 8.5. Consultation with appropriate physician groups would be essential. Implementation of the study design and consultation phase could begin immediately.

FINAL COMMENT ON IMPLEMENTATION

With the apparent demise of comprehensive health care reform, the climate for moving ahead on a reform agenda affecting primary care might seem to be unfavorable. Yet, as noted at the beginning of this report, the pace of change in the health care systems of communities around the country remains very rapid. In those changes and the restructuring being proposed for Medicare and Medicaid, opportunities exist to pursue a strategy that holds promise for making the American health care system more effective and efficient. Important parts of the primary care agenda and strategy for implementation proposed in this report do require federal actions. For many elements, however, the key decisionmakers are more diffusely located across the states and communities of the nation, health care plans, educational institutions, and professions. The great private foundations, are also well suited to undertake some parts of this agenda and to engage in collaborative efforts with the other interested parties.

Many of these groups are already committed to a renewed emphasis on primary care. In this situation, opportunities for coalition building and for implementation are at hand and should be exploited. That fact alone is one important reason that the committee has recommended establishment of the primary care consortium.

This is a time when creative effort and collaboration can influence the forces driving health care change to take the directions defined by this committee. It will not be a time for weak hearts or quick fixes—but the promise of improving health care for Americans should be motivation enough to stay the course set out in this report.

Appendixes

A

Site Visits

Location, dates, organizations, and groups with whom the committee met are listed below.

Minneapolis/St. Paul and Rochester, Minnesota: November 13–16, 1994

Minneapolis/St. Paul

Park Nicollet Medical Center
Institute for Clinical Systems Integration
University of Minnesota Institute of Health Services Research and Policy
Hennepin County Medical Society
Health Data Institute
Group Health

Rochester

Mayo Clinic and Foundation

Los Angeles and San Diego, California: February 21–24, 1995

Los Angeles

Kaiser Permanente
Kaiser Center
Center for Corporate Innovation Incorporated

Department of Health Services Facility
San Antonio Health Clinic
Watts Health Foundation
Department of Health Services Facility
Hubert H. Humphrey Comprehensive Health Center
Sepulveda Veterans Administration Medical Center
El Proyecto del Barrio
Los Angeles County Medical Society
Venice Family Clinic
FHP
Mullikin Medical Center—Pioneer Hospital

San Diego

Sharp—Clinical Work Station
Sharp—The Birthplace
Sharp—Gateway Medical Group
Department of Public Health/Children's Hospital

El Paso, Texas, and Albuquerque, New Mexico: April 10–13, 1995

El Paso

Clinica Guadalupana
Kellogg Community Health Education Center
Tigua Clinic, Tigua Indian Reservation
Thomason Hospital

Albuquerque

Ben Archer Health Center
Cuba Health Center
Guadalupe County Hospital
Indian Health Service
Jemez Clinic
University of New Mexico
    Family Practice
    Rural Outreach Committee

North Carolina: April 19–20, 1995

Dinner Meeting with Directors of the North Carolina Office of Rural Health and
Resource Development

Scotland Neck

Our Community Hospital, Inc.

Jackson

Rural Health Group, Inc.

Boston, Massachusetts: July 27–28, 1995

Boston

Boston City Hospital-Boston University
    Center for Primary Care
Harvard Medical School
    Department of Ambulatory Care and Prevention
    Primary Care Residency Program
New England Medical Center
    Tufts University School of Medicine
    The Primary Care Outcomes Research Institute
    Department of Medicine
    Department of Pediatrics
    Division of Clinical Decision Making
    Primary Care/Managed Care
    The Health Institute

East Boston

East Boston Neighborhood Health Center

Brookline

The Center for Physician Development
Harvard Pilgrim Health Plan
PruCare

Framingham

Cigna Health Care of Massachusetts

B

Public Hearing

COMMITTEE ON THE FUTURE OF PRIMARY CARE

8:30 a.m.–4:30 p.m.
December 5, 1994

Mirage I Ballroom
Holiday Inn Georgetown
2101 Wisconsin Avenue, N.W.
Washington, D.C. 20007

AGENDA

8:30 a.m.–8:45 a.m.	Opening Comments and Introduction, Neal A Vanselow of the Institute of Medicine President's Welcome, Kenneth I. Shine
8:45 a.m.–9:40 a.m.	**Panel I**
8:45 a.m.	American Academy of Family Physicians C. Earl Hill
8:50 a.m.	National Board of Medical Examiners Donald E. Melnick
8:55 a.m.	American Society of Internal Medicine Philip T. Rodilosso
9:00 a.m.	Association of State and Territorial Health Officials E. Liza Greenberg
9:05 a.m.	Group Health Association of America Bruce Davis
9:10 a.m.–9:40 a.m.	Committee Discussion

9:45 a.m.–10:40 a.m.	**Panel II**
9:45 a.m.	Association of American Medical Colleges
	Jordan J. Cohen
9:50 a.m.	American College of Obstetricians and Gynecologists
	Ganson Purcell, Jr.
9:55 a.m.	American College of Nurse-Midwives
	Deanne Williams
10:00 a.m.	FHP International, Inc.
	Robert Larsen
10:05 a.m.	Health Insurance Plan of Greater New York
	Jesse Jampol
10:10 a.m.–10:40 a.m.	Committee Discussion
10:45 a.m.–11:00 a.m.	Break
11:00 a.m.–11:55 a.m.	**Panel III**
11:00 a.m.	North American Primary Care Research Group
	Larry Culpepper
11:05 a.m.	Society of General Internal Medicine
	Eric B. Larson
11:10 a.m.	Health Care Financing Administration
	Sam S. Shekar
11:15 a.m.	Agency for Health Care Policy and Research
	Carolyn Clancy
11:20 a.m.	American College of Preventive Medicine
	Michael Parkinson
11:25 a.m.–11:55 a.m.	Committee Discussion
12:00 p.m.–1:00 p.m.	Lunch Break
1:00 p.m.–1:55 p.m.	**Panel IV**
1:00 p.m	American Board of Internal Medicine
	Harry R. Kimball
1:05 p.m.	National Association of Community Health Centers
	H. Jack Geiger
1:10 p.m.	American Academy of Physician Assistants
	Ann Davis

1:15 p.m.	American Osteopathic Association Edward A. Loniewski
1:20 p.m.	American College of Physicians David Babbott
1:25 p.m.–1:55 p.m.	Committee Discussion
2:00 p.m.–2:55 p.m.	**Panel V**
2:00 p.m.	American Academy of Pediatrics Joseph R. Zanga
2:05 p.m.	American Medical Student Association Anne Olinger
2:10 p.m	American Academy of Ophthalmology Fora Lum
2:15 p.m.	American Geriatrics Society David B. Reuben
2:20 p.m.	American Dental Association Kevin J. McNeil
2:25 p.m.–2:55 p.m.	Committee Discussion
3:00 p.m.–4:00 p.m.	**Panel VI**
3:00 p.m.	American Physical Therapy Association Marilyn Moffat
3:05 p.m.	American College of Nurse Practitioners Marilyn Edmunds
3:10 p.m.	American Psychiatric Association James Griffith
3:15 p.m.	American Medical Association Richard A. Cooper
3:20 p.m.	American Association of Colleges of Nursing Geraldine Bednash
3:25 p.m.	American Nurses Association Marilyn Chow
3:30 p.m.–4:00 p.m.	Committee Discussion
4:00 p.m.–4:30 p.m.	Comments from Observers If Time Allows
4:30 p.m.	Closing Remarks from the Committee Chair
4:30 p.m.	Adjourn

WRITTEN TESTIMONY RECEIVED FOR PUBLIC HEARING ON THE FUTURE OF PRIMARY CARE

Academy of General Dentistry
Ambulatory Pediatric Association
American Academy of Allergy and Immunology
American Academy of Family Physicians
American Academy of Neurology
American Academy of Ophthalmology
American Academy of Orthopaedic Surgeons
American Academy of Otolaryngology
American Academy of Pediatric Dentistry
American Academy of Pediatrics
American Academy of Physician Assistants
American Association of Colleges of Nursing
American Association of Colleges of Osteopathic Medicine
American Association of Dental Schools
American Association of Public Health Dentistry
American Board of Family Practice
American Board of Internal Medicine
American Board of Pediatrics
American College of Allergy and Immunology
American College of Medical Genetics
American College of Nurse-Midwives
American College of Nurse Practitioners
American College of Obstetricians and Gynecologists
American College of Occupational and Environmental Medicine
American College of Osteopathic Obstetricians and Gynecologists
American College of Osteopathic Pediatricians
American College of Physicians
American College of Preventive Medicine
American College of Rheumatology
American Dental Association
American Dental Hygienists' Association
American Geriatrics Society
American Group Practice Association
American Medical Association
American Medical Informatics Association
American Medical Student Association/Foundation
American Nurses Association
American Optometric Association
American Osteopathic Association
American Pharmaceutical Association

American Physical Therapy Association
American Psychiatric Association
American Public Health Association
American Public Health Association—Oral Health Section
American School Health Association
American Society of Clinical Oncology
American Society of Hematology
American Society of Internal Medicine
American Speech-Language Hearing Association
American Thoracic Society
American Urological Association
Association of American Medical Colleges
Association of Medical School Pediatric Department Chairmen, Inc.
Association of Professors of Medicine
Association of Program Directors in Internal Medicine
Association of State and Territorial Directors of Nursing
Association of State and Territorial Health Officials
Association of Teachers of Preventive Medicine
Council on Resident Education in Obstetrics and Gynecology
Department of Defense—the Air Force
Department of Defense—the Navy
Department of Health and Human Services—Agency for Health Care Policy and
    Research
Department of Health and Human Services—Substance Abuse and Mental Health
    Services Administration
FHP International
Group Health Association of America
Group Health Cooperative of Puget Sound
Health Insurance Plan of Greater New York
Healthy Mothers, Healthy Babies Coalition
Henry Ford Health System
International Hearing Society
National Alliance of Nurse Practitioners
National Association of Community Health Centers
National Association of Pediatric Nurse Associates & Practitioners
National Board of Medical Examiners
National Governors' Association
National Institute of Mental Health
National Institute on Alcohol Abuse and Alcoholism
National Institute on Drug Abuse
National Public Health and Hospital Institute
National Safe Kids Campaign
North American Primary Care Research Group

Society for Academic Emergency Medicine
Society of Adolescent Medicine
Society of General Internal Medicine
Society of Teachers of Family Medicine
World Organization for Care in the Home and Hospice

C

Workshops

I
AGENDA
Invitational Workshop
THE SCIENTIFIC BASE OF PRIMARY CARE
Institute of Medicine
National Academy of Sciences
Lecture Room
2101 Constitution Avenue, N.W.
Washington, D.C. 20418

January 24–25, 1995

TUESDAY, JANUARY 24, 1995

8:00–8:30 a.m.   Continental Breakfast

8:30–8:40 a.m.   Introductory Comments and Introduction of Dr. Karen Hein
Neal A. Vanselow, M.D. (IOM)
Chair, IOM Committee on the Future of Primary Care
Welcomes
Karen Hein, M.D. Executive Officer, IOM

8:40–10:50 a.m.   SESSION 1
THE NATURE OF PRIMARY CARE
Moderator: *Neal A. Vanselow, M.D.*

8:40–9:00 a.m.   Defining Primary Care: The IOM's Interim Report
Neal A. Vanselow, M.D.

9:00–9:30 a.m.   Keynote: Relationship-Centered Health Care
Thomas S. Inui, Sc.M., M.D. (IOM)
Professor and Chairman
Department of Ambulatory Care and Prevention
Harvard Medical School and Harvard Community Health
  Plan

9:30–10:00 a.m.   What Do We Know About the Content of Primary Care?
Henk Lamberts, M.D., Ph.D. (IOM)
Professor and Chair
Department of General Practice
University of Amsterdam

10:00–10:30 a.m.   A Framework for Research in Primary Care
Barbara Starfield, M.D., M.P.H. (IOM)
Professor and Head
Division of Health Policy
Johns Hopkins University
School of Hygiene and Public Health

10:30–10:50 a.m.   Discussion

10:50–12:00 p.m.   SESSION 2
PRIMARY CARE AND THE LIFE CYCLE:
OPPORTUNITIES FOR INQUIRY
Moderator: *Sheila A. Ryan, Ph.D. (IOM)*
Dean, School of Nursing
Director, Medical Center Nursing
University of Rochester

10:50–11:00 a.m.   Children
Robert J. Haggerty, M.D. (IOM)
Professor of Pediatrics Emeritus
University of Rochester

11:00–11:10 a.m.   Adolescents
Renee R. Jenkins, M.D.
Professor and Chairman
Department of Pediatrics and Child Health
Howard University College of Medicine

11:10–11:20 a.m.   Adults—Women
Vicki Seltzer, M.D.
Professor and Chair
Department of Obstetrics and Gynecology
Long Island Jewish Medical Center

11:20–11:30 a.m.   Adults—Men
Jeremiah A. Barondess, M.D (IOM)
President
New York Academy of Medicine

11:30–11:40 a.m.   The Elderly (Over Age 70)
                   Robert L. Kane, M.D.
                   Minnesota Chair in Long-Term Care and Aging
                   University of Minnesota

11:40–12:00 p.m.   Workshop Participant Discussion

12:00–1:00 p.m.   LUNCH (Refectory)

1:00–1:45 p.m.   SESSION 3
                   PRIMARY CARE AND SPECIAL POPULATIONS:
                   OPPORTUNITIES FOR INQUIRY
                   Moderator: R. Heather Palmer, M.B., B.Ch., M.S.
                   Director, Center for Quality of Care Research and
                     Education
                   Harvard University School of Public Health

1:00–1:10 p.m.   The Urban Poor
                   Roderick Seamster, M.D., M.P.H.
                   Associate Medical Director
                   Watts Health Foundation, Los Angeles

1:10–1:20 p.m.   Rural Populations
                   Marjorie A. Bowman, M.D., M.P.A. (IOM)
                   Professor and Chair
                   Department of Family and Community Medicine
                   Bowman Gray School of Medicine

1:20–1:45 p.m.   Workshop Participant Discussion

1:45–3:15 p.m.   SESSION 4
                   ESSENTIAL FIELDS OF INQUIRY:
                   OPPORTUNITIES FOR RESEARCH
                   Moderator: *Henk Lamberts, M.D., Ph.D. (IOM)*

1:50–2:00 p.m.   Biomedicine—Translating Research to Clinical Practice in
                     Primary Care
                   Catherine D. DeAngelis, M.D.
                   Vice Dean for Academic Affairs
                   Johns Hopkins University
                   School of Medicine

2:00–2:10 p.m.   Health Promotion and Evidence-Based Medicine,
Population-Based and Preventive Medicine
Robert S. Lawrence, M.D. (IOM)
Senior Scientist
The Rockefeller Foundation

2:10–2:20 p.m.   The Whole Person—The Patient's History
Mack Lipkin, Jr., M.D.
Associate Professor of Clinical Medicine and
Director Division of Primary Care
New York University School of Medicine

2:20–2:30 p.m.   The Whole Person—Shared Decision Making
Elizabeth A. Mort, M.D., M.P.H.
Massachusetts General Hospital

2:30–2:40 p.m.   Primary Care in a Systems Context
David R. Nerenz, Ph.D.
Director, Center for Health System Studies
Henry Ford Health System

2:40–3:15 p.m.   Workshop Participant Discussion

3:15–3:30 p.m.   BREAK

3:30–5:00 p.m.   General Discussion (Workshop Participants and Guests)

WEDNESDAY, JANUARY 25, 1995

8:00–8:30 a.m.   Continental Breakfast

8:30–10:15 am   **SESSION 5**
CLINICAL REASONING IN PRIMARY CARE
Moderator: William L. Winters, Jr., M.D.
Clinical Professor of Medicine
Baylor College of Medicine

8:30–8:50 a.m.   *Harold C. Sox, Jr., M.D. (IOM)*
Chairman, Department of Medicine
Joseph M. Huber Professor of Medicine
Dartmouth-Hitchcock Medical Center

8:50–9:10 a.m.   *Walter W. Rosser, M.D.*
                   Professor and Chair
                   Department of Family and Community Medicine
                   University of Toronto

9:10–9:30 a.m.   Reactors
                   Marjorie A. Bowman, M.D., M.P.A. (IOM)
                   Professor and Chair
                   Department of Family and Community Medicine
                   Bowman Gray School of Medicine

                   Rhetaugh G. Dumas, Ph.D., R.N. (IOM)
                   The Lucille Cole Professor of Nursing and
                       Vice Provost for Health Affairs
                   University of Michigan

                   L. Gregory Pawlson, M.D., M.P.H.
                   Chairman
                   Department of Health Care Sciences
                   George Washington University

9:30–10:15 a.m.   Workshop Participant Discussion

10:15–10:30 a.m.   BREAK

10:30–11:45 a.m. SESSION 6
                   A RESEARCH AGENDA FOR PRIMARY CARE
                   Moderator: Henry W. Foster, Jr., M.D. (IOM)
                   Senior Scholar-in-Residence
                   Association of Academic Health Centers

                   Summary of Promising Directions for Research and
                       Overlooked Questions
                   Gail J. Povar, M.D., M.P.H.
                   Clinical Professor of Health Care Sciences and Medicine
                   George Washington University

                   Developing a Research Agenda: Workshop Participants

11:45–12:45 p.m.   LUNCH

12:45–3:15 p.m. **SESSION 7**
BUILDING CAPACITY IN PRIMARY CARE RESEARCH
Moderator: Larry A. Green, M.D. (IOM)
Professor and Woodward-Chisholm Chairman of Family Medicine
University of Colorado Health Sciences Center

12:50–1:00 p.m. Building Capacity for Primary Care Research
Carolyn Clancy, M.D
Primary Care Division
Agency for Health Care Policy and Research

1:00–1:10 p.m. *Mary O. Mundinger, R.N., Dr.P.H. (IOM)*
Dean, School of Nursing
Columbia University

1:10–1:20 p.m. *Paul A. Nutting, M.D., M.S.P.H. (IOM)*
Director, Ambulatory Sentinel Practice Network
Denver, Colorado

1:20–1:30 p.m. *Kurt C. Stange, M.D., Ph.D.*
Assistant Professor
Family Medicine, Epidemiology & Biostatistics, and Sociology
Department of Family Medicine
Case Western Reserve University

1:30–3:15 p.m. General Discussion (Workshop Participants and Guests)

3:15–3:30 p.m. Synopsis
Larry A. Green, M.D. (IOM)

3:30 p.m. Adjourn

II
AGENDA

Invitational Workshop on Roles
Institute of Medicine
STUDY OF THE FUTURE OF PRIMARY CARE

Yorba Room
Four Seasons Hotel
Newport Beach, California

June 12–14, 1995

MONDAY, JUNE 12, 1995

8:00 a.m.–9:00 a.m.	CONTINENTAL BREAKFAST

9:00 a.m.–12:00 p.m. **SESSION 1**
**INTRODUCTION AND PRESENTATIONS OF
ISSUES ON ROLES**
Moderator: Neal Vanselow, M.D.

9:00 a.m.–9:05 a.m. **Welcome and Purposes of the Workshop**
*Neal Vanselow, M.D., Chair of IOM Study
Committee*

9:05 a.m.–9:15 a.m. **Comments on the Clinicians' Perspectives on
Roles**
*Joel Alpert, M.D.
Jean Johnson, RN-C, Ph.D.
Co-chairs of the IOM Subcommittee on Roles*

9:15 a.m.–9:30 a.m. **Introductions of Participants and Observers**

9:30 a.m.–9:50 a.m. **The IOM Study on the Future of Primary Care
and the Committee's Definition of Primary
Care**
Neal A. Vanselow, M.D.

9:50 a.m.–10:15 a.m. **Keynote Presentation**
Roles in Primary Care: Issues and Challenges
Fitzhugh Mullan, M.D.
Director, Bureau of the Health Professions
Public Health Service

10:15 a.m.–10:30 a.m. **Discussion by Participants**

10:30 a.m.–10:45 a.m. BREAK

10:45 a.m.–11:10 a.m. **Reconfiguration of the Health Workforce**
in a Changing Health Care Environment
Richard Scheffler, Ph.D.
Professor of Health Economics and Policy
School of Public Health
University of California at Berkeley

11:10 a.m.–12:00 p.m. **Discussion by Participants to Identify Issues to**
Be Addressed During Workshop

12:00 p.m.–1:00 p.m. LUNCH

1:00 p.m.–5:00 p.m. **SESSION 2**
ROLES AND RELATIONSHIPS OF
PROVIDING COMPREHENSIVE PRIMARY
CARE
Moderator: Jean Johnson, RN-C, Ph.D.

1:00 p.m.–3:00 p.m. **Roles and Relationships in Providing**
Comprehensive Primary Care:
Family Practitioners, General Pediatrics, General
Internal Medicine, Osteopathy, Nurse
Practitioners, Physician Assistants, Other Nurses,
and Primary Care OB-GYNs

How Health Professionals and Other Health
Workers Are Being Used in Real Primary
Care Environments:
Including Examples of Cooperative Models and
Teams

Presentation of Several Case Studies and Vignettes

3:00 p.m.–3:15 p.m.	BREAK

3:15 p.m.–5:00 p.m. **Issues Around the Primary Care Team and the Provision of Comprehensive Primary Care: Directions for the Future**

Discussion

5:00 p.m. ADJOURN

6:00 p.m. DINNER

TUESDAY, JUNE 13, 1995

8:00 a.m.–9:00 a.m. CONTINENTAL BREAKFAST

9:00 a.m.–12:00 p.m. **SESSION 3**
THE ROLES OF MEDICAL SPECIALISTS IN PRIMARY CARE
Moderator: Peter Ellsworth

9:00 a.m.–10:45 a.m. **The Roles of Medical Specialists in Primary Care**
— Mixed Practice
— Principal Physician
— Consultation and Referral

Vignettes and Discussion

10:45 a.m.–11:00 a.m. BREAK

11:00 a.m.–12:00 p.m. **Direct Access by Patients to Specialists for "First Contact"**
Care of Problems
— Differences between First Contact and Primary Care

Discussion

12:00 p.m.–1:00 p.m. LUNCH

1:00 p.m.–3:00 p.m.   **SESSION 4**
ROLES AND RELATIONSHIPS OF OTHER "FIRST CONTACT" PROFESSIONALS IN PRIMARY CARE
Moderator: Richard Scheffler, Ph.D.

Examples of Dentistry and Optometry

3:00 p.m.–3:15 p.m.   BREAK

3:15 p.m.–4:00 p.m.   **SESSION 5**
ROLE OF THE PATIENT AS ACTIVE PARTICIPANT IN PRIMARY CARE
Moderator: carolyn Brown, M.D.

Vignettes
Discussion

4:00 p.m.–5:30 p.m.   **SESSION 6**
IMPLICATIONS OF DISCUSSIONS OF ROLES
Moderator: Joel Alpert, M.D.
— Demand for Health Professionals
— Education and Training
— Organization, Financing, and Infrastructure
— Patterns of Cooperation, Referral, and Coordination
— Legal and Credentialing Issues
(Discussion to be continued on Wednesday morning)

5:30 p.m.   ADJOURN

6:00 p.m.   DINNER

WEDNESDAY, JUNE 14, 1995

7:30 a.m.–8:30 a.m.　　　CONTINENTAL BREAKFAST

8:30 a.m.–10:00 a.m.　　**SESSION 6 CONTINUED**
　　　　　　　　　　　　IMPLICATIONS OF DISCUSSIONS OF
　　　　　　　　　　　　　ROLES

10:00 a.m.–10:15 a.m.　　BREAK

10:15 a.m.–11:15 a.m.　　**SESSION 7**
　　　　　　　　　　　　OBSERVATIONS ON THE WORKSHOP
　　　　　　　　　　　　Moderator: Neal Vanselow, M.D.

　　　　　　　　　　　　Michael Whitcomb, M.D.
　　　　　　　　　　　　Vice President, Division of Education Policy
　　　　　　　　　　　　American Association of Medical Colleges

　　　　　　　　　　　　Catherine Gilliss, D.N.Sc.
　　　　　　　　　　　　Professor and Chair
　　　　　　　　　　　　Department of Family Health Care Nursing
　　　　　　　　　　　　University of California, San Francisco

　　　　　　　　　　　　Karl Yordy
　　　　　　　　　　　　Study Director
　　　　　　　　　　　　Institute of Medicine Study of the Future of
　　　　　　　　　　　　　Primary Care

11:15 a.m.–11:30 a.m.　　**Final Comments and Observations by**
　　　　　　　　　　　　　Participants

11:30 a.m.　　　　　　　ADJOURN

D

Mental Health Care in the Primary Care Setting

Frank deGruy III, M.D., MSFM[1]

INTRODUCTION

In this paper I will make the case that a major portion of mental health care is rendered in the primary care setting, and always will be, sometimes despite strong disincentives; that a sensible vision of primary health care must have mental health care woven into its fabric; that the primary care setting is well suited to the provision of most mental health services; that despite suboptimal recognition and management of mental disorders and attention to mental health, the structure and operation of primary care can be modified so as to greatly augment the provision of these services; and that the efforts under way in the United States to reform the health care system offer an opportunity to find the most effective of these modifications and to discover fruitful collaborative structures both within the primary care setting and between primary care clinicians and mental health professionals.

Most likely this country will retain a parallel primary mental health system. Among the most interesting and complex issues we face are those having to do with the complementarity and integration of services between these two systems, the proportion and makeup of the population that will avail themselves of these respective systems, the factors that affect the interface between primary care and

[1]Frank deGruy is Associate Professor, Department of Family Practice and Community Medicine at the University of South Alabama College of Medicine, Mobile.

specialty mental health care, and the relative cost and effectiveness of mental health care rendered by clinicians within these different systems.

THE RANGE AND COMPLEXITY OF PRIMARY CARE

A Paradigm Problem: The Indivisibility of Mental and Physical Health

I will be speaking of mental health, mental disorders, and mental diagnoses throughout this paper. This convention of language is convenient and powerful and is thoroughly ingrained into contemporary conceptual formulations. It is also fundamentally wrong to speak of mental health as though it were distinct from physical health or health in general; this convention can mislead the unwitting into dangerous and expensive errors. A definitive treatment of this problem would begin with a critique of *Meditations on First Philosophy*, published in 1641 by Rene Descartes, in which he divided reality into two domains, the physical and the mental. Even if such a critique were within my competence, my purpose here is more concrete and practical, and such an excursion would not be justified. Therefore, I will deal with more practical implications. Whether or not it is inherently impossible to portray accurately the clinical reality of primary care within a Cartesian dualism, one of the consistent consequences of this dualism is inattention to the *relationships* between these two domains. In primary care these relationships pervade all aspects of the clinical enterprise. Two implications of this disintegration of the psyche from the soma are salient.

First, let us consider the clinical relationship between physical and mental problems. Mental distress, symptoms, and disorders are usually embedded in a matrix of explained or unexplained physical symptoms, as well as acute and chronic medical illnesses.[1-3] Generally, primary care clinicians deal with mental symptoms as *part* of something—part of a larger, more general problem. The nature of primary care, as we will see in a moment, is integrative. The more pronounced the physical symptomatology, whether or not the symptoms have a physical explanation, the greater the likelihood that a primary care patient has a mental diagnosis.[2] In other words, mental symptoms and disorders are concentrated in precisely those patients who are visiting their primary care clinician for other reasons—physical disease or at least biomedical problems. Conversely, psychologically distressed patients experience increased physical symptomatology.[4] This means that mental illness itself produces symptoms likely to lead one to a primary care clinician. The relationship between physical and mental symptoms is complex and interesting, but I need to note here only that it is inextricable—inevitable. Systems of care that force the separation of "mental" from "physical" problems consign the clinicians in each arm of this dichotomy to a misconceived and incomplete clinical reality that produces duplication of effort, undermines comprehensiveness of care, hamstrings clinicians with incomplete data, and ensures that the patient cannot be completely understood.

The second implication involves patient health beliefs and care preferences. Primary care patients do not view their "mental diagnoses," such as we apply them, as a thing apart from their general health, and they will not tolerate our doing so. One-third to one-half of primary care patients will refuse referral to a mental health professional;[5,6] those who refuse tend to be high medical utilizers with unexplained physical symptoms, but refusers cut across all demographic and diagnostic groups.[7] Securing the consent of primary care patients for clinical trials of treatment by mental health professionals for mental disorders is even more problematic, unless the primary care clinician participates in the protocol.[8] In other words, a certain large proportion of primary care patients prefer to receive mental health care in medical settings, and this is in part because it is not construed as "mental health care."

Thus, one can describe the range of mental disorders that occur in primary care, and this description is accurate inasmuch as it counts symptoms and diagnoses that are actually present. But when seen from the inside, these symptoms and diagnoses are embedded in a matrix of *physical* symptoms, disorders, and diseases; other *mental* symptoms and disorders; and *social* predicaments and stressors. This context completely changes the meaning and consequences of the identified mental disorders and profoundly affects the manner in which the clinician approaches patients who harbor these disorders. It also changes the strategies of the researcher who wishes to gain an insider's understanding of how primary care patients with "mental" disorders appear to those caring for them. Breaking a patient's predicament into a string or list of problems is acceptable only if one continuously takes account of the relationship between the problems, sees the problems as only a part of what the person is, and understands that the patient's clinical predicament cannot be represented by even a complete list of her or his problems. There is an interaction term between every pair of problems. We need never to forget that the whole is greater than the sum of the parts.

I have belabored this at such length because it has important implications for who manages mental disorders, how they are classified, how primary care clinicians are trained to see and manage them, and how we restructure primary care to make incentives and resources available to deal with these problems. It actually has something to do with a core attribute of primary care, despite its bewildering forms: the primary care clinician has a moral responsibility to the person who is the patient. To the whole person. That person *must* be taken as a whole; whether we wish it otherwise or not, that means taking responsibility for mental as well as physical well-being. One aspect of this can be called comprehensive care, and another aspect can be called continuity—continuity in the sense that a physician sees a patient regularly until an understanding of the patient's individuality has taken place. Recognition of this inherent inseparability of mind and body also helps account for the vehement reaction primary care clinicians sometimes have to the news that mental disorders are prevalent and largely undiagnosed in their setting; this implies that they are not taking care of their patients, without acknowledgment of the relatively enormous domains into which they are extending excellent care. This is not to argue that specific mental symptoms or diagnoses do not demand a correspondingly specific set of responses—they do—but these responses are always modified and reordered according to the personal context in which they occur. Mental health care cannot be divorced from primary medical care, and all attempts to do so are doomed to failure. Primary care cannot be practiced without addressing mental health concerns, and all attempts to do so result in inferior care.

The Range of Problems Seen in Primary Care

That being said, there is value in breaking a clinical predicament into its constituents and understanding the constituent problems that are causing such high mischief when they interact: let us step outside the complex web of primary care and break the work of the primary care clinician into component problems. We see from Figure D-1 that no single problem or task accounts for a large proportion of time or resources. This is in sharp contrast to most of the specialties and subspecialties. In other words, one defining feature of primary care medicine is the range, diversity, and sheer number of different problems. I am presenting this figure to draw out three implications:

1. This range has a marked effect on diagnostic behavior. It creates the need for diagnostic categories as inclusive as possible while retaining management specificity—generalists are "lumpers."

2. This range of problems also can degrade the value of diagnostic tests, compared with their value in the hands of specialists, by lowering the pretest or prior probability, and therefore lowering predictive values. This is a warning about applying diagnostic assumptions generated in one setting to another setting.

3. Mental health care is but a small proportion of the range of problems faced by the primary care clinician. By the NAMCS data presented here, less than 3 percent of the average caseload is mental health care. We will see in a moment that this is a gross underestimate, but the point still stands: mental health care is only a part of primary care practice. Most of the patients with diagnosable mental disorders appear under a different diagnostic label and are receiving care for problems other than mental illness. In other words, the primary care clinician is laboring under the burden of competing demands during every encounter; this concept of competing demands will be developed more fully as we explore the adequacy of care rendered to patients with mental diagnoses.

Another piece comes into focus when we "transpose the matrix," as it were, and look at the problem list for each patient. The primary care patient has an active problem list containing an average of six problems.[9] This means not only that primary care clinicians are dealing with many problems other than mental health ones but also that each individual patient is dealing with many problems, some of which are mental in nature.

The concept of comorbidity has come into currency to deal with this phenomenon, and in some measure it does. But comorbidity is merely a list of concurrent diagnoses, which does not adequately account for the interactions between these diagnoses. These interactions increase geometrically with the number of comorbid conditions. Sometimes a more comprehensive, fundamental formulation is necessary to understand adequately the constituent problems and the relationship between them. This has implications for how diagnostic and management formulations are transferred into primary care from mental health specialty settings.

The Range of Mental Problems Seen in Primary Care

A great deal of research has gone into describing the psychological problems of primary care patients; I will summarize the most salient features of this research.

Some 10–20 percent of the general population will consult a primary care clinician for a mental health problem in the course of a year.[10,11]

About 40–50 percent of primary care patients who are high utilizers exhibit significant psychological distress.[4,12] The proportions of pediatric primary care patients with significant psychosocial or psychosomatic problems are about 15 and 8 percent respectively[13,14]

Some 10–40 percent of primary care patients have a diagnosable mental disorder. The PRIME-MD validation study diagnosed 26 percent of primary care patients with at least one of 18 possible diagnoses in the III–R edition of the Diagnostic and Statistical Manual for Mental Disorders (DSM–III–R) (site range, 18–38 percent) and an additional 13 percent with a subthreshold diagnosis associated with significant functional impairment (site range 10–14 percent).[15] The World Health Organization (WHO) Collaborative Study found a prevalence of 21 percent for at least one of their eight possible International Classification of Diseases disorders (site range, 8–53 percent).[16] Mood, anxiety, substance abuse, and somatoform diagnoses account for more than 90 percent of the diagnoses in adults[15,16] Both the PRIME-MD and the WHO studies cited above documented extensive mental comorbidity: nearly one-third of subjects in the PRIME-MD study had three or more mental diagnoses, whereas in the WHO study all but one of the specific mental diagnoses had comorbidity rates above 50 percent.

The Phenomenology of Mental Problems in Primary Care

When a patient having a mental disorder presents to a primary care clinician, she or he usually does so with a physical complaint[1,3] Such presentation results in

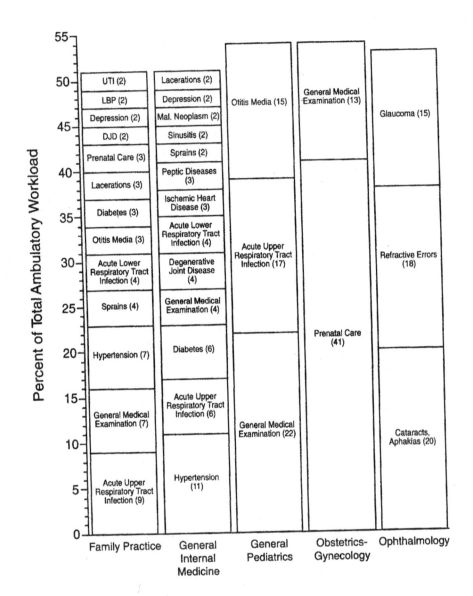

FIGURE D-1 Diagnostic profiles of the 10 largest physician specialities based on all nonreferred ambulatory visits, NAMCS, 1989–1990. All relative standard errors are <30 percent. Values in parentheses are percentages of all visits to the indicated specialty for that diagnostic cluster. Diagnosis cluster key: Acne = acne and diseases of sweat and sebaceous glands; cholelith = cholelithiasis and cholecystitis; depression = depression, anxiety, and neuroses; diabetes = diabetes mellitus; DJD = degenerative joint disease;

Orthopedic Surgery	Dermatology	General Surgery	Psychiatry	Cardiology
Bursitis, Synovitis, and Tenosynovitis (9)	Skin Keratoses (12)	Diabetes (2)	Schizophrenia (34)	General Medical Examination (5)
		Skin Neoplasm (2)		
		Sprains (2)		Hypertension (16)
		URI (2)		
		GME (2)		
		Cholelith (2)		
Sprains (16)	Dermatitis, Eczema (13)	Acne (3)	Depression (47)	
		Hypertension (3)		
		Hemorrhoids (3)		
		Nonfungal Skin Infections (3)		
		Surgical Aftercare (3)		
		Lacerations (3)		
All Fractures and Dislocations (25)	Acne (25)	Chronic Cystic Breast Disease (4)		Ischemic Heart Disease (32)
		Benign Neoplasm (4)		
		External Abdominal Hernias (6)		
		Malignant Neoplasm (7)		

GME = general medical examination; lacerations = lacerations, contusions, and abrasions; LBP = low back pain; schizophrenia = schizophrenia and affective psychosis; skin neoplasm = malignant neoplasms of skin; sprains = acute sprains and strains; URI = upper respiratory tract infection; and UTI = urinary tract infection. SOURCE: Rosenblatt RA. Identifying primary care disciplines by analyzing the diagnostic content of ambulatory care. *J Am Board Fam Pract.* 1995;8(1):41. Reprinted with permission.

recognition of the underlying mental diagnosis about half the time, whereas for the small proportion of patients in whom the presenting complaint is emotional distress or a psychological symptom, the mental diagnosis is correctly ascribed in more than 90 percent of cases.[1]

The mental disorders seen in primary care are probably less severe than those seen in specialty mental health settings; this has been documented most extensively for depression.[17–20]

Primary care patients with mental diagnoses—even subthreshold mental diagnoses—show profound functional impairment. Wells first demonstrated this with the Medical Outcomes Study (MOS) study, in which depressed patients were seen to have functional impairment comparable to patients with chronic medical conditions such as chronic obstructive pulmonary disease, diabetes, coronary artery disease, hypertension, and arthritis.[21] The PRIME-MD data set offers a look at patterns of impairment by specific mental diagnosis and affords a comparison between the relative contributions to impairment of physical and mental disorders. Figures D-2 and D-3 illustrate these findings. One can see that

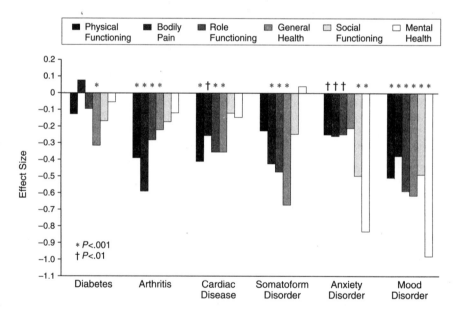

FIGURE D-2 Unique association of common mental and general medical disorders with Short-Form General Health Survey health-related quality-of-life scales. SOURCE: Spitzer et al. Health-related quality of life in primary care patients with mental disorders. *JAMA.* 1995;274(19):1513. Copyright 1995 by the American Medical Association. Reprinted with permission.

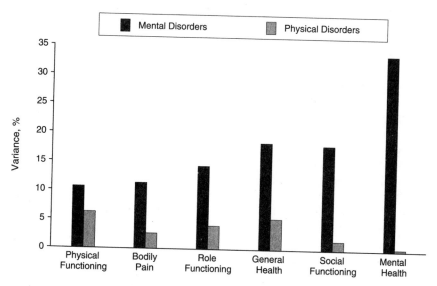

FIGURE D-3 Proportion of variance in Short-Form General Health Survey (SF-20) health-related quality-of-life scales uniquely accounted for by mental disorders and physical disorders (i.e., general medical disorders). SOURCE: Spitzer et al. Health-related quality of life in primary care patients with mental disorders. *JAMA.* 1995;274(19):1513. Copyright 1995 by the American Medical Association. Reprinted with permission.

different disorders produce different patterns of impairment, but they are generally much more severe than those arising from physical disorders.

Patients with mental diagnoses show consistently higher utilization of medical resources than their unaffected counterparts, generally on the order of twice the baseline utilization rates.[22–24] In some cases, such as with somatization disorder, the increased utilization is quite extraordinary—nine times the national norm.[25]

Confounding these differences between the phenomenology of mental disorders in the primary care and the mental health specialty settings are probable demographic differences between patients who seek care in these respective systems: the old, the less educated, the poor, and the non-white—in other words, the vulnerable—are more likely to appear for care in the primary care setting.[21]

Classification: The Web of Comorbidity, Threshold, and the Breakdown of Diagnostic Categories

Up to now, primary care clinicians have lacked an adequate classification system for mental disorders, but quite a bit of work is under way in this area. At this point it is useful to make a distinction between a classification system and a diagnostic system. A classification system establishes categories into which conditions are placed, but the means by which conditions are assigned to one or another of the categories is not necessarily specified. The ICD-9-CM is an example of a classification system; since ICD-9-CM codes are required by all payers for reimbursement of services, it is safe to say that all primary care clinicians use this system. But this system is of little value in advancing our understanding of the nature of mental disorders in primary care, because it contains neither diagnostic criteria nor a systematic framework for clinical decision rules to guide clinicians and researchers in making diagnostic judgments.

On the other hand, the *Diagnostic and Statistical Manual for Mental Disorders (DSM)* is a diagnostic system. It was developed and published by the American Psychiatric Association. The DSM system, currently in its fourth edition (DSM-IV), is the de facto standard in mental health settings; it is also used by many mental health professionals working in medical settings. This diagnostic system has revolutionized the field of psychiatry and has caused an explosion in our knowledge about mental illness, largely by virtue of its explicit, measurable diagnostic criteria. DSM-IV is linked to the ICD system for billing purposes. However, DSM-IV (and its predecessors) has significant limitations when it is used in the primary care setting, and it is rarely used there. The principal limitation is that the DSM-IV is large, complex, and difficult to navigate. It contains much material that is utterly irrelevant to primary care. It does not address with acceptable simplicity mixed syndromes, subthreshold conditions, and the extensive comorbidity found in the primary care setting. Moreover, the natural history and effectiveness of treatment of many mental syndromes in the primary care setting are incompletely studied; it is not at all clear that it is always worthwhile to identify and treat DSM-IV-defined conditions.

A number of diagnostic systems that are specifically for use in primary care are under development. Two of these are worth mentioning: ICD-10-PHC, based on ICD-10, and DSM-IV-PC, based on DSM-IV. It is too early in the development of these systems to assess their utility, but both are enjoying widespread dissemination, and will most likely evolve into forms more congenial to the demands, constraints, and phenomenology of mental distress in primary care. Specifically, these systems are far less detailed and impenetrable than their parent systems; additionally, DSM-IV-PC is organized into algorithms that begin with presenting complaints.

As described in the introductory paragraphs, some of the problems with mental diagnoses in primary care settings are more fundamental than simply deciding which categories to lump together or which criterion symptoms work best in this setting. In some instances it appears that no combination of DSM criteria adequately captures the nature and extent of mental disturbance that occurs in people appearing for care in the primary medical setting. For example, in a study of somatizing patients in three family practices, deGruy and colleagues identified a group of patients who met the diagnostic threshold for no DSM-III-R conditions but who had symptoms across several categories (e.g., mood, anxiety, and somatoform) and suffered significant functional impairment.[26] These patients had been abused and had generally grown up in dangerous, violent families. These patients have important relationship problems, including with their primary care clinician, and frequently appear for medical care. These are patients who require entirely new diagnostic formulations in order to benefit from appropriate research inquiry and clinical ministrations.

A particularly important diagnostic problem in primary care has to do with the comorbidity between mental and medical illnesses. Two-thirds of primary care patients with a psychiatric diagnosis have a significant physical illness.[1,15] It is well established that chronic medical illnesses, taken as a whole, increase the likelihood of depression by two- to threefold.[27] Certain disorders, such as parietal cerebrovascular accidents, are associated with an even higher risk of depression.[28] Depression in a patient who has suffered a stroke is probably different from that which appears in the absence of concomitant physical disease. It is not at all clear that the condition should be labeled depression in both instances. Moreover, as demonstrated in the PRIME-MD validation study, the mere presence of physical symptoms—explained or unexplained—increases the likelihood of a mental diagnosis.[2] Thus, we need diagnostic formulations that take into account this interplay between the biomedical and the psychological and that allow us to address the question of whether conditions should be regarded and managed differently when they occur in the presence of physical illness.

Distress is what usually causes a patient to seek out a primary care clinician, and relief of this distress can be viewed as the hallmark of a successful clinical encounter. Distress has been shown to correlate imperfectly with mental diagnoses. For example, Katon and colleagues showed that only 52 of 119 distressed high utilizers in a large primary care setting met the criteria for a DSM-III-R diagnosis, although 73 percent met the criteria for abridged somatization disorder.[29] This interesting finding underscores the need for careful attention to the patients in the "off-diagonals"—those patients who are distressed without a mental diagnosis (whom clinicians are compelled to care for) and those who are not distressed but who meet the diagnostic criteria for a mental diagnosis (whom clinicians can easily overlook and who may well not benefit from disorder-level therapeutic ministrations).

No matter how refined diagnostic categories and criteria ultimately become, proper management of patients with mental disorders always requires more than diagnostic information. Appropriate management takes into consideration such factors as patterns of functional impairment and patient treatment preferences.[30]

In summary, the current diagnostic systems for mental disorders, developed for use in mental health care systems, are difficult for primary care clinicians to use and are inadequate to characterize the phenomenology of mental illness as it occurs in primary care settings. Although such efforts as DSM-IV-PC and the

ICD-10-PHC appear to address some of these shortcomings, mental health care in the primary medical setting will continue to be problematic until a thoroughly congenial diagnostic system has been developed and management formulations routinely include patient-specific information beyond diagnosis.

The Varieties of Primary Care Practices

Although it is possible to describe the core responsibilities of a primary care clinician and to describe the range of activities and distribution of diagnoses made and managed in this setting, we should note here that such pooled data can conceal the diversity of practice structures and the actual content of practice across these practices. Some primary care practices deal with children only, some deal with adults only, whereas others deal with both; some practices are in urban areas with a wealth of ancillary resources available nearby, whereas others are rural and self-contained; some practices are made up of large groups with in-house resources such as consultant and laboratory support, social workers, and patient educators, whereas others consist of solo practitioners and an assistant or two; some primary care clinicians have practices that emphasize obstetrics, adolescent medicine, geriatrics, or sports medicine; some practices are family-oriented and some are community-oriented; some practices emphasize procedures whereas others refer all patients needing procedures; some are organized around unique cultural needs; some are organized around occupational concerns; some are organized around teaching programs. This bewildering variety does not even take into account the practice variation caused by variations in reimbursement systems, which are discussed below; nor does it take into consideration the differences that follow from physician preferences and a perceived ability to manage mental health problems.

This extraordinary range of practice content and styles reflects creative local solutions to local problems and interests. This diversity of practice content also applies to the provision of mental health care: some practices offer extensive mental health services, whereas others offer few, and the content of the actual offerings is sometimes very different across practices. Any consideration of the future of primary care will need to be inclusive and accommodating of the plurality of individual practices; a narrow, rigid definition of primary care will most likely injure the ability to fit the practice to the problems at hand.

THE ADEQUACY OF MENTAL HEALTH SERVICES RENDERED IN THE PRIMARY CARE SETTING

Diagnosis

More than a dozen studies have examined the rate of recognition of mental disorders in primary care.[31] Even though these studies have used different settings (e.g., community practices versus residency training programs), different patient groups (e.g., adults versus children), different diagnostic criteria, and very different criteria for what constitutes recognition, they converge somewhat on the fact that one-half to two-thirds of patients meeting the criteria for a mental disorder are unrecognized. This rate of nonrecognition is considerably higher when patients present with a somatic rather than a psychologic complaint and when the diagnostic criteria are stringent.[1,3]

Why is the rate of recognition so low? A number of factors have been identified. Badger and deGruy studied the factors related to the recognition of depression among 47 community-based primary care practitioners using a panel of standardized patients and discovered that almost no physicians knew or used the DSM diagnostic criteria for depression.[32] This finding is especially noteworthy in light of the fact that depression is the best known and most widely studied mental disorder in primary care. Thus, insufficient knowledge of diagnostic criteria is one factor related to the low rate of recognition. A correct diagnosis was associated with longer interviews, and with certain patient-centered interviewing behaviors, but not with general interest in psychosocial issues.

There are other factors as well, such as the physician's perception that treatment is effective and that he or she has the time and resources to manage depression effectively.[33]

Rost and colleagues recently published a fascinating paper on the deliberate misdiagnosis of depression in primary care,[34] in which they reported that half of 444 primary care physicians surveyed had deliberately miscoded at least one depressed patient in the previous 2 weeks. The most common reasons for this astounding behavior are worth noting carefully: diagnostic uncertainty, problems with reimbursement, jeopardizing future insurability, and stigma associated with a mental diagnosis. These physicians usually coded a presenting physical complaint rather than the underlying depression. Thus, even when suspected, mental diagnoses are sometimes not recorded because of pressure from insurers and patients not to do so.

Management

Purely on the basis of the rate of underdiagnosis, one could infer that the mental health needs of primary care patients are not being adequately addressed. But the problem is deeper than diagnosis alone; at least a half dozen studies have documented that even when they are recognized and treated, mental disorders (at least depressive disorders) are treated inadequately, both in terms of dosage and duration of antidepressant medication.[35,36] Moreover, several naturalistic primary care studies have shown no difference in clinical outcomes between depressed patients who are recognized and treated and depressed patients who are not recognized; this may be because of the inadequacy of treatment or of the low severity and responsiveness of patients spontaneously recognized.[37–40] In any event, it is clear that simple recognition, although perhaps necessary, is insufficient to ensure adequate care.

There is very little evidence assessing the adequacy of treatment of mental disorders other than depression in primary care. Clinical guidelines for treatment in primary care exist only for depression.[41] We can, therefore, conclude that for depression, treatments that have been shown to be effective for some patients in primary care are underutilized; for other mental diagnoses, treatments shown to be effective in other settings are underutilized, but their effectiveness in the primary care setting has not been demonstrated and may in fact not exist.

Competing Demands and the Tasks of the Primary Care Clinician

One of the major impediments to the successful integration of mental health care into the primary care setting has been the assumption that diagnostic skills (or aids) and management protocols are sufficient to correct this problem. This assumption leads to particularly unpleasant consequences. Primary care clinicians are busy; their days are full; and they are under continuous demand to provide new or additional clinical services. Often, a clinician's inattention to a problem represents not negligence or unwillingness but a rational setting of priorities among a list of competing demands. After all, the average primary care visit lasts 13 minutes,[42] patients have an average of six different problems on their problem list, and they come in with a presenting complaint that demands attention. This is a zero-sum game: there is no room for the provision of new services without either eliminating another service or adding resources to do the additional work. Some glimpse into this predicament can be gained by considering the provision of preventive services. Although family physicians endorse an average of 87 percent of the U.S. Preventive Services Task Force Guidelines, they perform only 20 to 60 percent of them.[43–46] The pressure to render more and more services without compensatory augmentation of resources or elimination of competing demands is particularly demoralizing: 25 percent of rural physicians say they are likely or very likely to leave their practices within the next 2 years, principally because the demands of practice are too overwhelming. Thus, this problem of underdiagnosis and undertreatment cannot be remedied by simple provision of guidelines and protocols, no matter how elegant; it will require a reordering of the actual structure and process of primary care.

Incidentally, this equation might be modified by the demonstration that attention to and management of mental disorders resulted in the expenditure of less time or resources for a given benefit to the patient's health.

The Organization of Services and Incentives

At the present time, there is a rather extraordinary set of forces that collude to inhibit provision of mental health care in the primary care setting. Some of these have been discussed above and will simply be listed here so their collective effect can be weighed.

- Patient resistance to accepting the stigma of a mental diagnosis.
- Somatic presentation of mental distress—patient somatization.
- Inadequate knowledge and skills on the part of the primary care clinician.
- The pace of primary care practice. It has been customary for primary care clinicians to see four or five patients per hour. The enormous weight of prevailing custom, reimbursement, patient expectation, and generalist-specialist relations conspire to maintain this pattern. This leaves insufficient time for detailed psychological assessment or management of mental symptoms. Clinicians may deal with this problem by scheduling frequent return visits for the patient with such symptoms or scheduling occasional longer visits, both solutions that themselves create problems.
- The somatic, biological orientation of medical education. Both undergraduate and residency educational programs tend to emphasize the biomedical, technical aspects of tertiary care. Psychosocial material is devalued as unscientific and irrelevant, or at least of secondary importance.
- Specialist somatization—the insistence upon extensive diagnostic workups for somatic complaints and the pursuit of incidental findings in those patients referred for consultation.
- Psychiatry itself, in its recent preoccupation with brain biology and psychopharmacology, has evolved in a way that is rather unhelpful to generalists. This is not to minimize the enormous value of this orientation, but to point out the vacuum that it has created. Primary care clinicians have lost a theoretical framework for understanding the human predicament and giving meaning to symptoms. Today, there is no coherent medical psychology that is taught in every medical school. With certain important exceptions, psychiatrists are most often called into service to prescribe or monitor psychotropic drugs or to make difficult diagnostic decisions about seriously disturbed patients. This leaves the primary care clinician without support when she or he is trying to understand and deal with the "ordinary" mental distress, disorders, and illnesses encountered in the daily practice of primary care.
- Diagnostic systems that do not fit the clinical phenomenology.
- Insurer somatization—in some instances, reimbursement is forthcoming for biomedical diagnoses but not mental diagnoses.
- Finally, the general manner in which patient services are structured and reimbursed can seriously undermine the capacity to render integrated primary mental health care. These service system-level factors will be discussed in detail in the next section.

Capitation, Managed Care, and Gatekeeping

As our health care system undergoes a fundamental transformation, we find innumerable variations in the structure, resources, and incentives that provide natural experiments for judging the effects on patient outcomes and the health system as a whole. Although we can expect these natural experiments to eventually produce voluminous data, at this time there is much more conjecture and hypothesis than knowledge about the effects of variations in the organization of services. The first task is to outline some of the more salient variations in the organization of services and incentives and to describe their effects on the provision of mental health services in primary care.[47]

The most basic distinction is between fee-for-service, capitated, and salaried clinicians. Within each of these general categories lies an enormous set of variations.

Salaried clinicians represent the simplest category: these people have no incentive to diagnose and manage mental disorders, but neither do they have an incentive to avoid doing so. A complicated or extended patient visit can be accommodated by displacement of subsequent patient visits without financial penalty—unless, of course, the employer controls the scheduling or sets the visit rates. Here we might see high variation in practice style across clinicians, according to their interest in mental health issues and especially according to the productivity incentives that are attached to their basic salaries.

Two features characterize clinicians working under a fee-for-service system: the first is that the system itself is disappearing, particularly for primary care providers. The second is that the effects on the provision of mental health services depend entirely upon what fees are paid for which services. If mental diagnoses are not reimbursable codes, then primary care physicians have no financial incentive to identify, refer, or treat these conditions. If the fee-for-service structure favors procedures over time-intensive talking work, as it has in almost all cases in the past, then again clinicians will be motivated to ignore or avoid mental diagnoses and, when this is not possible, to refer patients having them elsewhere. If the amount of time spent and the complexity of problems addressed are the bases for reimbursement, as they have recently become in the Medicare Resource-based Relative-Value Scale system, then the incentive tips somewhat toward the identification and management of mental disorders. At this point I have located no evidence that addresses the actual effect of this change.

Finally, we come to capitated systems of care and their manifold variations. Capitation has become the de facto standard reimbursement system under managed care and will most likely remain so for the forseeable future. In its most basic form, without any supplemental incentives, clinicians would be motivated not to identify mental health problems in their patients and if identified, would refer them elsewhere for care; if treatment is rendered by the primary care clinician, this system favors low-intensity, short-duration treatments. This presumes, of course, that the cost of identifying and treating mental disorders is greater than any savings in patient care costs to the primary care clinician that might result from these disorders remaining undiagnosed and untreated. There is an active literature on this so-called cost-offset effect, which at this time is inconsistent and controversial; some evidence suggests that identification and treatment save the system money,[48] whereas other findings suggest that it costs money to identify and treat mental disorders in primary care.[49,50] There is little controversy about the cost to the primary care provider, however—such savings as accrue tend to result from lower hospitalization and emergency services, and perhaps specialist visits, but not from a lowering of primary care visits. (There are exceptions to this general rule, such as the finding of Smith and colleagues that a specific management of primary care patients with somatization disorders lowers the use of the primary care clinician's services.[51]) Thus, with some exceptions, identification of mental disorders in primary care is locally expensive, and under a system of straight capitation, the primary care physician will be motivated to avoid this effort.

Of course, the situation is much more complicated than this. Two levels of complexity deserve more detailed discussion. The first is the superimposition of incentives upon the basic capitation structure. The two most common incentives are productivity and quality of care. It is clearly in the best interest of a managed care system to retain clinicians who can see many patients. The "carrot" approach to promoting this end is to offer a financial reward to clinicians who exceed a given volume of patient visits; the "stick" approach is to penalize those who fall below a minimum productivity standard. In both cases this number sometimes undergoes a case-mix adjustment for the complexity of the cases being seen. This incentive structure works against the discovery and management of mental disorders, unless the case-mix adjustment explicitly makes allowance for this added level of complexity. Incentives for quality of care have recently made their appearance; although providing the highest quality of care admittedly costs more money than providing substandard care, it allows managed care organizations to market truthfully their services as being of the highest quality. The organization will generally publish standards of care and measure clinician conformance to these standards. Any condition or set of conditions can be targeted for quality improvement; moreover, there have been innumerable strategies by which the standards are developed and implemented, with important implications for the quality of care rendered. Discussion of these issues is beyond the scope of this paper.

Although there is controversy concerning the cost of identifying and treating mental disorders, there is no such controversy about the value to the affected patients of identifying and treating at least certain mental disorders (such as major depression). Plans that offer the primary physicians an incentive to do this are offering their panel the probability of improved health.

The second level of complexity in capitated systems mentioned above has to do with the manner in which mental health services are organized in relation to primary care services. One option is to *carve out* the resources for mental health care and organize them under a separate system. A mental health carve-out has the advantage of preserving resources for mental health care that might be displaced into other services in an integrated system. Such a system may consist of contracts with private mental health professionals or of a unified, plan-wide mental health center consisting of a team of psychiatrists, psychologists, family and other therapists, counselors, group leaders, social workers, and so forth. All patients identified with mental health problems are referred. The mental health professionals working under such a system may themselves be capitated or may work on a fee-for-service basis; their fees may come from the primary clinician's capitation or directly from the plan. The source and structure of such payment obviously affect the nature and extent of services rendered. For example, a primary care clinician would be loath to refer a patient to an unknown mental health provider for an unknown number of visits if he or she were paying for the referral; conversely, if the mental health carve-out is itself capitated, the mental health professionals have an incentive to function more as consultants and educators for the primary care clinician than as a simple referral resource. Such self-evident hypothesized relationships have as yet little empirical corroboration and will not be discussed further, with one exception. The concept of gatekeeper assumes salience under such circumstances. If primary care clinicians must pay other providers for mental health services to their patients, they have a strong incentive to not recognize mental symptoms, and their role has become that of gatekeeper in the worst sense of the word.

Mental health carve-out systems have major drawbacks and in fact can subvert certain core principles and values of primary care—comprehensiveness and continuity. Carve-out providers have no incentive to reduce general medical costs and may in fact try to shift costs into the general medical sector. Moreover, as mentioned in the opening paragraphs, one-third to one-half of patients referred for mental health services fail to accept the referral, and the refusals generally come from patients who are high utilizers. This creates a cohort of untreated patients purely as an artifact of the system's unwillingness to accommodate them in the primary care setting. Disruption of continuity has been shown to result in less adequate treatment for depression[52] and to result in more expensive and less satisfactory primary care in general.[53] This should serve as a reminder that the artifact of annual enrollment periods, with their characteristic disruption of continuity, injures the quality of care and should be discouraged.

A further useful perspective on this issue can be gained by examining the content of mental health referrals by primary care clinicians. One-half are for V-code diagnoses (usually family relationship problems), and another one-fourth are for uncomplicated mood and anxiety diagnoses. This leads to a fundamental question: Can these problems be managed adequately in the primary care setting? At this time, there is simply no evidence comparing similar patients under carve-out and integrated systems; some data should emerge soon from the enormous numbers of natural experiments now under way with Medicaid populations. However, the MOS sheds some light on this issue, containing as it does 550 patients with severe depression, 44 percent of whom were managed by primary care physicians, 31 percent by psychiatrists, and 25 percent by other mental health professionals.[35] Analysis of these cohorts revealed that the quality of care was significantly higher for the patients treated by psychiatrists than for those treated by generalists, that the cost of care was significantly less in the general medical sector, and that the most cost-effective care could be achieved by shifting some patients from the specialty to the general medical sector and instituting quality improvement measures. This analysis assumed that it was possible to effect a significant improvement in detection and increase the appropriate use of antidepressants. The authors assumed that this would require incentives and resources. But even given these, is it possible to improve significantly the mental health care rendered in the primary care setting? The answer, as discussed in the next section, is an unambiguous "yes."

The alternative to mental health carve-outs is integrated care. As Mechanic argues[54] with the possible exception of patients who are seriously mentally ill, basic mental health services can be successfully managed in the primary care setting. Certainly, integrated primary care has been shown to be cost-effective in general principle. Take, for example, the Pike Street Clinic Project.[55] This was an integrated, multidisciplinary clinic offering services to indigent elderly in Seattle. All services were coordinated through the primary care physician, who functioned as the case manager. The same services were available to neighbors, but the primary care coordination was not there. With comparable outcomes, Pike Street cost $1,000 per patient per year less. In this instance, the primary care was more expensive, specialty care and social services cost the same, whereas emergency care and inpatient care were much less expensive. With respect to mental health outcomes, the most compelling evidence is again related to the management of depression: both Schulberg and colleagues[56] and Katon and colleagues[36] have demonstrated that integrating mental health professionals into the primary care setting to accomplish selected aspects of mental health care results in impressive improvements in patient outcomes, sometimes at minimal net cost. The critical factors related to successful outcomes seem to be application of protocol-level standards of care, the maintenance of the relationship between the patient and the primary care physician, and operation of the mental health professionals within the constraints of the primary care setting itself. These studies are the first of many to come; projects addressing a variety of mental diagnoses and symptoms with an even larger variety of collaborative models of care are under way. At this moment the field is ripe for discovering who to integrate into the primary care team, how to integrate them, and to which problems the team should address itself. These research efforts are necessary to convince payers that such integration is more effective and less expensive than the alternatives.

In summary, most mental health care will be rendered in the primary care medical setting or it will not be rendered at all. Primary care clinicians are recognizing and treating only a fraction of the mental health needs of their patients. The reasons for this are good; the competing demands of primary care are such that additional resources (which already exist and which function outside the primary care system) must be brought to bear on this problem. There is evidence that such resources, if organized properly, could result in dramatic improvement in the functional health of primary care patients, at little additional cost to the system.

THE MENTAL HEALTH SERVICES SYSTEM AND THE PLACE WITHIN IT OF PRIMARY CARE

In some ways we in primary care regard specialty mental health clinicians just as we regard other medical specialists: we each deal with a subset of the other's domain, and each deals with that subset somewhat differently; we view them as resources for consultation and referral for patients with complicated problems, as educators in our training programs, and as colleagues in the general effort to improve the health of the people. These similarities allow us to apply the lessons we learn in our relationships with mental health professionals to our relationships with other specialists. For example, we might expect to see differences in the presentation, natural history, recognition rate, and optimum management for a given diagnostic entity across specialties; we might expect the problem of subthreshold conditions and extensive comorbidity to be an issue; we might expect management recommendations developed in specialty settings to be difficult to implement or downright inappropriate in the primary care setting; we might expect multidisciplinary primary care teams to be useful in augmenting and extending the capacities of the primary care system; and so on.

The mental health system is in some ways unique. To a much larger extent than with any other specialty, there is a primary mental health care system parallel to the primary medical care system. The point of entry into this system is usually either community mental health centers or private mental health professionals, which provide primary mental health care for patients who identify their problem as principally mental. Some of these patients have little or no medical symptomatology, and there is no reason to think that these patients would benefit from having their care integrated into a primary medical setting. Others may have serious or persistent mental illness. These patients are best served by facilities offering multidisciplinary, specialized services such as case workers, psychiatric social workers, and psychopharmacologists. It does not make sense to integrate these resources into ordinary primary care settings, as they would be used too infrequently. However, these patients have a very high burden of medical illness, and their medical care is often haphazard and fragmentary. This is a place where integrating a primary care clinician into the mental health setting makes sense.

The overall care may best be coordinated by the mental health professional, with the primary care clinician serving as a consultant/team member. The concept of a mental health maintenance organization makes sense in this context.[57]

The relationship between primary care and consultation/liaison (C/L) psychiatry is particularly interesting. C/L psychiatrists work in medical settings and thus provide a vital link between psychiatry and the rest of medicine. But very few psychiatrists work in ambulatory medical settings, and even as primary care clinicians are beginning to understand the nature of mental symptoms and disorders in their patients, there is a need for a corresponding psychiatric understanding of these patients that should converge on a single perspective. Given the sheer burden of mental illness in primary care, such inattention can be regarded as surprising. (It must be said that of the few mental health professionals conducting research inside primary care settings, a number of them are producing knowledge of truly outstanding quality.) Formulations conceived from within the context of psychiatric practice are altogether inadequate—the view from within primary care practice is an absolute prerequisite.

Several years ago Strain, Pincus, and colleagues undertook an ambitious survey of the psychiatric training of general medical practitioners.[58] This survey described a rich variety of relationships between the two disciplines, but what was missing was a sense that they were converging on agreement about what was being observed, what needed to be learned, who should teach it, and how the relationship between them should be configured.

Finally, it makes sense to administer some treatments in the primary care setting, but not by primary care clinicians. For example, primary care patients with a preference or an indication for high-intensity services such as cognitive-behavioral therapy or family therapy, patients with chronic diseases requiring extensive patient education and support and perhaps case management, and somatizing patients may benefit from the coordinated, collaborative care of a primary care clinician and a psychologist, family therapist, counselor, social worker, case manager, or other mental health professional. These collaborative arrangements have enormous appeal and offer compelling theoretical advantages, but they must withstand the rigors of systematic evaluation before they can be endorsed without reservation.

SUMMARY OF IMPLICATIONS

Research

We have learned a lot recently about the mental health of our citizens and about the services that we can bring to bear on their mental health problems. However, very little of the research leading to this knowledge has been conducted in the primary care setting. A conspicuous exception to this general statement is the Primary Care Research Program in the Services Research Branch of the

National Institute of Mental Health, which has produced impressive advances in the state of our knowledge for a relatively modest outlay. Since most mental health care occurs in the primary care setting, we have had a profoundly unbalanced mental health research agenda. At this time, the single most effective strategy for improving the mental health of the people of this country and one of the most effective strategies for improving the overall health of these same people would be to make a significant investment in primary care mental health research. The systems are already in place, awaiting our informed modifications and augmentations, to deal with much of the unmet mental health needs in the United States. What follows is a sampling of the kind of knowledge we need to realize this improvement.

- Descriptive work and the need for a new taxonomy, including the following:

—So-called subthreshold syndromes.
—High comorbidity syndromes, such as post-traumatic stress disorder, somatizing syndromes, and mixed anxiety-depression.
—Medical–mental interactions. The relationship between medical illnesses and mental symptoms is bidirectional, or circular, and extremely complex. Since most mental disorders in primary care occur in patients having medical illness, this problem deserves particularly high priority. Unfortunately, untangling these relationships will require expensive, longitudinal cohort studies.
—Expansion of our preoccupation with mental disorders to include other psychosocial factors and syndromes, such as the relational diagnoses.
—Attention to patients with high levels of distress or functional impairment, but without a mental diagnosis.

- The natural history of detected and undetected disorders. There is some evidence that detection of certain mental disorders in primary care does not necessarily result in improved patient outcomes.[37–40] This surprising finding needs to be explored in terms of detection bias, treatment bias, and treatment fidelity to ensure that our attentions are appropriate and effective.
- Development and refinement of outcome indicators, including:

—Health-related quality of life and patterns of impairment.
—Disease-specific outcome measures for mental syndromes common to primary care.
—Patient satisfaction and its relation to cost and function.
—The measurement of continuity, in all its varieties, and the assessment of its effects.
—Utilization, especially beyond primary care services.
—Indirect costs.

—Modifier effects of comorbid conditions.

- Models of service delivery. This should involve observational studies during the innumerable natural experiments now under way, as well as effectiveness trials. We need tests of the effectiveness and cost-effectiveness of different collaborative and consultative modes between mental health professionals and primary care clinicians. These need to be condition specific and also need to take into account local variations, such as rurality, ethnic considerations, and prevailing customs. Wide-angle studies that look at the larger trade-offs involved in augmented mental health services are needed.

Finally, testing the transferability of clinical guidelines and therapies shown to be effective in mental health settings into the primary care setting needs to be done. This has been done for depression, and now needs to be done for the other common primary care mental disorders.

Educational

One of the most pressing needs is for the development of a coherent, consistent medical psychology that can be taught to all future clinicians. This should be in the undergraduate curriculum, as should material on the doctor-patient relationship and communication skills. A demonstrated capacity to communicate effectively with patients should be a prerequisite to the practice of primary care, since the essence of our work involves offering a safe, dependable clinical relationship in which any complaint can be received and evaluated. At the level of postgraduate residency training, there is still no agreement on what constitutes a behavioral science curriculum, how much time should be devoted to it, who should teach it, or how and where it should be taught. This is not to suggest that all programs should have identical, indistinguishable curricula, but that we are suffering for lack of a set of core knowledge and skills we can assume are present in all primary care clinicians. Educational leaders across all primary care disciplines should sit down together and draw up a master document dealing with this issue.

Until now we have depended extensively on specialists to educate us. It is clear that this education will be inappropriate unless we educate mental health educators themselves about how mental health and mental health care is different in the primary care setting as compared to the specialty setting. This is, therefore, a call for the placement of mental health educators and trainees in primary medical settings as a principal site of service. This applies to undergraduate medical education as well as resident training.

As managed care plans develop more stringent expectations about the provision of mental health services in primary care, clinicians will have to change their practice habits. This will require a coherent, sustained educational effort. We have no idea about the most effective way to accomplish this.

Clinical

We must come to terms with what we have learned about mental health in primary care—we cannot unlearn what we have discovered. We must either mobilize our clinical resources to address mental problems or explicitly acknowledge that their prevalence and salience are insufficient to justify the expense and effort that it takes to address them. In some cases, for some disorders, this is probably the best course of action, but the evidence suggests that reordering primary care to accommodate the mental distress of patients would be a good investment.

Therefore, we must proceed to provide the incentives and resources necessary to force a restructuring of primary care along these lines. Nobody knows how to do this yet. For some years this will most likely involve experiments with modified caseloads, interjection of new personnel into the primary health care team, acquisition of skills and tasks by current members of the primary health care team, and new collaborative and consultative relationships with mental health professionals. It will involve the development of clear, explicit clinical expectations coupled with the knowledge, skills, and attitudes necessary to accomplish the expected clinical care. Management guidelines and diagnostic instruments are being developed for the most common mental diagnoses in primary care; now we must learn how to implement these tools into our routine clinical activities. This process will need to transpire under the eye of services researchers, economists, mental health professionals, and primary care clinicians—but mostly patients themselves should decide who will do what to whom.

REFERENCES

1.   Bridges KW, Goldberg DP. Somatic presentation of DSM III psychiatric disorders in primary care. *J Psychosom Res.* 1985;29:563–569.

2.   Kroenke K, Spitzer RL, Williams JB, et al. Physical symptoms in primary care. Predictors of psychiatric disorders and functional impairment. *Arch Fam Med.* 1994;3:774–779.

3.   Kirmayer LJ, Robbins JM, Dworkind M, Yaffe MJ. Somatization and the recognition of depression and anxiety in primary care. *Am J Psychiatry.* 1993;150:734–741.

4.   Katon W, Von Korff M, Lin E, et al. Distressed high utilizers of medical care. DSM-III-R diagnoses and treatment needs. *Gen Hosp Psychiatry.* 1990;12:355–362.

5.   Orleans C, George L, Houpt J, Brodie H. How primary care physicians treat psychiatric disorders: A national survey of family practitioners. *Am J Psychiatry.* 1985;142:52–57.

6.   Von Korff M, Myers L. The primary care physician and psychiatric services. *Gen Hosp Psychiatry.* 1987;9:235–240.

7.   Olfson M. Primary care patients who refuse specialized mental health services. *Arch Intern Med.* 1991;151:129–132.

8.   Schulberg HC, Block MR, Madonia JJ, Rodriguez E, Scott CP, Lave J. Applicability of

clinical pharmacotherapy guidelines for major depression in primary care settings. *Arch Fam Med.* 1995;4:106–112.

9. Lamberts H. Unpublished data from The Transition Project; 1995.

10. Hankin J, Oktay JS. Mental disorder and primary medical care: An analytical review of the literature. *D. No. 5.* Washington, D.C.: National Institute of Mental Health; 1979.

11. Schulberg HC, Burns BJ. Mental disorders in primary care: Epidemiologic, diagnostic, and treatment research directions. *Gen Hosp Psychiatry.* 1988;10:79–87.

12. Ormel J, Giel R. Medical effects of nonrecognition of affective disorders in primary care. In: Sartorius N, Goldberg D, deGirolamo G, Costa e Silva J, Lecrubier Y, Wittchen U, eds. *Psychological Disorders in General Medical Settings.* Toronto: Hogrefe & Huber; 1990:146–158.

13. Office of Technology Assessment, U.S. Congress. Children's mental health: Problems and services. A background paper. Washington, D.C.: Government Printing Office; 1986.

14. Costello E. Diagnosis and management of children in an organized primary health care setting. Bethesda, Md.: National Institute of Mental Health; 1987.

15. Spitzer RL, Williams BW, Kroenke K, et al. Utility of a new procedure for diagnosing mental disorders in primary care. The PRIME-MD 1000 study. *JAMA* 4;272:1749–1756.

16. Ormel J, VonKorff M, Ustun B, Pini S, Korten A, Oldehinkel T. Common mental disorders and disability across cultures. Results from the WHO collaborative study on psychological problems in general health care. *JAMA.* 1994;272:1741–1748.

17. Coyne JC, Fechner-Bates S, Schwenk TL. Prevalence, nature, and comorbidity of depressive disorders in primary care. *Gen Hosp Psychiatry.* 1994;16:267–276.

18. Katon W, Schulberg H. Epidemiology of depression in primary care. *Gen Hosp Psychiatry.* 1992;14:237–247.

19. Johnson D, Mellor V. The severity of depression in patients treated in general practice. *J R College Gen Pract.* 1977;237.

20. Sireling L, Paykel ES, Freeling P, Rao BM, S.P. P. Depression in general practice: Case thresholds and diagnosis. *Br J Psychiatry.* 1985;147:113–119.

21. Wells KB, Stewart A, Hays RD, et al. The functioning and well-being of depressed patients. *JAMA.* 1989;626:914–919.

22. Shapiro S, Skinner EA, Kessler LG, et al. Utilization of health and mental health services: Three epidemiologic catchment area sites. *Arch Gen Psychiatry.* 1984;41:971–978.

23. Williams P, Tarnopolsky A, Hand D, Shepherd M. Minor psychiatric morbidity and general practice consultation: the West London Survey. *Psychol Med.* 1986:1–37.

24. McFarland BH, Freeborn DK, Mullooly JP, Pope CR. Utilization patterns among long-term enrollees in a prepaid group practice health maintenance organization. *Med Care.* 1985;23:1221–1233.

25. Smith GR. The course of somatization and its effects on utilization of health care resources. *Psychosomatics.* 1994;35:263–267.

26. deGruy FV, Dickinson L, Dickinson P, Hobson F. NOS: Subthreshold conditions in primary care. *The Eighth Annual NIMH International Research Conference on Mental Health Problems in the General Health Care Sector.* McLean, Va.: National Institute of Mental Health; 1994.

27. Weyerer S. Relationships between physical and psychological disorders. In: Sartorius N, Goldberg D, de Girolamo G, Costa e Silva J, Lecrubier Y, Wittchen U, eds. *Psychological Disorders in General Medical Settings.* Toronto: Hogrefe & Huber; 1990:34–46.

28. Wells KB, Golding JM, Burnam MA. Psychiatric disorder in a sample of the general population with and without chronic medical condition. *Am J Psychiatry.* 1988;145:976–981.

29. Katon W, Von Korff M, Lin E, et al. A randomized trial of psychiatric consultation with distressed high utilizers. *Gen Hosp Psychiatry.* 1992;14:86–98.

30. Brody DS, Lerman CE, Wolfson HG, Caputo GC. Improvement in physicians' counseling of patients with mental health problems. *Arch Intern Med.* 1990;150:993–998.

31.   Higgins ES. A review of unrecognized mental illness in primary care: Prevalence, natural history, and efforts to change the course. *Arch Fam Med*. 1994;3:908–917.

32.   Badger LW, deGruy FV, Hartman J, et al. Psychosocial interest, medical interviews, and the recognition of depression. *Arch Fam Med*. 1994;3:899–907.

33.   Main D, Lutz L, Barrett J, Matthew J, Miller R. The role of primary care clinician attitudes, beliefs, and training in the diagnosis and treatment of depression. *Arch Fam Med* 1993;2:1061–1066.

34.   Rost K, Smith GR, Matthews DB, Guise B. The deliberate misdiagnosis of major depression in primary care. *Arch Fam Med*. 1994;3:333–337.

35.   Sturm R, Wells KB. How can care for depression become more cost-effective? *JAMA*. 1995;273:51–58.

36.   Katon W, Von Korff M, Lin E, et al. Collaborative management to achieve treatment guidelines: Impact on depression in primary care. *JAMA*. 1995;273:1026–1031.

37.   Schulberg H, McClelland M, Gooding W. Six month outcome for medical patients with depressive disorders. *J Gen Intern Med* 1987;2:312–317.

38.   Schulberg H, Block M, Madonia M, Scott C, Lave J, Rodriguez E, Coulehan J. The "usual care" of major depression in primary care practice. *Arch Intern Med*. In press.

39.   Ormel J, Koeter M, van den Brink W, van de Willige G. Recognition, management and course of anxiety and depression in general practice. *Arch Gen Psychiatry*. 1991;48:700–706.

40.   Simon G, Von Korff M. Recognition, management, and outcomes of depression in primary care. *Arch Fam Med*. 1995;4:99–105.

41.   Panel DG. Depression in primary care. Rockville, Md.: Agency for Health Care Policy and Research; 1993.

42.   Bryant E, Shimizu I. Sample design, sampling variance, and estimation procedures for the National Ambulatory Medical Care Survey. Vital and Health Statistics. Public Health Service; 1988.

43.   Lewis CE. Disease prevention and health promotion practices of primary care physicians in the United States. *Am J Prev Med*. 1988;4(Suppl.):9–16.

44.   Bass MJ, Elford RW. Preventive practice patterns of Canadian primary care physicians. *Am J Prev Med*. 1988;4(Suppl.):17–23.

45.   Woo B, Woo B, Cook EF. Screening procedures in the asymptomatic adult: a comparison of physicians' recommendations, patients' desire, published guidelines, and actual practice. *JAMA*. 1985;254:1480–1484.

46.   Romm FJ, Fletcher SW, Hulka BS. The periodic health examination: comparison of recommendations and internists' performance. *South Med J*. 1981;74:265–271.

47.   Pincus HA. Assessing the effects of physician payment on treatment of mental disorders in primary care. *Gen Hosp Psychiatry*. 1990;12:23–29.

48.   Richman A. Does psychiatric care by family practitioners reduce the cost of general medical care? *Gen Hosp Psychiatry*. 1990;12:19–22.

49.   Hankin JR, Kessler LG, Goldberg ID, Steinwachs DM, Starfield BH. A longitudinal study of offset in the use of nonpsychiatric services following specialized mental health care. *Medical Care*. 1983;21:1099–1110.

50.   Von Korff M, Katon W, Lin E, et al. Evaluation of cost and cost offset of collaborative management of depressed patients in primary care. *The Eighth Annual NIMH International Research Conference on Mental Health Problems in the General Health Care Sector*. McLean, Va.: National Institute of Mental Health; 1994.

51.   Smith GR, Rost K, Kashner TM. A trial of the effect of a standardized psychiatric consultation on health outcomes and costs in somatizing patients. *Arch Gen Psychiatry*. 1995;52:238–243.

52.   Rogers WH, Wells KB, Meredith LS, Sturm R, Burnam MA. Outcomes for adult outpatients with depression under prepaid or fee-for-service financing. *Arch Gen Psychiatry*. 1993;50:1002–1003.

53.   Wasson JH, Sauvigne AE, Mogielnicki RP, et al. Continuity of outpatient medical care in elderly men: A randomized trial. *JAMA*. 1984;252:2413–2417.

54.   Mechanic D. Integrating mental health into a general health care system. *Hosp Community Psychiatry*. 1994;45:893–897.

55.   Baldwin L, Inui TS, Steinkamp S. The effect of coordinated, multidisciplinary ambulatory care on service use, charges, quality of care, and patient satisfaction in the elderly. *J Community Health*. 1993;18:95–108.

56.   Schulberg HC, Madonia MJ, Block MR, et al. Major depression in primary care practice: Clinical characteristics and treatment implications. *Psychosomatics*. 1995;36:129–137.

57.   Scheffler R, Grogan C, Cuffel B, Penner S. A specialized mental health plan for persons with severe mental illness under managed competition. *Hosp Community Psychiatry*. 1993;44:937–942.

58.   Strain JJ, Pincus HA, Gise LH, Houpt JL. The role of psychiatry in the training of primary care physicians. *Gen Hosp Psychiatry*. 1986;8:372–385.

E

Life in the Kaleidoscope: The Impact of Managed Care on the U.S. Health Care Workforce and a New Model for the Delivery of Primary Care

Richard M. Scheffler, Ph.D.

ABSTRACT

Market forces are producing dramatic changes in health care financing and delivery mechanisms. Payment systems are rapidly moving away from fee for service to capitation and risk sharing between payers and providers. These changes are likely to result in a major reconfiguration of the health care workforce over the next few decades. In the world before managed care, individual physicians and hospitals were the system's principal billing units and workforce research focused primarily on physicians. In the world after managed care, group practices and organized delivery systems are the principal billing units and physicians are one of a number of clinicians on a team of health care professionals. Application of managed care organization staffing ratios to the entire delivery system implies significant physician surpluses (particularly specialists) and short-

Supported in part by the Bureau of Health Professions, Resources and Health Services Administration, Department of Health and Human Services.

Richard S. Scheffler is professor of health economics and public policy at the School of Public Health and the Graduate School of Public Policy, University of California, Berkeley. Dr. Scheffler earned a Ph.D. in economics at New York University. His published research includes studies of health care workforce policy, managed care, the economics of preventive health measures, and mental health care delivery systems. Dr. Scheffler is currently a member of the Institute of Medicine Committee on the Future of Primary Care and co-author (with Norman S. Waitzman) of a forthcoming book on the physician workforce in the era of managed care.

ages of nurse practitioners and physician assistants. Successful development of the team delivery concept will require development of economic incentive systems that reward team effort. To stimulate thought about the challenges that a team concept produces, this paper presents an innovative model of team health production. Finally, the workforce modification suggests the need for an ambitious research agenda: one that deals with micro- and macro-issues of team and workforce composition, organizational forms and incentives, practice context, and overall health care policy.

INTRODUCTION

In response to the projected excess supply of physician specialists,[1] the rapid growth of managed care,[2] and continued pressure to limit increases in health care costs, the organization of the U.S. health care workforce is likely to undergo dramatic change over the next few decades. Virtually all of the major workforce components are subject to reconfiguration. In broad terms, what will this reconfiguration look like? What are the implications of this reconfiguration for the previously established ideas about how to assess health workforce needs? What should a research agenda for the next few decades look like at this stage of the reconfiguration?

This paper addresses these questions with a special emphasis on primary care as defined by the Institute of Medicine (Institute of Medicine, 1994). The IOM definition emphasizes the integration of services and supports the team delivery of primary care.[3]

> Primary care is the provision of integrated, accessible health care services by clinicians who are accountable for addressing a large majority of personal health care needs, developing a sustained partnership with patients, and practicing in the context of family and community (Institute of Medicine, 1994, p. 1).

---

[1] Although most recent forecasts of physician supply have predicted a surplus of physician specialists (Gamliel et al., 1995; Kohler, 1994), some researchers believe that advancements in medical technology and other factors will create shortages of physicians (Schwartz, Sloan, and Mendelson, 1988; Schwartz and Mendelson, 1990). As explained elsewhere in this paper, projections of the size and composition of the future health care workforce are sensitive to assumptions about patient utilization patterns, use of nonphysician clinicians, and other factors.

[2] For the purposes of this paper, managed care is defined as health plans and products that involve the integration of health care financing and delivery systems.

[3] Although this definition does not explicitly mention teams, Chapter 2 of the 1994 IOM report discusses the importance of team structures in primary care (Institute of Medicine, 1994). "Team" is a broad term that connotes a collaborative grouping of individuals whose clinical, managerial, and interpersonal skills can be brought to bear on individual or family health. The composition of the team will vary according to the type of individual or population served. Although teams are often organized in a hierarchical manner, IOM conceives of teams as more democratic, interdisciplinary structures in which clinicians rotate leadership and accountability depending on the patient situation.

Integration is the key term because it reflects ongoing structural changes in the health care system (Physician Payment Review Commission, 1995). However, this term has multiple meanings. It can connote the integration of primary care and specialty care, the merger of inpatient and outpatient treatment, or a combination of organizational structures and financial incentives such as group practice with capitation (Shortell and Hull, 1995; Shortell, Gillies, and Anderson, 1994). Economists typically view integration in efficiency terms: how do we organize the health workforce in an efficient way without sacrificing quality of care? This is an ambitious goal, but one for which governments, employers, and the public are striving.

It is useful to classify relationships among workforce components in terms that turn on the notion of skills: (1) What is the set of skills unique to each type of clinician? (2) What set of skills can more than one clinician use? (3) What sets of skills are interdependent (i.e., skills that require more than one health care worker)? The first set contains specific skills, the second contains substitutional skills, and the third contains complementary skills. Skill, as defined here, involves clinical, interpersonal, and organization or management competencies.

The relative economic returns to each type of skill since the 1980s after managed care (AMC) are likely to be much different than those prior to the 1980s before managed care (BMC). BMC, the health care workforce functioned in a fee for service (FFS), patient self-referral, and physician-specialty-dominated system. AMC, the health care workforce copes with capitated payment and managed-patient referrals, and strives to integrate primary care and specialty care.

THE HEALTH CARE WORKFORCE BMC AND AMC

BMC, the health system was characterized by few payer restrictions on patient choice of providers, independent provider billing units, and open-ended FFS payment. Patients freely chose the providers whom they believed would provide the best care; freestanding physicians, hospitals, and other providers did the billing; and insurance plans paid virtually all provider bills (Enthoven, 1987; Pauly, 1970). Because insurance payment schedules favored highly specialized, procedure-based skills, this system rewarded specialty over primary care (Delbanco, Meyers, and Segal, 1979; Roe, 1981).

The health system BMC supported nonphysician clinicians to a limited degree. In the 1970s it began to train and license significant numbers of nurse practitioners (NPs) and physician assistants (PAs).[4] However, because of physician resistance, legal restrictions, and other barriers, NPs and PAs were delegated

---

[4]Another important category of nonphysician clinicians is certified nurse-midwives (CNMs). This paper emphasizes the role of NPs and PAs in primary care because the literature on CNMs is relatively limited (Scheffler, 1995).

a very limited set of clinical tasks and payment systems ignored complementary skills. NP and PA substitution also did not generate significant economic rewards for physicians, because substitution could result in smaller payments. However, substitution did make economic sense where there were shortages of physicians or, in some rare circumstances, where increased throughput could offset reduced payments (Safriet, 1992; U.S. Congress, Office of Technology Assessment, 1986).

Workforce policy debates of the 1960s, 1970s, and 1980s focused primarily on physician supply issues (Fein, 1967; Ginzberg, 1978; Ginzberg and Ostow, 1984; Scheffler et al., 1978; Schwartz, Sloan, and Mendelson, 1988). The debate dealt with numbers: How many more doctors did we need? Was there a surplus or shortage of primary care doctors or specialists? BMC, the emphasis on physicians made sense, particularly from an economic perspective. However, as discussed later, the focus on physicians is attenuated in the AMC world.

In the AMC world, the predominant payment mode is capitation, patient choice of providers is more restricted, and payers or primary care case managers control access to specialists and hospitals. Under managed care, the financing and delivery of care are integrated, and the billing unit is more likely to be a group practice or network of providers, rather than a solo-practice physician or individual hospital (Physician Payment Review Commission, 1995; Shortell and Hull, 1995).

A long-run-oriented managed care organization under capitation has a strong incentive to find the most efficient combination of health care professionals to deliver quality care to an enrolled population.[5] As explained below, in the AMC world collaborative practice among diverse teams of clinicians, rather than a physician specialist orientation, begins to make economic sense. Consequently, PAs and NPs could have a much more important role to play in the AMC health care system.[6]

---

[5]Although virtually all HMO plans receive capitated payments from employers and other health care purchasers, the methods that organizational billing units use to reallocate financial risks to individual physicians are not well understood. Surveys suggest that approximately 35 to 40 percent of HMOs still pay their primary care physicians by FFS. Also, preferred provider and point-of-service plans, which are growing more popular, currently tend to use modified FFS to pay physicians (Gold et al., 1995). Under FFS, incentives for physician practices to use NPs and PAs may be reduced. Nevertheless, managed care physician payment systems appear to be moving away from FFS toward greater use of capitation, particularly in the larger managed care markets (InterStudy, Inc., 1995).

[6]In their discussion of redesigned nursing care processes, Schneller and Ott (1996) note the advantages of a multiprofessional division of labor that is based on continuous quality improvement and total quality management principles.

THE SUPPLY OF PAs AND NPs

PAs have generally been physician substitutes supervised by physicians. As of 1993, roughly 27,000 persons had graduated from PA training programs; 23,000 were actually engaged in practice (Bureau of Health Professions, U.S. Department of Health and Human Services, 1994). About 1,600 individuals graduated from U.S. PA training programs in 1992 (Cawley, 1993). Health maintenance organizations (HMOs) currently employ 8 percent of PAs, and if clinic settings are included, almost two-thirds of all PAs work in some type of ambulatory care setting (Bureau of Health Professions, U.S. Department of Health and Human Services, 1994). As of 1992, approximately 43 percent of PAs worked in primary care (family practice, general internal medicine, and general pediatrics). Since the late 1970s the proportion of PAs working in specialty areas has steadily increased. The fastest growth has been in surgical subspecialties, where 22 percent of all PAs now work (Cawley, 1993).

As of 1992, approximately 28,000 NPs were certified by a national organization (such as the American Nurses Association) or a state, and 27,000 of these NPs were employed in nursing positions (Moses, 1994). NPs are increasingly receiving master's-level preparation, and in 1992 approximately 1,500 NPs graduated from U.S. nursing schools with master's degrees (Aiken, Gwyther, and Whelan, 1994). Although an additional 20,000 noncertified NPs also appear to have some level of formal training, the total number of certified and noncertified nurse practitioners is difficult to determine, because licensing and educational requirements vary significantly across the states (Morgan, 1993; Washington Consulting Group, 1994). NPs work in some arenas as physician substitutes and in other arenas as complements providing services such as health prevention, patient education, and counseling. In nine states NPs can establish independent practices[7] (Birkholz and Walker, 1994; Henderson and Chovan, 1994; Pearson, 1994). Almost 11 percent of NPs now have hospital admitting privileges and one-third have hospital discharge privileges. About 29 percent work in private practices or HMOs, 23 percent work in hospital outpatient departments, 11 percent work in hospital inpatient departments, and 23 percent in public or community health centers (Washington Consulting Group, 1994). Approximately 42 percent of NPs render primary care (family/general practice, general internal medicine, or general pediatrics) (Physician Payment Review Commission, 1994).

PRODUCTIVITY AND QUALITY OF PAs AND NPs

Given the economic incentives associated with capitation, health care deliv-

---

[7]"Independent" practice is permitted within a context that provides for consultation, collaborative management, and referral between physicians and NPs (Henderson and Chovan, 1994).

ery organizations should employ PAs and NPs to the extent that they improve the competitive position of the organizations: by improving productivity, enhancing quality of care, and increasing patient satisfaction.[8] This section summarizes the key findings from the literature on productivity and quality of care.

Productivity

Simply put, productivity is output per unit of input. In the context of workforce policy, researchers are interested in comparing the productivity *levels* of physicians, nonphysician clinicians, and entire teams of clinicians, as well the *gains* in productivity that might be realized through reconfiguration of the delivery system. It is important to know how many patients can be treated or how many services can be delivered per unit of time (per hour, per day, per month, per year), how this might vary by clinician or team, and how reconfiguration of the delivery system changes the numbers. For example, are PAs or NPs more productive in staff model HMOs than in other settings? How does their productivity compare with those of physicians in different settings? What is the impact on team productivity from adding a second or a third PA or NP to a practice that already employs at least one?

Most productivity studies of PAs and NPs have focused on opportunities for physician substitution (Reinhardt, 1975, 1991). A typical study will ask, "How many tasks currently performed by a physician could be performed by a PA or NP?" The tasks that PAs and NPs can perform in their roles as a physician substitute can vary greatly (Ross, Bower and Sibbald, 1994).[9] Table E-1 summarizes key findings from selected productivity studies of PAs and/or NPs over a recent 15-year period and also illustrates the variety of approaches used by researchers to measure PA and NP inputs and outputs.[10] Some clear, long-standing patterns have emerged from empirical investigations of PA and NP productivity. Studies generally indicate that the substitution rate of PAs and NPs for physicians is somewhere between one-half and three-fourths; that is, PAs and NPs can substitute for some (but not all) physician roles at that rate. For example, Schneider and Foley (1977) found that the addition of roughly 13 NPs allowed an HMO to reduce its staffing of physicians by 6.72 physicians, a substitution ratio

---

[8]Whether the organization is a for-profit or nonprofit organization influences how it responds to economic incentives (Pauly, Hillman, and Kerstein, 1990). However, both types of organizations will focus on productivity, quality, and patient satisfaction.

[9]During its visits to selected primary health care delivery organizations around the United States, the IOM Committee on the Future of Primary Care observed that in response to managed care cost pressures, some of the organizations had transferred certain triage-related tasks from clinicians to nonclinicians. For instance, one of the organizations visited by the committee trained its telephone assistants in the use of a structured patient interview protocol for initial screening of urinary tract infections.

[10]The Gravely and Littlefield study (1992) listed in Table E-1 also examined the productivity of teams that included clinical nurse specialists other than NPs.

TABLE E-1 Key Findings from Selected Non-Physician Provider (NPP) Productivity Studies, 1979–1993

Study	Time per Q			Effect on TQ		
	NPP	MD	Team	NPP	MD	Team
Scheffler (1979)	—	—	—	63.0% (1)	—	—
Mendenhall (1980)	16.4 (2)	11.2 (2)	11.3 (2,4)	11.1 (3)	21.4 (3)	18.9 (3,4)
Salkever (1982)	13.4 (2)	9.3 (2)	—	—	—	—
Cintron (1983)	—	—	—	−85.0% (5)	—	—
Buchanan (1990)	—	—	—	−50.0% (5)	—	—
Tirado (1990)	—	—	—	10.8% (6)	11.6% (6)	22.5% (6)
Spisso (1990)	—	—	—	−13.0% (5)	—	—
Gravely (1992)	2.0 (7)	1.7 (7)	1.0 (7)	—	—	—
Knickman (1992)	—	—	—	45.6% (8)	—	—
Hooker (1993)	2.61 (9)	2.39 (9)	—	—	—	—

NOTE: NPP = non-physician practitioner; MD = physician; Q = unit of output; time = absolute level of productivity; effect = marginal impact on total productivity; and TQ = total practice output.

(1) = NPP workload as percent of physician's; (2) = minutes per direct patient encounter; (3) = direct patient encounters per day; (4) = NPP-supervising physician only; (5) = change in total hospitalization days after NPP; (6) = percent total workload contribution ; (7) = appointments per hour; (8) = NPP workload as percent of MD residents; and (9) = internal medicine patient visits per hour.

of 50 percent. They found a similar substitution rate of NPs for pediatricians. In another study, Scheffler calculated the marginal rate of substitution of PAs for physicians to be 63 percent (Scheffler, 1979). Record et al. (1980) reviewed a large number of productivity studies and concluded that the rate of task delegation (i.e., the percentage of physician tasks that a PA or NP can perform) is typically 0.75 for large practices (four or more providers) and 0.40 for small practices in adult care. In pediatric care, the delegation figures were 0.90 and 0.45, respectively. Because of scale economies, large practices are more likely to use PAs and NPs and tend to delegate a larger proportion of medical services. In a small practice, the volume of services that can be handled by a PA or NP may not be large enough to fill up his or her time (Record et al., 1980).

Comparing productivity levels in different types of settings is complicated by a variety of factors. Some early studies assumed that the patient mix in physician practices did not change with the introduction of PAs or NPs and that the substitutions were representative of all types of medical practices (U.S. Congress, Office of Technology Assessment, 1986). However, if NPs and PAs treat less serious or less risky cases than physicians, simple comparisons of substitution ratios and productivity levels may be misleading. Furthermore, PAs or NPs may add costs to a physician practice that go beyond their salaries and fringe benefits. For example, NPs and PAs might order more tests than physicians or prescribe more drugs, and they may require additional space, supervision, equipment, malpractice insurance, and training. Thus, productivity studies must examine changes in total practice resources, not just salaries.[11]

Quality of Care and Patient Satisfaction

PAs and NPs have demonstrated that they are able to deliver care in a manner acceptable to patients, and research shows that they deliver more preventive and educational services than physicians. Studies show that PAs and NPs deliver health care services that are comparable, in terms of clinical outcomes, to the care provided by physicians, and the care provided by the nonphysician practitioners is often superior in terms of patient satisfaction and process measures (Brown and Grimes, 1993; U.S. Congress, Office of Technology Assessment, 1986). Furthermore, recent studies that have looked at geriatric care, neonatal intensive care unit care, and colposcopy show that not only primary care but specialty care is in the purview of advanced practice nurses (APNs) such as NPs (Burl and Bonner, 1991; Burl, Bonner, and Rao, 1994; Carzoli et al., 1994; Hartz, 1995). Additionally, the U.S. Department of Health and Human Services has examined National Practitioner Data Bank malpractice reports for APNs, showing them to be much

---

[11]Abbott (1988), Begun and Lippincott (1993), and Kindig (1993) also provide useful discussions of physician substitution issues.

less frequently reported than physicians (Birkholz, 1995). However, a major limitation of the medical literature on PAs and NPs is the absence of recent (1986 or later), methodologically rigorous studies comparing NPs or PAs with physicians or each other (Scheffler, 1995).

The following appear to be reasonable conclusions regarding quality of care at this time:

• Nonphysician clinicians who have received training equivalent to that of physicians in a technical procedure can perform the procedure as well as physicians.

• Nonphysician clinicians can supply high-quality care for simple acute problems and chronic stable ones. Studies are not adequate to determine whether these providers may occasionally miss a rare diagnosis (and fail to seek consultation[12]), nor are they adequate to determine whether nonphysician clinicians can treat complicated cases as well as physicians can.

• There is no evidence to support the assertion that independent practice by nonphysician clinicians results in quality of care comparable to that of collaborative practice or that of physician-only care. Neither is there evidence against this assertion. Studies have not been conducted, in part, because of the paucity of such independent practices (Scheffler, 1995).

HEALTH CARE WORKFORCE CONFIGURATION STUDIES

This section and the two sections that follow describe several investigations of PA and NP staffing and productivity, the potential impacts of PAs and NPs on the overall health workforce, and two case studies of mature staff-model HMOs. This discussion emphasizes (1) the variations in managed care organizations' workforces that have emerged in recent years and (2) the adjustments necessary to compare workforces across organizations.

Recently, several noteworthy studies of PAs and NPs have appeared. Hooker (1993) studied PA and NP staffing in Kaiser Permanente's Northwest Region (KPNW), which provides prepaid medical care to 380,000 members in the Portland, Oregon, metropolitan area. During 1992, KPNW had 2.5 million patient encounters and employed 520 full-time-equivalent physicians. Hooker analyzed clinical staffing patterns and productivity by specialty. In internal medicine, KPNW used 100 physicians, 13 PAs, and 15.5 NPs, the highest number of nonphysician providers (NPPs) in any specialty other than mental health. KPNW also used significant numbers of NPPs in family practice and obstetrics-gynecol-

---

[12]If such studies were performed, it would be important to compare the nonphysician provider rate of failing to appropriately seek consultation with the failure rate for primary care physicians in comparable settings.

ogy (OB-GYN), although the ratios of NPPs to physicians were higher in several other specialties. The physician/NPP staffing ratios in family practice and OB-GYN differed from each other, with OB/GYN using more NPs and certified nurse-midwives. Hooker also reported that although physicians and PAs saw similar types of patients NPs delivered almost twice the amount of preventive service and three times the amount of prenatal services. NPs performed most routine physical exams, which suggests that more complex patients were seen by physicians and PAs. That study indicates that KPNW patients' quality ratings (based on patient satisfaction) of NPs and PAs were comparable to the ratings of physicians.

Hooker's study must be viewed in context, as the KPNW model might not be generalizable. KPNW has a long tradition of using NPs and PAs (Hooker, 1993), and Oregon has a relatively liberal medical practice act that allows NPs (but not PAs) to prescribe medication (Henderson and Chovan, 1994). Furthermore, within the Kaiser system the use of NPs and PAs varies dramatically. For example, Kaiser's Northern California Region employs 360 NPs but only a handful of PAs, whereas the Southern California Region has more than 500 PAs and NPs on staff. Many factors apparently influence the differences in NP and PA use, including the supply of physicians, the locations of NP and PA training programs, legal liability considerations, management opinion, physician beliefs about NP and PA effectiveness, and acceptance of nonphysician clinicians by enrollees (Hooker, 1993).

Although not translatable to a non-hospital-based practice environment, Knickman et al. (1992) conducted an important investigation of the potential for substituting nonphysicians for resident physicians at two New York City hospitals. Using a time-motion study, Knickman and his colleagues analyzed physicians' clinical tasks under two different models: a traditional model in which the physician resident is the primary medical manager and an alternative model in which a nonphysician clinician such as an NP performs baseline patient care monitoring. In the traditional model, residents spent almost half of their time on tasks that they could *not* delegate. However, using the alternative practice model the study found that only 20 percent of the residents' time was nondelegatable.[13]

Other studies have shown that NPs can work effectively in trauma units (Spisso et al., 1990), geriatric care settings (Burl, Bonner, and Rao, 1994), and neonatal intensive care units (Carzoli et al., 1994). Although it is not possible to quantify productivity gains from these studies, they suggest that the potential for efficiency gains exists in a variety of clinical settings.

---

[13]That study also has important implications for the size of the future physician resident workforce (Physician Payment Review Commission, 1993).

POTENTIAL IMPACT OF PAs AND NPs ON THE
OVERALL HEALTH CARE WORKFORCE

The studies described above suggest that NPs and PAs can make major contributions to the health care system. However, estimates of the overall impacts of NPs and PAs on the size and composition of the future health workforce vary widely because of the different assumptions that forecasters make about patient utilization rates, physician delegation rates, the extent to which managed care organizations are willing to use NPPs, and other variables. The varying assumptions about managed care organizations reflect the fact that so far, researchers have been able to obtain detailed data on physician and nonphysician staffing patterns for only a handful of HMOs and staffing patterns vary widely among those HMOs that have made data accessible to researchers (Weiner, 1993, 1994).

In 1980, the Graduate Medical Education National Advisory Committee (GMENAC) published its report to the secretary of the U.S. Department of Health and Human Services on the future national supply and requirements for physicians, concluding that there would be a surplus of 70,000 physicians by 1990 (15 percent more than needed) and 145,000 by the year 2000 (30 percent more than needed) (Health Resources Administration, 1981a). These projections were developed by a panel of experts by combining current utilization patterns, projected numbers of medical school graduates and international medical graduates, population trends, and other data. The GMENAC approach to forecasting physician requirements was based on need ("needs-based"): the basic premise was that the requirements should be based on an assessment of the total burden of disease and disability for all people (McNutt, 1981).

Although GMENAC did consider the possibilities for delegating certain physician tasks to NPs and PAs (Health Resources Administration, 1981b), it did not anticipate the subsequent rapid enrollment growth in managed care organizations. Steinwachs and his colleagues (1986) compared actual staffing patterns in three large HMOs in the early 1980s with the national requirements for physicians in 1990 projected by GMENAC. They concluded that compared with the projections of GMENAC, after making adjustments for demographic and other differences between HMO patients and the overall U.S. population, 20 percent fewer primary care physicians for children and 50 percent fewer primary care physicians for adults would be needed to meet national primary care needs. Interestingly, that study found that GMENAC's assumed percentages of primary care encounters that could be handled by nonphysicians (12 percent of adult health care encounters and 15 percent of child health care encounters) were substantially *higher* than the actual HMO percentages. Nevertheless, the authors' estimates of overall national physician requirements were still lower than the GMENAC projections, primarily because the patient utilization rates reported by the HMOs were lower than GMENAC's needs-based estimates (Weiner, Steinwachs and Williamson, 1986).

An unpublished 1991 study by Marder, Gaumer, and Minkovitz, using a GMENAC-type model which incorporates clinical experts' judgments about appropriate patient utilization patterns rather than actual FFS or HMO utilization rates, estimated that NPs and PAs could assume responsibility for 630 million visits or slightly more than one-third of the 2.1 billion annual U.S. primary care visits. Marder and his colleagues employed a delegation rate for adult medicine of 30 percent and one for pediatrics of 33 percent. Conservatively, that study indicated that there is a potential shortfall of about 75,000 PAs and NPs *in primary care alone*. The increased use of PAs and NPs in specialty care suggested by recent trends would exacerbate the shortfall (Cawley, 1993). That study also concluded that there would be surpluses of most types of primary care physicians in the United States by the year 2010 (Marder, Gaumer, and Minkowitz, 1991).

In a more recent study, Weiner extrapolated HMO staffing levels to the entire U.S. physician workforce, adjusting for demographic and other differences between HMOs' enrolled populations and the overall U.S. population. He estimated that national physician requirements in the year 2000 under two reform scenarios that provided for staffing based on HMO patterns would range from 137.5 to 143.8 physicians per 100,000: 58.7 to 59.2 primary care physicians per 100,000 and 78.8 to 84.6 specialists per 100,000. Weiner concluded that (1) there will be an overall surplus of about 165,000 physicians by the year 2000, (2) supply and demand of primary care physicians will be in relative balance, and (3) the supply of specialists will exceed the requirements by more than 60 percent. Although Weiner did not project the demand for NPs and PAs, he observed that, in general, HMOs appear to use more NPs and PAs than the overall U.S. health system (23.0 per 100,000 lives in HMOs versus 19.6 per 100,000 lives overall). Thus, his study also implies that demand for NPs and PAs will increase in the AMC world (Weiner, 1994).

STAFFING PATTERNS:
CASE STUDIES OF TWO MATURE HMOS

As part of the IOM study on the future of primary care, clinical staffing data were collected on two mature, West Coast-based HMOs (see Table E-2[14]). These simple case studies illustrate the large staffing variations that apparently exist in the HMO industry and the implications of these variations for the future size and composition of the U.S. health workforce.

---

[14]Table E-2 presents 1994 staffing data for each HMO plan. I also analyzed staffing for 1992 and 1993 and found that staffing patterns in each plan had been fairly stable over a 3-year period.

TABLE E-2 1994 Staffing Patterns in Two West Coast Staff Model HMOs

	HMO # 1	HMO # 2
Total Enrollment	<500,000	>500,000
% of Enrollees age 65 and older	12.18%	9.33%
PHYSICIANS PER 100,000 ENROLLEES		
Primary Care	66.42	46.01
OB-GYN	9.68	12.52
Specialty	100.89	126.43
Subtotal	176.99	184.96
PAs PER 100,000 ENROLLEES		
Primary Care	17.87	0.01
OB-GYN	6.20	0.70
Specialty	6.99	14.42
Subtotal	31.06	15.13
NPs PER 100,000 ENROLLEES		
Primary Care	3.96	5.28
OB-GYN	0.53	8.57
Specialty	37.25	21.59
Subtotal	41.74	35.44
TOTAL CLINICIANS	249.79	235.53
Specialty MDs as % of All Physicians	57.00%	68.36%
Specialty MDs as % of All Clinicians	40.39%	53.68%
Specialty Clinicians as % of All Clinicians	58.10%	68.97%
Total Physicians per NP and PA	2.43	3.66

NOTE: NP = nurse practitioner; PA = physician assistant.

HMO #1

HMO #1 is a West Coast-based staff model plan. In 1994, this HMO had 177 physicians per 100,000 enrollees.[15] In addition, HMO #1 used 31 PAs and 42 NPs per 100,000 enrollees. Thus, HMO #1 used 2.4 physicians for each PA or NP.

---

[15]Note that OB-GYN clinicians are listed separately from specialists. Furthermore, approximately 12 to 15 percent of HMO # 1 physicians are retained by contract. I assumed that these contract physicians were distributed among the practice categories in the same way as employed physicians, since actual counts of contract physicians by specialty were not available.

TABLE E-3 Projected U.S. Health Workforce Based on Selected HMO
Staffing Patterns*

	Based on HMO #1	Based on HMO #2
Physicians:		
Primary Care	171,364	118,706
OB-GYN	24,974	32,302
Specialty	260,296	326,189
Total Physicians	456,634	477,197
Physician Assistants:		
Primary Care	46,105	26
OB-GYN	15,996	1,806
Specialty	18,034	37,204
Total PAs	80,135	39,035
Nurse Practitioners:		
Primary Care	10,217	13,622
OB-GYN	1,367	22,111
Specialty	96,105	55,702
Total NPs	107,689	91,435
TOTAL CLINICIANS	644,458	607,667

NOTE: NP = nurse practitioner; PA = physician assistant.

*Based on estimated total 1993 U.S. resident population of 258 million (U.S. Bureau of the Census, 1994).

In 1994, physician specialists in HMO #1 accounted for 57 percent of the total physician staff and 40 percent of the total clinical staff. Adding specialist PAs and NPs to physician specialists, we observe that 58 percent of HMO #1's clinicians were involved in specialty care.

If HMO #1's clinical staffing ratios are directly applied to the entire U.S. population (see Table E-3), there would be a need for approximately 457,000 total active patient care physicians in the United States, approximately 75,000[16] fewer nonfederal physicians than were actually involved in patient care in 1993.[17] Moreover, if the entire United States (like HMO #1) used 31 PAs and 42 NPs per 100,000 population, there would be a current need for approximately 80,000 PAs

---

[16]Adjustments for demographic differences between HMO #1's population and the entire U.S. population would probably not significantly change this estimate, as the age and sex distribution of HMO #1's enrollees is similar to the distribution in the entire U.S. population.

[17]As of January 1, 1993, 531,659 U.S. nonfederal physicians were active in patient care (American Medical Association, 1994).

and 108,000 NPs, resulting in a nationwide shortfall of 57,000 PAs and 81,000 NPs. As noted previously, there are currently 23,000 and 27,000 active certified PAs and NPs, respectively, in the United States.

HMO #2

The second HMO case study also involves a West Coast-based staff model plan. In 1994, HMO #2 had a younger population than HMO #1: 9 percent of HMO #2's enrollees were 65 and older, compared with 12 percent of HMO #1's enrollees (see Table E-2). Despite its younger patient population, HMO #2's overall physician staffing ratio was somewhat higher than HMO #1's ratio (185 versus 177 physicians per 100,000 enrollees, respectively), and it also did not use NPs and PAs to the same extent as HMO #1. In 1994, HMO #2 used 15 PAs and 35 NPs per 100,000 enrollees,[18] compared with 31 PAs and 42 NPs in HMO #1. Overall, HMO #2 used 3.7 physicians for each PA or NP, about 50 percent higher than HMO #1's physician to PA or NP ratio.

Staffing in HMO #2 was more oriented toward physician specialists. In 1994, 68 percent of HMO #2's physicians (exclusive of OB-GYNs) were specialists, versus 57 percent in HMO #1. Furthermore, 54 percent of HMO #2's overall clinical staff consisted of specialty physicians, compared with 40 percent for HMO #1. Adding specialist PAs and NPs to physician specialists, we observe that 69 percent of HMO #2's clinicians were involved in specialty care, compared with 58 percent in HMO #1.

Projecting HMO #2's staffing ratios over the entire U.S. population (see Table E-3) suggests the need for 477,000 total physicians, resulting in a surplus of 55,000 physicians. The overall need for PAs and NPs in the United States amounts to 39,000 and 91,000, respectively. Thus, even based on HMO #2's staffing patterns (which rely much more on physician specialists than HMO #1), there would be a nationwide shortfall of 16,000 certified PAs and 64,000 certified NPs in relation to the current supply of active professionals.

RESULTS OF COMPARISON OF HMOs

This simple comparison of staffing patterns in two mature HMOs illustrates some important lessons and indicates the need for more research into the underlying causes of staffing variations in managed care organizations. First, merely counting physicians and specialist physicians does not provide a useful staffing analysis in a managed care world. Researchers must also examine the use of PAs, NPs, and other nonphysician clinicians. Second, researchers cannot merely com-

---

[18]HMO #2 uses a variety of other nonphysician health professionals and para-professionals, including psychologists, social workers, audiologists, occupational therapists, and optometrists.

pare the number of health professionals used by a plan to the total plan enrollment in order to make inferences about productivity. They need to investigate differences in enrollee and other plan characteristics (enrollee age and sex distribution, severity of patient illness, patient outcomes, staff productivity, and the organizational structure of the clinical practice). Third, there are certain health care workforce parameters that staffing numbers alone cannot reveal, such as complementarity and substitution possibilities within health care teams.

ELEMENTS OF A NEW MODEL OF
TEAM HEALTH PRODUCTION

The 1978 IOM definition of primary care and the new (1994) definition both support the delivery of primary care in the context of a collaborative format (Institute of Medicine, 1994). Although there is a substantial body of literature on primary care team models, most of this literature is based on research conducted in FFS settings prior to the 1980s (Baldwin, 1994). What is missing is a conceptual framework for team delivery of primary care in contemporary managed care environments that explicitly considers the role of economic incentives in the health production process.[19] This section presents a model that is consistent with the new IOM definition of primary care.

Implicit in the discussion that follows is the notion that current managed care payment incentives may not always produce optimal outcomes in terms of quality of care, patient satisfaction, or efficient use of resources. Whether payment[20] incentives can produce optimal outcomes depends on a variety of factors. For example, health care purchasers (e.g., employers and purchasing cooperatives) must be willing and able to balance incentives for high quality and low cost. Even though purchasers are increasingly demanding both high quality and low cost and are developing tools for comparing risk-adjusted costs and outcomes across provider organizations (Giacomini, Luft, and Robinson, 1995; Report Card Project, 1995; U.S. General Accounting Office, 1994b; Winslow, 1995), these tools currently have significant limitations (Epstein, 1995; Giacomini, Luft, and Robinson, 1995; U.S. General Accounting Office, 1994a). This is an important consideration because some physicians may respond to capitation by withholding beneficial treatment (Pauly, 1992; Rodwin, 1993). Furthermore, the effects of current managed care payment incentives on access to care for vulnerable subpopulations such as the poor, the severely mentally ill, and the chronically ill are

---

[19]Also absent from most of this literature is any discussion of how to educate health professionals in team-building skills. As Schneller and Ott (1996) observe, health professionals often have difficulty adapting to the team concept, and interprofessional conflicts are common.

[20]Although it is beyond the scope of this discussion, it should be noted that nonpayment incentives (such as utilization review and selective contracting) can also affect outcomes (Robinson, 1993).

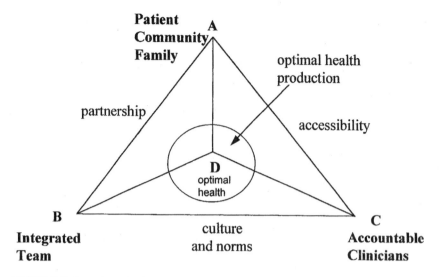

FIGURE E-1 Optimal health production.

not well understood (Davis and Rowland, 1991; Lurie et al., 1992; Safran, Tarlov, and Rogers, 1994).

Optimal Production of Health

This model begins with three basic premises: (1) the ultimate goal of primary care is the optimal health of the patient, produced with the least-cost combination of inputs; (2) the optimal health outcome is achievable; and (3) patients, individual clinicians, and health care teams each contribute certain unique, critical inputs to the health production process.[21]   For example, patients must comply with medical advice and engage in preventive health behaviors; team members must share information to maintain continuity of care.

In Figure E-1 the circle represents the optimal production of health. The circle varies in size depending on how exact or inexact the measure of a health outcome may be. The more exact the measure of the health outcome, the smaller the circle. Attainment of an optimal health outcome (point D) requires a mix of inputs: from the patient, community, and family (vertex A of the triangle), the integrated team (vertex B of the triangle), and/or individual clinicians who are accountable for the patient's health outcomes (vertex C of the triangle). The

---

[21]The "force-field paradigm" developed by Henrik Blum of the University of California, Berkeley (1983), influenced my thinking in this area.

location of the optimal production circle can change depending on whether a particular treatment or disease requires more inputs from the patient, community, and family (the circle would move toward vertex A), individual accountable clinicians (toward vertex C), or the team (toward vertex B). For example, treatment of a simple fracture might find the circle located far away from vertex B because an individual clinician and the patient can accomplish this task with few inputs from the team. In contrast, a treatment regimen for heart disease would require a variety of complex inputs from individual clinicians, the team, and the patient. Therefore, in this situation the circle would be located in the center of the triangle.

The sides of the triangle show the relationships among the three points of the triangle. The role of each accountable clinician is to facilitate *access* to care: side AC. Optimal access occurs when an individual clinician (e.g., physician, PA or NP) assumes responsibility for the patient's health outcome. Side AB represents the *partnership* between the patient, the family, and the community, in accordance with the 1994 IOM definition of primary care. Patient outcomes need to be evaluated in the context of this partnership. Finally, the team and the individual clinicians must commit to a patient-centered culture and set of norms that encourage optimal health outcomes and efficient delivery of care. Accordingly, side BC represents *culture and norms*. Each of these sides may vary in length, depending on the amount of inputs contributed by each element.

Patient goals must be aligned with economic incentives to achieve optimal health outcomes (Dranove and White, 1987). Thus, economic incentives should elicit the least-cost combination of inputs from the patient, community, family, accountable clinicians, and the team that achieves the optimal health outcome. In Figure E-1, the lines from each of the vertices to point D represent the amount of each input: line AD represents the contribution by the patient, community, and family to the production of his or her own health, line CD is the contribution of individual clinicians, and line BD is the contribution provided by the team (above and beyond individual contributions). This joint effort should clearly define mutually determined accountability as well as rewards for the members of the team. In this example the contributions intersect at point D, the optimal health outcome.

Nonoptimal Production of Health

If economic incentives do not work properly, the payment system may elicit a mix of inputs that are too costly for the task at hand and/or that fail to achieve an optimal health outcome. For example, if the incentives stimulate the right amount of inputs from the patient and individual clinicians but fail to adequately reward team collaboration when it is needed, the optimal patient outcome may not be achieved (i.e., point D is outside the circle), as shown in Figure E-2. Alternatively, if the incentives stimulate the right amount of inputs from the

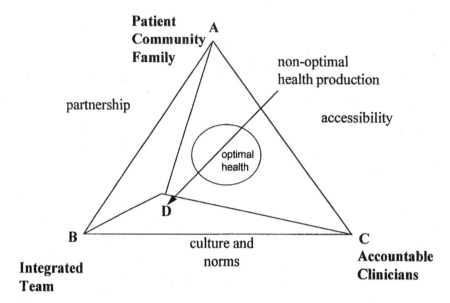

FIGURE E-2 Nonoptimal health production.

patient, family, and community but do not generate the right amount of inputs from both the individual clinicians and team, a suboptimal patient outcome (i.e., point D is outside the circle) may also be achieved, as shown in Figure E-3.

Improperly designed financial incentives could elicit an excessive rather than an insufficient amount of inputs from individual clinicians and teams. Figure E-4 illustrates a situation in which excessive payments have stimulated too many of these types of inputs: the health system relies too much on inputs from clinicians and not enough on the patient, family, and community. For example, a patient's expensive treatment plan for bronchitis fails because he does not receive adequate family and community support for smoking cessation.

To summarize, the challenge for the health care system is to generate an appropriate mix of patient involvement, contributions from individual clinicians, and teamwork. The system requires a balance, in the sense that the patient, the individual providers, and the team must provide just the right level and combination of inputs, so that optimal health outcomes are achieved. The economic reward structure must encourage this balance, but this is not easily accomplished. Heretofore, rewards generally emphasized individual clinicians; rewards for team performance have been rare and rewards (other than intrinsic) for patient participation in the process have been almost nonexistent. In essence, the system seems to have produced the outcome shown in Figure E-4. The challenge for health policymakers who are trying to develop the AMC workforce will be to design economic incentives that produce the optimal health outcome for the patient,

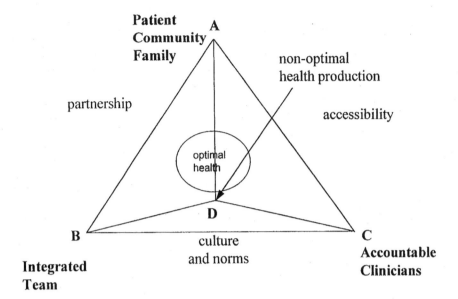

FIGURE E-3 Nonoptimal health production.

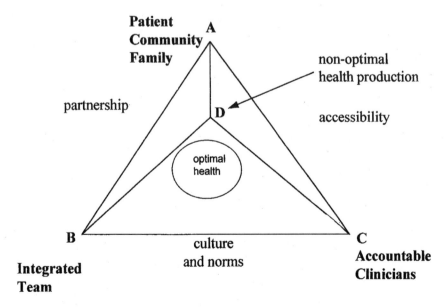

FIGURE E-4 Nonoptimal health production.

shown in Figure E-1. An additional challenge will be to design work-forces that are economically feasible but that also meet the diverse needs of different populations.

A NEW HEALTH CARE WORKFORCE RESEARCH AGENDA

This paper has shown that the AMC world will probably be a much different place than the BMC world. If the nation is to develop a health care workforce policy that meets the needs of this new world, policymakers must develop a workforce research agenda attuned to these needs. This section identifies the major gaps in the current health workforce research literature.

Productivity

Productivity studies in the BMC world focused primarily on opportunities for physician substitution: primary care physicians for specialists and PAs and NPs for physicians. The traditional emphasis on substitution has intuitive appeal, but it also has substantial limitations. A key research priority in the AMC world will be to improve and extend our knowledge about complements as well as substitutions. Researchers will also need to identify institutional barriers to productivity, because some practices may be organized in a manner that does not permit realization of the potential productivity gains from PAs and NPs. For example, some practices may simply be too small to efficiently utilize indivisible inputs such as PAs and NPs (Record et al., 1980; Steinwachs, 1992), whereas others may lack adequate information systems to measure costs and patient outcomes (Shortell and Hull, 1995). Also, effective substitution may require redeployment of physicians so that when substitution occurs the physician can perform other, more productive tasks. If there are already too many physicians, substitution of NPs and PAs for physicians may produce less in the way of benefits than we might otherwise expect.[22]

Legal Restrictions on NPs and PAs

Legal restrictions may adversely affect the ability of NPs, PAs, and other nonphysician clinicians to practice at levels commensurate with their training and skills (Sekscenski et al., 1994). Lack of uniformity among the states and arbitrary

---

[22]Researchers also need to consider who reaps the benefits of productivity improvements in a health care system that is increasingly market-driven. This depends on the structure of market competition and the relative bargaining power of providers, payers, consumers, and other actors in the market. For example, in markets characterized by a surplus of physicians and little or no competition among health plans, plans could realize substantial financial gains from physician productivity improvements but not feel compelled to share these gains with consumers.

(i.e., not based on well-established differences in clinical skills or patient outcomes) limitations prevent full utilization of PAs and NPs in many settings (Bureau of Health Professions, U.S. Department of Health and Human Services, 1994; Henderson and Chovan, 1994; Jones and Cawley, 1994; Safriet, 1994). An additional tension exists between sets of providers when legal accountability for all actions falls on the physician. Thus, an expanded scope of practice for nonphysician clinicians may require changes in legal liability principles (Chiarella, 1993).

Workforce research in the AMC world could play an important role in shaping the public policy debate about the appropriate role of nonphysician clinicians in the health care delivery system. Although the health policy literature provides many examples of how scope-of-practice laws and payment barriers constrain the effectiveness of non-physician professionals in traditional FFS settings, no recent analyses of controlled or natural experiments clearly establish a cause and effect relationship between specific practice barriers and clinical or economic outcomes. Furthermore, virtually no studies compare the impact of practice barriers on PAs or NPs who work in organized delivery systems with the impact of such barriers on nonphysician professionals who work in FFS settings (Scheffler, 1995). Federal and state practice barriers may have fewer adverse effects on nonphysician practitioners in organized delivery systems, because these systems are less dependent on FFS revenues and may have more flexible work rules or collegial relationships that enhance the effectiveness of all practitioners. For example, recent case study data suggest that health professionals in some organized care settings are able to work around state legal barriers affecting prescriptive authority (Physician Payment Review Commission, 1994).

Quality of Care

As noted above, a significant body of research shows that the quality of care provided by NPs and PAs appears to be comparable to that provided by physicians in terms of clinical outcomes and is often superior in terms of patient satisfaction and process methods. However, there remains a paucity of recent, methodologically rigorous studies comparing the quality of care provided by nonphysician clinicians and physicians. Furthermore, most of the current literature on quality of care is based on research conducted in traditional FFS environments or hospitals rather than managed care environments (Scheffler, 1995; U.S. Congress, Office of Technology Assessment, 1986).

In addition to problems with nonrandom assignment and the possible confounding effects of gender, the following methodological issues should be addressed by future research comparing the quality of care provided by physician and nonphysician clinicians:

- Adequate sample size of patients *and* clinicians, with use of power analysis to determine sample size and use of statistical significance testing.
- Use of a representative sample of settings and clinicians, not just academic medical center-related sites and providers.
- Allowance for the time factor: if nonphysician clinicians spend twice as much time with patients, for example, it is likely that the patients will report greater satisfaction or improved outcomes.
- Calculation of the percentage of a population of patients for whom nonphysician clinicians seek physician consultation over time, not simply the percentage of visits for which such consultation is requested.

CONCLUSIONS

As this paper has shown, the AMC world will demand much more cooperation between physicians and other health professionals, beginning with the teaching of team skills, as well as research into the new methods of professional collaboration. The health care workforce in the BMC world emphasized the physician and promoted specialists over primary care physicians; the AMC world emphasizes efficiency and economy, and it is much more likely to reward delivery organizations that substitute primary care physicians for specialists and NPs, PAs, and other health professionals for physicians. This paper has outlined a variety of studies that indicate the potential for the large-scale substitution of NPs and PAs for physicians.

The AMC world could turn into a zero sum game that pits physicians and other health professionals against one another (Rodgers, 1994; Scherer, 1994), particularly given the absence of a tradition and an educational system that emphasizes collaborative team provision of medical care and the development of professional complements. PAs and NPs were initially accepted by physicians and health policymakers in the 1960s and 1970s, when there was a perceived shortage of physicians. However, we may now have a surplus of physicians, particularly in a number of specialties (Schroeder, 1994a,b). If expanded use of NPs and PAs results in lower incomes for physicians, physician resistance to NPs and PAs may intensify.[23] Under these circumstances, some physicians may campaign for additional restrictions on PAs' and NPs' practices, just as they have campaigned for "any-willing-provider" laws in response to selective contracting by managed care organizations (Caldwell, 1995). On the other hand, with appropriate economic incentives and reorganized methods of delivering health care, the world that evolves after managed care could produce a more cooperative

---

[23]A current example of a health profession's controversy is the American Medical Association's recent proposal for direct physician supervision of NPs, similar to the traditional relationship of PAs to physicians (Rodgers, 1994).

health care team delivery model. This paper has outlined one way of thinking about the development of such a team concept, a team production of health model, as a stimulus that can be used to consider the potential benefits available from a synergistic approach. Studies of economic incentive systems and organizational frameworks that promote teamwork, balanced health production inputs, and optimal participation could produce great returns.

The AMC world is still evolving and promises to change quite rapidly over the next two decades. This means that workforce research itself may require a new model: The change may be so rapid that researchers will have to become part of the health production and management teams that they have elected to study. Although this requires researchers to take on a new role, they must maintain their neutrality.

Some of the more important topics for a new health workforce research agenda are identified below:

- What federal and state policies will promote an effective market response to the team provision of primary care?
- How will the team delivery of primary care affect funding for and training of health professionals?
- How do micro workforce policies (team composition) and macro workforce policies (training and funding) interrelate?
- What is the potential for development of new models for health care teams in primary care?
- How will the composition of a team vary by patient demographics, culture, and case mix severity?
- What types of payment and incentive programs can be designed and tested to promote the team delivery of primary care?
- What are appropriate measures of productivity and performance for the health care team?
- To what extent do federal and state laws and regulations impede the evolution of innovative health care teams?
- How does the health care team relate to organizational form (staff and group HMOs, IPA, FFS, preferred provider organizations) and the market for health care services?
- What data and information should we collect and disseminate in order to monitor performance and to promote effective decisionmaking?

ACKNOWLEDGMENTS

This paper was supported in part by the Bureau of Health Professions. Valuable guidance was provided by Neal A. Vanselow, Karl D. Yordy, and Molla S. Donaldson of the IOM, as well as Fitzhugh Mullan, Robert M. Politzer, and Edward Sekscenski of the Bureau of Health Professions. In addition, Linda

Aiken, Joel Alpert, Jean Johnson, Eugene Jones, David A. Kindig, Kathleen N. Lohr, Thomas G. Rundall, and Eugene S. Schneller provided helpful comments on an earlier draft of the paper.

Special thanks to John M. Hillman (Agency for Health Care Policy and Research predoctoral fellow) and Susan Ivey (National Institute for Mental Health postdoctoral fellow) for their assistance in revising the paper and significantly improving its value. Finally, I appreciate the conceptual contributions of Stephen E. Foreman and Norman S. Waitzman.

REFERENCES

Abbott, A. 1988. *The System of Professions: An Essay on the Division of Expert Labor.* Chicago: University of Chicago Press.

Aiken, L.H., Gwyther, M.E., and Whelan, E. 1994. *Advanced Practice Nursing Education: Strategies for the Allocation of the Proposed Graduate Nursing Education Account.* Philadelphia: Center for Health Services and Policy Research.

American Medical Association. 1994. *Physician Characteristics and Distribution in the U.S.* G. Roback et al., eds. Chicago: American Medical Association.

Baldwin, D. 1994. *The Role of Interdisciplinary Education and Teamwork in Primary Care and Health Care Reform.* Rockville, MD: Bureau of Health Professions, U.S. Department of Health and Human Services.

Begun, J., and Lippincott, R.C. 1993. *Strategic Adaptation in the Health Professions.* San Francisco: Jossey-Bass.

Birkholz, G. 1995. Malpractice Data from the National Practitioner Data Bank. *Nurse Practitioner* 20(3):32–35.

Birkholz, G., and Walker, D. 1994. Strategies for State Statutory Language Changes Granting Fully Independent Nurse Practitioner Practice. *Nurse Practitioner* 19(1):54–58.

Blum, H.L. 1983. *Expanding Health Care Horizons* (Second Edition). Oakland, Calif.: Third Party Publishing.

Brown, S.A., and Grimes, D. 1993. *Nurse Practitioners and Certified Nurse-Midwives: A Meta-Analysis of Studies on Nurses in Primary Care Roles.* Washington, DC: American Nurses Publishing.

Buchanan, J.L., Bell, R.M., Arnold, S.B., et al. 1990. Assessing the Cost Effects of Nursing Home-Based Geriatric Nurse Practitioners. *Health Care Financing Review* 11(3):67–78.

Bureau of Health Professions, U.S. Department of Health and Human Services. 1994. Physician Assistants in the Health Workforce: Final Report of the Advisory Group on Physician Assistants and the Workforce. Washington, DC: U.S. Department of Health and Human Services.

Burl, J.B., and Bonner, A. 1991. A Geriatric NP/Physician Team in a Long-Term Care Setting. *HMO Practice* 5(4):139–142.

Burl, J.B., Bonner, A., and Rao, M. 1994. Demonstration of the Cost-Effectiveness of a Nurse Practitioner/Physician Team in Long-Term Care Facilities. *HMO Practice* 8(4):157–161.

Caldwell, B. 1995. Managed Care Stumbles Under Weight of State Laws. *Employee Benefit Plan Review* 49(8):28–30.

Carzoli, R.P., Martinez-Cruz, M., Cuevas, L.L., Murphy, S., and Chiu, T. 1994. Comparison of Neonatal Nurse Practitioners, Physician Assistants, and Residents in the Neonatal Intensive Care Unit. *Archives Pediatric and Adolescent Medicine* 148(12):1271–1276.

Cawley, J.F. 1993. Physician Assistants in the Health Care Workforce. In *The Roles of Physician Assistants and Nurse Practitioners in Primary Care.* D.K. Clawson and M. Osterweis, eds. Washington, DC, Association of Academic Health Centers.

Chiarella, E.M. 1993. Nurses' Liability in Doctor-Nurse Relationships. *Contemporary Nurse* 2(1):6–10.

Cintron, G., Bigas, C., Linares, E., Aranda, J.M., and Hernandez, E. 1983. Nurse Practitioner Role in a Chronic Congestive Heart Failure Clinic: In-Hospital Time, Costs, and Patient Satisfaction. *Heart and Lung* 12(3):237–240.

Davis, K., and Rowland, D. 1991. Financing Health Care for the Poor. In *Health Services Research: Key to Health Policy*. E. Ginzberg, ed. Cambridge, Mass.: Harvard University Press.

Delbanco, T.L., Meyers, K.C., and Segal, E.A. 1979. Paying the Physician's Fee: Blue Shield and the Reasonable Charge. *The New England Journal of Medicine* 301(24):1314–1320.

Dranove, D., and White, W.D. 1987. Agency Theory: New Insights Into the Health Care Industry. *Inquiry* 24(4):405–415.

Enthoven, A. 1987. The Health Care Economy in the U.S.A. In *Health Economics: Prospects for the Future*. G.T. Smith, ed. Kent, England: Croom Helm Ltd.

Epstein, A. 1995. Performance Reports on Quality: Prototypes, Problems, and Prospects. *The New England Journal of Medicine* 333(1):57–61.

Fein, R. 1967. *The Doctor Shortage: An Economic Diagnosis*. Washington, DC: Brookings Institution.

Gamliel, S., Politzer, R.M., Rivo, M.L., and Mullan, F. 1995. Managed Care on the March: Will Physicians Meet the Challenge? *Health Affairs* 14(2):131–142.

Giacomini, M., Luft, H.S., and Robinson, J.C. 1995. Risk Adjusting Community Rated Health Plan Premiums: A Survey of Risk Assessment Literature and Policy Applications. *Annual Review of Public Health* 16:401–430.

Ginzberg, E. 1978. *Health Manpower and Health Policy*. Montclair, NJ: Allanheld Osmun.

Ginzberg, E., and Ostow, M., eds. 1984. *The Coming Physician Surplus: In Search of a Policy*. Totowa, NJ: Rowman and Allanheld.

Gold, M., Nelson, L., Lake, T., Hurley, R., and Berenson, R. 1995. Behind the Curve: A Critical Assessment of How Little Is Known About Arrangements Between Managed Care Plans and Physicians. *Medical Care Research and Review* 52(3):307–341.

Gravely, E.A., and Littlefield, J.H. 1992. A Cost-Effectiveness Analysis of Three Staffing Models for the Delivery of Low-Risk Prenatal Care. *American Journal of Public Health* 82(2):180–184.

Hartz, L.E. 1995. Quality of Care by Nurse Practitioners Delivering Colposcopy Services. *Journal of the American Academy of Nurse Practitioners* 7(1):23–27.

Health Resources Administration. 1981a. *Report of the Graduate Medical Education National Advisory Committee to the Secretary, Department of Health and Human Services, September 1980*. Volume 1, GMENAC Summary Report. Hyattsville, Md.: Health Resources Administration, U.S. Department of Health and Human Services.

Health Resources Administration. 1981b. *Nonphysician Health Care Providers Technical Panel Report*. Volume 6, GMENAC Summary Report. Hyattsville, Md.: Health Resources Administration, U.S. Department of Health and Human Services.

Henderson, T., and Chovan, T. 1994. *Removing Practice Barriers of Nonphysician Providers: Efforts by States to Improve Access to Primary Care*. Washington, DC: Intergovernmental Health Policy Project, The George Washington University.

Hooker, R.S. 1993. The Role of the Physician Assistants and Nurse Practitioners in a Managed Care Organization. In *The Role of Physician Assistants and Nurse Practitioners in Primary Care*. D.K. Clawson and M. Osterweis, eds. Washington, DC: Association of Academic Health Centers.

InterStudy, Inc. 1995. *The InterStudy Competitive Edge 5.1*. Saint Paul, Minn.: InterStudy Publications.

Institute of Medicine. 1994. *Definition of Primary Care: An Interim Report*. M. Donaldson, K. Yordy, and N. Vanselow, eds. Washington, DC: National Academy Press.

Jones, P.E., and Cawley, J.F. 1994. Physician Assistants and Health System Reform: Clinical Capabilities, Practice Activities and Potential Roles. *Journal of the American Medical Association* 271(16):1266–1272.

Kindig, D.A. 1993. What Does the Literature Tell Us About the Potential and Feasible Substitution of Non-Physician Providers for Physicians? A Policy Perspective. Princeton, NJ: The Robert Wood Johnson Foundation.

Knickman, J.R., Lipkin, M., Finkler, S.A., Thompson, W.G., and Kiel, J. 1992. The Potential for Using Non-Physicians to Compensate for the Reduced Availability of Residents. *Academic Medicine* 67(7):429–438.

Kohler, P.O. 1994. Specialists/Primary Care Professionals: Striking a Balance. *Inquiry* 31(3):289–295.

Lurie, N., Moscovice, I.S., Finch, M., Christianson, J.B., and Popkin, M.K. 1992. Does Capitation Affect the Health of the Chronically Mentally Ill? *Journal of the American Medical Association* 267(24):3300–3304.

Marder, W.D., Gaumer, G.L., and Minkovitz, C.S. 1991. GMENAC Revisited: Updated Projections for Selected Specialties. Cambridge, Mass.: Abt Associates, Inc. Unpublished paper.

McNutt, D. 1981. GMENAC: Its Manpower Forecasting Framework. *American Journal of Public Health* 71(10):1116–1124.

Mendenhall, R.C., Repicky, P.A., and Neville, R.E. 1980. Assessing the Utilization and Productivity of Nurse Practitioners and Physician Assistants: Methodology and Findings on Productivity. *Medical Care* 18(6):609–623.

Morgan, W.A. 1993. Using State Board of Nursing Data to Estimate the Number of Nurse Practitioners in the United States. *Nurse Practitioner* 18(2):65–66, 69–70, and 73–74.

Moses, E. 1994. *The Registered Nurse Population: Findings from the National Sample Survey of Registered Nurses, 1992.* Washington, DC: U.S. Government Printing Office.

Pauly, M.V. 1970. Efficiency, Incentives and Reimbursement for Health Care. *Inquiry* 7(1):114–131.

Pauly, M.V. 1992. Effectiveness Research and the Impact of Financial Incentives on Outcomes. In *Improving Health Policy and Management: Nine Critical Research Issues for the 1990s.* S.M. Shortell and U. Reinhardt, eds. Ann Arbor, Mich.: Health Administration Press.

Pauly, M.V., Hillman, A.L., and Kerstein, J. 1990. Managing Physician Incentives in Managed Care: The Role of For-Profit Ownership. *Medical Care* 28(11):1013–1024.

Pearson, L. 1994. Annual Update of How Each State Stands on Legislative Issues Affecting Advanced Nursing Practice. *The Nurse Practitioner* 19(1):11–53.

Physician Payment Review Commission. 1993. Reforming Graduate Medical Education (Chapter 4). In *Annual Report to Congress, 1993.* Washington, DC: Physician Payment Review Commission.

Physician Payment Review Commission. 1994. Nonphysician Practitioners (Chapter 14). In *Annual Report to Congress, 1994.* Washington, DC: Physician Payment Review Commission.

Physician Payment Review Commission. 1995. Provider-Driven Integration (Chapter 11). In *Annual Report to Congress, 1995.* Washington, DC: Physician Payment Review Commission.

Record, J., McCally, M., Schweitzer, S., Blomquist, R., and Berger, B. 1980. New Health Professionals After a Decade and a Half: Delegation, Productivity, and Costs in Primary Care. *Journal of Health, Politics, Policy and Law* 5(3):470–497.

Reinhardt, U. 1975. *Physician Productivity and the Demand for Health Manpower.* Cambridge, Mass.: Ballinger Publishing Company.

Reinhardt, U. 1991. Health Manpower Forecasting: The Case of Physician Supply. In *Health Services Research: Key to Health Policy.* Cambridge, Mass.: Harvard University Press.

Report Card Project. 1995. Key Findings and Lessons Learned: 21 Plans' Performance Profiles. Washington, DC: National Committee for Quality Assurance.

Robinson, J.C. 1993. Payment Mechanisms, Nonprice Incentives, and Organizational Innovation in Health Care. *Inquiry* 30:328–333.

Rodgers, C. 1994. Nonphysician Providers and Limited License Practitioners: Scope of Practice Issues. *Bulletin of the American College of Surgeons* 79(2):12–17.

Rodwin, M.A. 1993. *Medicine, Money, and Morals: Physicians' Conflicts of Interest.* New York: Oxford University Press.

Roe, B. 1981. Sounding Board. The UCR Boondoggle: A Death Knell for Private Practice? *The New England Journal of Medicine* 305(1):41–45.

Ross, F.M., Bower, P.J., and Sibbald, B.S. 1994. Practice Nurses: Characteristics, Workload and Training Needs. *British Journal of General Practice* 44(378):15–18.

Safran, D.G., Tarlov, A.R., and Rogers, W.H. 1994. Primary Care Performance in Fee-for-Service and Prepaid Health Care Systems: Results from the Medical Outcomes Study. *Journal of the American Medical Association* 271(20):1579–1586.

Safriet, B. 1992. Health Care Dollars and Regulatory Sense: The Role of Advanced Practice Nursing. *The Yale Journal of Regulation* 9(2):149–220.

Safriet, B. 1994. Impediments to Progress in Health Care Workforce Policy: License and Practice Laws. *Inquiry* 31(3):310–317.

Salkever, D.S., Skinner, E., Steinwachs, D.M., and Katz, H. 1982. Episode-Based Efficiency Comparisons for Physicians and Nurse Practitioners. *Medical Care* 20(2):143–153.

Scheffler, R.M. 1979. The Productivity of New Health Practitioners: Physician Assistants and MEDEX. *Research in Health Economics* 1:37–56.

Scheffler, R.M. 1995. Report on Selected Nonphysician Practitioners in Primary Care: Physician Assistants, Nurse Practitioners, and Certified Nurse Midwives. Unpublished background paper prepared for the Institute of Medicine.

Scheffler, R.M., Weisfeld, N., Ruby, G., and Estes, E.H. 1978. A Manpower Policy for Primary Health Care. *The New England Journal of Medicine* 298(19):1058–1062.

Scherer, J.L. 1994. Union Uprising: California Nurses React Aggressively to Work Redesign. *Hospital and Health Service Networks* 68(24):36–37.

Schneider, D.P., and Foley, W.J. 1977. A Systems Analysis of the Impact of Physician Extenders on Medical Cost and Manpower Requirements *Medical Care* 15(4):277–297.

Schneller, E.S., and Ott, J.B. 1996. Contemporary Views of Change in the Health Professions. *Hospital and Health Services Administration.* In press.

Schroeder, S.A. 1994a. The Latest Forecast. Managed Care Collides with Physician Supply. *Journal of the American Medical Association* 272(3):239–240.

Schroeder, S.A. 1994b. Managing the U.S. Health Care Workforce: Creating Policy Amidst Uncertainty. *Inquiry* 28:266–275.

Schwartz, W.B., Sloan, F.A., and Mendelson, D.N. 1988. Why There Will Be Little or No Physician Surplus Between Now and the Year 2000. *The New England Journal of Medicine* 318(14):892–897.

Schwartz, W.B., and Mendelson, D.N. 1990. No Evidence of an Emerging Physician Surplus: An Analysis of Change in Physicians' Work Load and Income. *Journal of the American Medical Association* 263(4):557–560.

Sekscenski, E., Sansom, S., Bazell, C., Salmon, M., and Mullan, F. 1994. State Practice Environments and the Supply of Physician Assistants, Nurse Practitioners, and Certified Nurse-Midwives. *The New England Journal of Medicine* 331(19):1266–1271.

Shortell, S.M., Gillies, R.R., and Anderson, D.A. 1994. New World of Managed Care: Creating Organized Delivery Systems. *Health Affairs* 13(5):46–64.

Shortell, S.M., and Hull, K.E. 1996. The New Organization of the Health Care Delivery System: In Strategic Choices for a Changing Health Care System. S.H. ALtman and U.E. Reinhardt, eds. Chicago: Health Administration Press.

Spisso, J., O'Callaghan, C., McKennan, M., and Holcroft, J.W. 1990. Improved Quality of Care and Reduction of Housestaff Workload Using Trauma Nurse Practitioners. *Journal of Trauma* 30(6):660–665.

Steinwachs, D.M. 1992. Redesign of Delivery Systems to Enhance Productivity. In *Improving Health Policy and Management: Nine Critical Research Issues for the 1990s.* S.M. Shortell and U. Reinhardt, eds. Ann Arbor, Mich.: Health Administration Press.

Steinwachs, D.M., Weiner, J.P., Shapiro, S., Batalden, P., Coltin, K., and Wasserman, F. 1986. A Comparison of the Requirements for Primary Care Physicians in HMOs with Projections Made by the GMENAC. *The New England Journal of Medicine* 314(4):217–222.

Tirado, N.C., Guzman, M., and Burgos, F. 1990. Workload Contribution of a Physician Assistant in an Ambulatory Care Setting. *Puerto Rico Health Sciences Journal* 9(2):165–167.

U.S. Bureau of the Census. 1994. *Statistical Abstract of the United States: 1994* (114th edition.) Washington, DC: U.S. Government Printing Office.

U.S. Congress, Office of Technology Assessment. 1986. *Nurse Practitioners, Physician Assistants and Certified Nurse Midwives: A Policy Analysis, Health Technology Case Study.* Washington, DC: U.S. Government Printing Office.

U.S. General Accounting Office. 1994a. *Health Care Reform: "Report Cards" Are Useful But Significant Issues Need to Be Addressed.* Gaithersburg, Md.: U.S. General Accounting Office.

U.S. General Accounting Office. 1994b. *Health Care: Employers Urge Hospitals to Battle Costs Using Performance Data Systems.* Gaithersburg, Md.: U.S. General Accounting Office.

Washington Consulting Group. 1994. *Survey of Certified Nurse Practitioners and Clinical Nurse Specialists: December 1992 Final Report to the Bureau of Health Professions,* Washington, DC: U.S. Government Printing Office.

Weiner, J.P. 1993. The Demand for Physician Services in a Changing Health Care System: A Synthesis. *Medical Care Review* 50(4):411–449.

Weiner, J.P. 1994. Forecasting the Effects of Health Reform on U.S. Physician Workforce Requirement: Evidence from HMO Staffing Patterns. *Journal of the American Medical Association* 272(3):222–230.

Weiner, J.P., Steinwachs, D.M., and Williamson, J.W. 1986. Nurse Practitioner and Physician Assistant Practices in Three HMOs: Implications for Future U.S. Health Manpower Needs. *American Journal of Public Health* 76(5):507–511.

Winslow, R. 1995. Major Purchasers of Health Services Form Alliance to Evaluate HMO Care. *Wall Street Journal,* July 3.

F

Integrating Our Primary Care and Public Health Systems: A Formula for Improving Community and Population Health

William E. Welton, M.H.A., Theodore A. Kantner, M.D., and
Sheila Moriber Katz, M.D., M.B.A.

INTRODUCTION

As we redefine the role of primary care in a health system rapidly reorienting to a market-oriented managed care paradigm, we must understand and re-explore the current and future relationship between population-based or public health services and personal medical services at the primary care level. This question is no less than that of ensuring our ability as a society to ensure and improve the health of our diverse populations in a dynamically changing delivery, financing, and accountability environment.

This question is of increasing importance as private employers move ever more aggressively, developing managed care programs to decrease costs, to improve overall accountability for performance, and to improve service quality and access. The significance is even further emphasized as government-sponsored health programs at the federal, state, and local levels (e.g., Medicare, Medicaid, Federal Employees Health Benefits Program, CHAMPUS, as well as numerous state and local employee health benefit and worker's compensation programs) move just as aggressively to adopt managed care concepts. Increasingly, prag-

Mr. Welton is Acting Dean of the School of Public Health at the Medical College of Pennsylvania and Hahnemann University in Philadelphia, Pa., Dr. Kantner is the Chairman of the Department of Family Medicine at the University and Deputy Director of its Robert Wood Johnson sponsored Generalist Physician Initiative, and Dr. Katz is the Senior Associate Dean of the Proposed School of Public Health and former Dean of the Hahnemann University School of Medicine. The authors express their appreciation to Mary Neighbour for editorial assistance provided.

matic analysis requires a rethinking of traditional notions and paradigms of population (public) health.

This paper identifies current issues and offers suggestions for integrating concepts to support functional and practical improvement while ensuring population health maintenance and improvement and reasonable access to services in a context of controlled long-term per capita cost. To ensure these desired outcomes, we must expand our vision to encompass both *population-based* and *primary* medicine and health care services as a single integrated system; we must work to remove barriers to its formation; we must develop new operating paradigms to ensure its high-quality performance; and we must develop programs to focus its objectives and ameliorate its excesses.

This paper identifies and highlights significant requirements and challenges for leadership within the public health and primary care communities, and for educational and research leadership among academicians serving and supporting those communities. In the final analysis, many of these challenges must also be addressed and changes supported by visionary leaders within our political and health care delivery systems, if such integrated community health systems are to be created and their potential achieved.

In short, we must view both public health and primary care as two interacting and mutually supportive components of an increasingly complex integrated community health system, having the single common goal of improving the health of a community and its diverse populations.

BACKGROUND: PUBLIC HEALTH AND PRIMARY CARE

We noted with interest the relative paucity of published material directly addressing the intersection and interaction of population-based programs and services (public health) and primary care programs and services. It is significant that many of the seminal documents on the subject are in the form of special reports and studies commissioned by the Institute of Medicine (IOM), a small number of private foundations, and, more recently, the U.S. Public Health Service (USPHS). In short, the subject is rarely dealt with directly but more often is dealt with obliquely, perhaps indicating a need for new concepts to guide our thinking.

Relatively few of the small number of writings identified were written from the perspective of public health. Most were written from the perspective(s) of preventive medicine and family medicine (mostly community-oriented primary care [COPC]). Few were identified in the internal medicine and pediatric literature. In general, the COPC concept has not spread broadly throughout the world of primary care medical practice since being the subject of a 1984 IOM study (1). The COPC practice model appears to be most apparent in staff-model health maintenance organizations (HMOs) and in a relatively small number of academic community-based practices. This report and concept have been important in guiding our developing thoughts on the appropriate roles and relationships of both public health and primary care, however.

Over the past two decades, our understanding of public health and primary health care has gone through a number of important transitions. It is important to acknowledge, at this juncture, that public health and primary health care have each developed as distinct and largely unrelated (somewhat competitive) cultures over the past 80 years. It may now be important to develop a more integrated view of the two, however, because these distinct cultures are increasingly being forced to operate together as a result of a series of broader market reforms. Increasingly, these market reforms emphasize the development of competitive managed care programs and strategies to organize and provide integrated health care and preventive services at controlled cost and quality to defined populations, including most of those formerly cared for directly by local and state health departments. This can be seen by the increasingly rapid transition of Medicaid populations to a broad range of managed care programs over the past decade. In this context it is also important to acknowledge the seeming preference of our political system to seek market-oriented solutions to complex health care problems.

As a result, the public health of the past will increasingly become the population health of the future and the primary care of the past will increasingly become the clinical and preventive primary care and community-based medicine of the future. The combination of the two—working more closely (if not always in absolute harmony) in partnership with each other, with integrated health delivery systems, and with market-oriented financing systems to improve the health of the same populations—is increasingly likely to evolve toward the integrated community health system of the future.

In 1994 the IOM began its most recent exploration of primary care by clarifying its use of the term as one that "focuses on the delivery of personal health services" (2). This focus builds on the IOM's earlier conceptualization of COPC:

> [By 1984 the notion of] community oriented primary care . . . [had evolved as] . . . "a strategy whereby the elements of primary health care and of community medicine are systematically developed and brought together in a coordinated practice" [Abramson and Kark, 1983, p. 22]. [It was also] the provision of *primary care services* to a *defined community*, coupled with *systematic efforts to identify and address the major health problems of that community* through effective modifications in both the primary care services and other appropriate community health programs [italics added] (1, p. 2; 2, p. 12).

IOM's most recent formal definition of primary care combines concepts contained in both paragraphs, above:

> the provision of *integrated, accessible health care services* by *clinicians* who are *accountable* for addressing a large *majority of personal health care needs,* developing a *sustained partnership* with *patients,* and practicing in the *context of family and community* (2, p. 15).

During the period preceding this report, significant attention has also been given to developing a clearer understanding of the role of "public health" in our pluralistic, diverse, and often fragmented society. In 1988, the IOM published its report *The Future of Public Health* (3), which has provided significant guidance to the development of public health since that time. The study committee's core recommendations included the following: "the mission of public health (is defined) as fulfilling society's interest in assuring conditions in which people can be healthy" and "the core functions of public health agencies at all levels of government are assessment, policy development, and assurance" (3, p. 7). Additional implementation recommendations were made in areas involving the creation of the appropriate statutory authority, reorganizing all health functions into a single cabinet-level agency (separate from income maintenance functions) at the state level, definition of clear lines of public accountability for public health down through the local level, and strengthening public health ties to the related areas of mental health, environmental health, social services, and care of the indigent (3, pp. 8–13).

From a conceptual point of view the report outlines the basic public health functions of government as shown in Figure F-1.

Assessment involves the systematic collection and analysis of information on the health of the community; assurance involves ensuring that necessary services are provided to achieve agreed-upon (population health) goals; evaluation reviews the results of prior actions (or inactions) relative to previously determined policy goals and/or quality standards; and policy development is intended to guide the operation of the health system and resource allocation for its support,

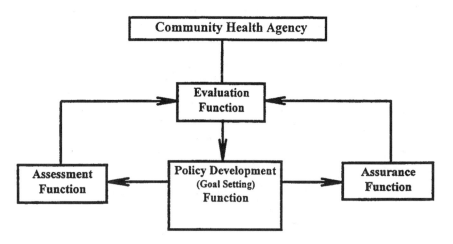

FIGURE F-1 Functions of public health. SOURCE: Adapted from Institute of Medicine (1988), with modifications and clarifications suggested by the authors.

while taking a strategic approach in the context of a democratic political process (3, p. 8).

Within this overall construct we can seek further clarification of the role of public health and its division of effort with primary care medicine in the increasingly important area of prevention as suggested by the Partnership for Prevention in 1993 (4). That report identified three essential elements of prevention: clinical preventive services, community-based health promotion and disease prevention, and public policy for health promotion and disease prevention. In many ways the area of prevention is the critical link between traditional notions of public health and personal and community health (4). In this paper we will assume that the responsibilities for providing and/or facilitating clinical preventive services reside principally within the primary care personal service arena. In this paper we will also assume that the principal responsibility for providing and/or ensuring the provision and coordination of community-based health promotion and disease prevention and public policy for health promotion resides principally within the public arena.

Emphasis is given to the importance of these elements and is eloquently emphasized by Lashof (5) and Schauffler (6) in their papers. We endorse the importance of these points and include them as a matter of definition and clarification in the model(s) set forth throughout this paper in the following manner. For the purposes of this paper, IOM's concepts of assessment and assurance (3) (Figure F-1) will be assumed to incorporate the appropriately determined public functions associated with community-based health promotion and disease prevention. Additionally, the policy development function will be assumed to incorporate the appropriately determined public policy functions required to support health promotion and disease prevention programs. It is significant that Schauffler goes further to propose the development of a new form of community-based organization, community-based health promotion and disease prevention. Such a public-private organization would be separate from the health department, would be based on collaborative and partnership principles within and across the community, and would assume significant responsibility for overseeing community-based programs of health promotion and disease prevention and for providing appropriate linkages between the world of primary and preventive services and public health policy (6).

A more recent and somewhat more functionally oriented definition of public health is provided in the 1994 USPHS *Report for a Healthy Nation: Returns on Investment in Public Health* (7). According to the report, public health (7, p. 1):

Prevents epidemics
Protects the environment, workplaces, housing, food, and water
Promotes healthy behaviors
Monitors the health status of the population
Mobilizes community action

Responds to disasters
Assures the quality, accessibility, and accountability of medical care
Reaches out to link high-risk and hard-to-reach people to needed services
Researches to develop new insights and innovative solutions
Leads the development of sound health policy and planning

Over the past two decades, the definitional refinements for primary care and for public health have taken place, for the most part, independently of each other. To date, there does not appear to be a single integrated definition that has as its explicit purpose the integration of the two into a single system with the common goal of improving the health of populations through a team approach.

This general issue was recently recognized by Joyce Lashof in 1991:

Bringing public health and primary care together is essential for the economically disadvantaged, but it is also increasingly important to all communities. What is lacking in this effort, however, is the organizational and financial mechanisms necessary to implement this approach on a larger scale (8).

Additionally, Thomas Rundall recently recognized the issue in the broader context of medicine and public health in his discussion of the need to seek their more effective integration (9):

[T]he effectiveness of our future system for improving the health of our citizens depends greatly on the reform and [effective] integration of our nation's public health and medical care systems . . . [where] "effective" means successfully achieving the functions the system is designed to perform . . . (and) functional integration ("unity or harmony within a system based upon the interdependence of specialized parts"—Theodorson and Theodorson, Modern Dictionary of Sociology, 1969). . . . The benefits to our nation's health of proceeding in this way, however, are enormous. As we move into the twenty-first century, an integrated system of public health and medical care services is our nation's best hope not only for improving the health of all of our citizens, but also for closing the "health gap" between socioeconomically disadvantaged groups and the rest of the population.

These definitional refinements have paralleled significant changes in our national health care system, as seen through the passage of the HMO Act of 1973 (and subsequent amendments), OBRA 1991 (diagnosis-related group reimbursement for hospitals), and subsequent legislation defining physician payment in terms of the Resource-Based Relative Value Scale. These major legislative initiatives, occurring in combination with the increasingly aggressive adoption of managed care programs by large employers and governmental programs, have begun to force a practical integration of personal and preventive services and the development of population-based management and assurance systems to support this integration. Unfortunately, as we will see, this often happens without utilizing our traditional public health systems, thus leading to additional confusion and inefficiency, with an inherent loss of effectiveness in achieving the larger goal of improving the health of the population.

Since the creation of Medicare and Medicaid in 1966, the focus of the nation's health and budgetary policy makers has increasingly turned to issues of cost-containment. Over the same period, the focus of the nation's major industries and employers has turned to issues of international competitiveness and cost control focusing on controlling the rapidly rising cost of health care. State and local governments are facing increasingly constrained resources to support rapidly rising health care costs and the competing needs of more effective social, educational, and crime prevention programs. Overall, the demands have increasingly focused on preventing premature death and disability and on achieving greater value for resources expended.

In 1993 McGinnis and Foege published a landmark study identifying the actual causes of death in the United States (10). In that study the authors concluded that

> Approximately half of all deaths that occurred among U.S. residents in 1990 could be attributed to the factors identified [tobacco, 19 percent; diet/activity patterns, 14 percent; alcohol, 5 percent; microbial agents, 4 percent; toxic agents, 3 percent; firearms, 2 percent; motor vehicles, 1 percent; illicit use of drugs, 1 percent]. Despite their approximate nature these estimates . . . hold implications for program priorities . . . (and) . . . they compel examination of the way the United States tracks its health status.

This conclusion underscores the fact that most of these deaths are behaviorally mediated and are therefore potentially preventable. They "are by definition premature and are often preceded by impaired quality of life . . . the public health burden imposed by these contributors offers both a mandate and guidance for shaping health policy priorities" (10).

In a similar vein the 1994 USPHS *Report for a Healthy Nation: Returns on Investment in Public Health* (7) noted

> An appropriate investment in public health will lead to substantial future savings in medical care. . . . The fulfillment of public and personal health objectives will increasingly require close collaboration between the changing medical care and public health systems . . . even a reformed medical care system cannot mount the appropriate actions to address many of the conditions responsible for death and disability in the United States today.

In his 1994 book *Medicine's Dilemmas: Infinite Needs Versus Finite Resources* (11), William L. Kissick observes these needs from the medical care perspective, providing the following insights:

> The golden rule of health care in our society is that everyone deserves the finest health care attainable, provided someone else pays. . . . In health care it is possible to spend more but get less value, if value is measured as health status for the population. . . . Increasing quality or access adds value, but then so does

lowering costs if what we seek is cost-effectiveness. Costs, like access and quality and, for that matter, health itself, are relative (11, pp. 2, 14).

The foregoing assessment, of course, begs the issue of the interacting and interdependent "systems" relationship of public (population) health and primary care. Increasingly, public health leaders are calling for an integrated view of population and personal health. Of special note is Philip Lee's delivery of the 1994 Shattuck Lecture to the Massachusetts Medical Society (12), in which he observed

> Today, perhaps the best linkage between the personal health care system and the public health system is in the area of clinical preventive services. While clinical preventive services provide one very significant link, applying the population based perspective of public health to the personal health care system in its totality is the next necessary step. . . . In spite of the intellectual underpinnings and the syntheses of ideas integrating public health and personal health care, public policy has continued to separate public health from the personal health care system, However, if we want to achieve the goals of increasing the span of healthy life for Americans and reducing the health disparities among Americans at an affordable cost, our nation must adopt . . . an approach that accentuates and promotes a close working relationship between the personal care and public health systems (12).

All of these factors force us to refocus on the practical questions of the prevention-effectiveness and cost-effectiveness of our somewhat idealized "integrated health care system," as distinguished from its medical and acute care subsystems with which we are more familiar today.

THE STARTING POINT: A SYSTEMS MODEL
FOR CLINICAL AND PREVENTIVE SERVICES

If one accepts the notion that public health and primary care are two facets of a complex system influencing personal, population, and community health status, the next steps are to synthesize a model for such a system and to identify areas for specific intervention and improvement to move our health care system to higher levels of effectiveness. The beginnings for such a synthesis have been suggested by Thompson et al. (13) in their article "Primary and Secondary Prevention Services in Clinical Practice: Twenty Years' Experience in Development, Implementation, and Evaluation." In that article, the authors describe their own and their HMO's experience with primary and clinical preventive services and provide their recommendations for the effective implementation of an integrated population health and primary care model. Their overall conclusion is that

> Systematic population-based approaches to the development and provision of clinical preventive services targeting the one-to-one level of primary care and multiple infrastructure levels of care are forging a synthesis of clinical medicine

and public health approaches. This approach will become pervasive as clinical information systems improve, risk information is captured routinely, and practitioners gain skills in the art of risk behavior change and population-based care (13).

The key elements and concepts of their general model are summarized below. Critical elements for an ideal preventive care provision model are as follows (13):

- Population-based planning.
- Directed toward major causes of morbidity and mortality, epidemiologically determined. This includes the epidemiology of "needs" (the diseases and the risks) and the epidemiology of the "wants" (the desires of the enrollees).
- Evidence for intervention effectiveness.
- Functioning at multiple levels, including one-to-one level of primary care, infrastructure level, organization level, and external community.
- Prospective and automated to the maximum extent feasible.
- Health is a by-product of a shared endeavor between practitioners and patients; informed discussion and consent are maximized.

Criteria used to examine primary and secondary prevention issues are as follows:

- Condition (disease/risk factor) is important.
- The disease or risk factor has a recognizable presymptomatic stage.
- Reliable methods for detecting the disease or factor exist (considering the sensitivity, specificity, and positive predictive values of the screening test).
- Modifications of the risk factor therapy in the presymptomatic disease stage reduces morbidity and mortality more than after symptoms appear.
- Facilities to address the identified risk factor or condition exist.
- The cost and potential benefits of implementing a state-of-the-art approach have been considered.

Thompson et al. (13) have used these concepts to develop an intervention model, summarized in Figure F-2, which specifies three groups of factors necessary to support behavioral change in health professionals and necessary to achieve effective integration of primary and preventive medical services when the professionals deliver those services from an integrated population and individual or personal health perspective. These factor groups include those that predispose a health professional to make a necessary behavioral change in his or her practice (predisposing factors), those that make necessary behavioral change possible (enabling factors at the community level, organization level, and practice environment level), and those that reward and strengthen behavioral change (reinforcing factors).

The model goes on to define an integrated professional and behavioral system supporting effective and efficient delivery of personal health services (pri-

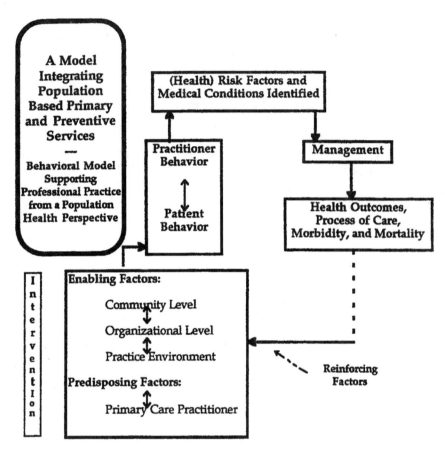

FIGURE F-2 A model integrating population-based primary and preventive services.
SOURCE: Adapted from Thompson et al. (1995).

mary and preventive care) in a population health context (an enrolled [defined] HMO population). The model has been developed and evaluated over a period of 20 years and has produced impressive results including

> a 32% decrease in late stage breast cancer (1989 to 1990); 89 percent of 2-year-olds with complete immunizations (1994); decrease in adult smokers from 25% to 17% (1985 to 1994); and an increase in bicycle safety helmet use among children from 4% to 48% along with a 67% decrease in bicycle-related head injuries (1987 to 1992) (13).

Although the work makes a significant theoretical and practical contribution to our understanding of the integration and actual delivery of population health and primary care concepts and its application to an organized primary care practice population, it begs the question of how this, or any model(s) of population-focused clinical and preventive services, can and should fit into an even broader and more integrated "systems" model supporting improvement of the health of the broader community.

Moving from the delivery model of clinical and preventive services within a staff model HMO, one might logically ask how this differs from the COPC model. The medical practice, as described, does not appear to be organized as a COPC model, although one could say that the staff model HMO is an ideal model for providing community-oriented medical care (COMC).

At the primary care level itself, the COPC concept and model attempt to extend the population-based clinical and preventive oriented primary care practice model described above by

- Defining and characterizing (a) "community" for which it has assumed responsibility to provide health care.
- Through local research the practice identifies the community's health problems.
- Modifying the (service) program in light of problems defined above.
- Monitoring the impact of the program's modification (14).

At this point one could simply conclude that community-oriented primary care is an excellent idea if the population of interest is clearly defined, if the medical practice is organized appropriately, if the financial incentives are appropriately aligned, if the policy support and community service coordination exist, if the staffing is affordable, and if the professionals are appropriately trained.

As noted earlier, the COPC model has not expanded its practice base substantially in this country beyond a relatively small number of academia-based urban practices and a number of staff-model HMOs (which place an increasing emphasis on the integration and delivery of clinical and preventive services at the primary care practice level). Observations on the state of the experiences of the COPC movement to date and shedding some light on its state are provided as follows:

A critical review of COPC applications in the United States shows that despite investigators' use of epidemiologic methods to identify important local health problems, the lack of a supportive policy environment has hampered local efforts to address these problems.

[T]he gap between knowledge about local problems and the power to achieve responsive policies has received scant attention in the COPC literature. While the efforts of COPC leaders deserve praise, optimism about the success of piecemeal approaches to local problems is less warranted than one might suppose. The situation is not likely to improve unless consistent and responsive national (state, and local) policies are put in place to support local actions (14).

Additionally, the W.K. Kellogg Foundation sponsored a demonstration project to begin 13 COPC rural practices in cooperation with the National Rural Health Association from 1989 to 1992. The Kellogg experience is summarized as follows:

the evaluation findings support previous reports in the literature of substantial impediments to the integration of COPC into primary care physician practices

for practices to play a substantial role in the COPC process, they may need to rethink their mission in very fundamental ways

another important finding relates to the (substantial) time and resources required to carry out the different elements in the COPC process

the experience of the demonstration also suggests that communities, with the support of local practices, can accomplish many COPC objectives, although this goal requires modification of COPC as it is generally conceptualized (15, pp. 489–501).

Despite substantial efforts to demonstrate its applicability and utility COPC has encountered significant obstacles to its spread, including the lack of generalized adoption as the practice and training model of choice across all primary care specialties (or at least more than family medicine alone); we should note that no one has suggested that the COPC model is inappropriate, simply suggest that the barriers to its effective implementation appear to have been too great to ensure widespread, rapid expansion to date.

Although there has been somewhat limited success of the COPC movement, one must conclude that there is still no viable model for integrating the population-based primary care practice effectively into a single population-based integrated community health care system at the general population level of the broader community, with the exception of the community-accountable and community-oriented staff model HMO, committed to the provision of COMC. Unfortunately, these models are few and far between.

MOVING TOWARD AN INTEGRATED COMMUNITY HEALTH SYSTEM: UNDERSTANDING PUBLIC HEALTH AND PRIMARY CARE INTERACTIONS

In general, there does not appear to be an effective and integrated working partnership between public health practitioners and community-based primary care practitioners in the local community. This, we believe, is not very surprising for two main reasons: (a) the historical cultures of public health and primary care medicine have not placed a value on building and maintaining this relationship and (b) the historical paradigms are shifting dramatically to one of managing the per capita cost and outcomes of enrolled populations under conditions of financial risk and market competitiveness. These two observations present both a large problem and a large opportunity for the public health and primary care communities, both of which bear significant shared responsibility for the health of populations within the community.

Because not much research has been conducted nor has much been written on the subject of this paper, we initiated discussions with a range of primary care and preventive medicine practitioners and educators and with public health practitioners and educators locally.[1] Most recently, this collaboration took the form of a roundtable discussion focusing on the relationship and relative roles of primary care and public health. The resulting insights are, we believe, sufficiently significant to suggest a direction for future investigation, synthesis, and policy evaluation in this important area. The observations and conclusions of the panel are important in that they provide early practical insight into a somewhat murky area. The conclusions may not be generalizable to all communities, but on the basis of other, similar discussions, we believe that the observations will provide guidance for others.

For background information, a summary of primary care and public health perspectives is presented below, organized by general areas of concern.

Primary Care Practitioner Perspective: General Comments

There is a conceptual gap between the primary care physician and the public health professional:

- Primary care physicians are providing care to individual patients and families.
- They do not routinely stay in touch with the local health department.
- Reportable diseases are generally reported through clinical laboratories.
- Incidence and prevalence of diseases of significance to the primary care practitioner and his (her) individual practice community are often not reportable (e.g. asthma, diabetes, coronary heart disease, etc.).
- Often, therefore, the local health department does not communicate information of practical importance to the primary care practitioner's practice.
- Neither group seems to talk about the same subject, community, or population at the same time.
- Many times it seems that each interrupts the other's work flow and, in fact, makes that work even more difficult and less efficient than it already is.

---

[1]The panel included (in addition to the authors) Richard Baron, MD (general internal medicine and medical director of a large Medicaid HMO; Trude Haecker, MD (pediatrician); Russell Maulitz, MD (general internal medicine and medical informatics); and Michael Spence, MD MPH (public health, preventive medicine, and obstetrics). Transcript editing was completed by Nancy Desmond.

It is, therefore, often difficult to believe that both are focusing on a common objective: improving the health of the same population.

Primary Care and Public Health Professionals in the Community

Both primary care practitioners and public health professionals are often marginalized in the broader health community. Knowledge-based, research-driven traditional medicine often focuses on finding and applying improved technical solutions to difficult technical problems and has attracted significant funding and public support, so it has become the focus of medical education and professional esteem. Neither primary care nor public health professionals have that focus. Both will need to recognize that they must build the better organizational, informational, and systems solutions of the future—as a team, however. These solutions will, of course, involve creation of a more efficient and effective population-focused health delivery system, integrated with more effective systems and methods for delivering primary and preventive services to individuals in a systems context.

Primary care physicians and public health professionals will need to understand that they often have much in common with each other as they develop the necessary systems solutions to difficult organization problems and as they provide the necessary leadership in these important areas to their communities and to their colleagues within the specialty medical community.

Integration of Public Health and Medicine in Education and in Practice

Integration of public health and primary care through a shared population perspective has been neither a primary focus nor an inherent value in either the primary care or public health educational and practice cultures. In practice, over many decades, neither public health nor primary care professionals have concentrated on constructing systems of mutual benefit aimed at supporting the work of the other. Both seem to have defined their own roles and methods independently of the other.

Achieving integration in community-based ambulatory medical practice requires resources (time, staff, easy and comprehensive information access, etc.) and organization that most practitioners do not have and cannot afford. Economic drawbacks to integration often make it simpler to continue to do what has been done before.

Integration of services and functions at the health department often appears nonexistent, and the system often appears to be completely compartmentalized. The shift toward a holistic outlook has already begun in primary care, but it has not yet begun in public health. Public health is still very fragmented, which is frustrating to generalist primary care physicians. Public health appears to be a series of subspecialties as well.

If the focus of both primary care medicine and public health move to a common and synchronized educational base and operate with and from common information and support systems, providing benefit for both and for their common patients, clients, and constituents within the same population(s), we will begin to eliminate this fragmentation.

Clinical Decision Making, Public Health, Primary Care, and Managed Care

A large concern of primary care physicians has to do with the de facto determination of health policy and standards of medical practice through individual health plan or HMO reimbursement policies. Ultimately, physicians are likely to be influenced by what they are paid for. Who is determining these policies and who is accountable to the public interest for the quality of their decision making? Who resolves policy conflicts among payers in favor of the public interest? The practicing physician and the patients are often caught in the middle. Generally, the payer with the most muscle or the one who gets there first will determine de facto clinical standards through early reimbursement policies. Perhaps the determination of general standards and the monitoring of performance against those standards of payers, professionals, and institutions should be a role of tomorrow's public health professionals, ensuring population health.

Information to Support Population Health Improvement, Health System Efficiency, and Health System Effectiveness

The increasingly rapid move to managed care in most larger metropolitan markets is forcing the management perspective of health systems, managers, and physicians to the population level. Information is the currency necessary to manage a population's health status efficiently and effectively. Population-based information is absolutely essential to define standards, to monitor performance against those standards, and to ensure public accountability over time. Managed care systems are playing the leadership role today, and state and local health departments are often sitting on the sidelines.

The community and its health providers often operate in a Tower of Babel because no one is standardizing record-keeping and information systems. This situation helps no one, particularly patients. Many providers feel that the state and local health departments or affiliated and newly formed nonprofit organizations chartered and operating in the public interest should be playing a community-wide role in leading this development. There are related roles in standardizing information systems across health plans and integrated health delivery systems and in supporting patients and families over time as they change health plans and move through their life cycles. This sort of information tracking will be increasingly important as the population ages and as management of chronic disease and the prevention of disability become increasingly important. In short, a kinship and potential for shared perspective and values exist between public health in this context and primary care practitioners.

Information to Ensure Market Function and Health Plan Accountability

Just as broad-based population health information is essential for ensuring the quality of care—currently and longitudinally—to populations and communities, it is also essential to improve market function and the public accountability of health plans offered in the market. In short, there are issues of consumer protection that are of great consequence. If, as a matter of policy, our society continues its movement to an even greater emphasis on competitive markets for health plans, and if one of the effects of such a policy is to deemphasize the traditional public and community accountability of the not-for-profit hospital system (deemphasizing their historical community accountability role through increased reliance on nationally owned insurance-driven health plans), who will step in at the local level to assure quality and access? Many believe that this role will be increasingly important for state and local health departments or community health agencies affiliated with the health departments. It is likely to require both a major shift in perspective and a Manhattan Project to develop community standards for community health information systems, however.

Public Health, Community Services, and Primary Care

The complexity of problems seen by primary care practitioners is growing, and many problems require coordination of a complex array of community-based social, educational, support, and transportation services. It is not uncommon for primary care practitioners to interact with utility companies to ensure that a patient's home will have heat. Public health can help primary care in this area by attempting to coordinate community-based medical support, social, educational, and transportation services with the primary care community. Even simple and inexpensive steps in this area are likely to show significant improvement at the patient, family, and individual practice levels. Coordination and standardization of information flows across all of these boundaries will only help patients of primary care practitioners who are also citizens of the community (and who also vote for the mayor or governor).

Community-Oriented Primary Care, Public Health, and the Primary Care Practitioner

Today, 10 years after the publication of the IOM study on COPC, it is interesting to note the relatively small number of primary care practices and graduate medical education training programs serving a relatively small number of mostly underserved urban communities. At the same time it is significant to note a growing number of influential multispecialty group practices and staff model HMOs around the country (Kaiser, Henry Ford, Group Health Cooperative, Harvard Community Health Plan, etc.) that are increasingly incorporating COPC—like clinical and preventive patient services and management models and strategies into their primary care practices. Perhaps the message is that the focus must be broad medically, community-wise, policy-wise, educationally, and financially. This stands to reason since communities are complex and diverse themselves.

One additional note at this point must take into account the focal emphasis on COPC in a portion of the family medicine community and its relative absence in the internal medicine and pediatrics communities. Rhetorically, how can we move to COPC unless the primary care disciplines standardize training and practice models and integrate those standardized models appropriately with current systems of economic incentives and organizational design and accountability?

Primary Care Office Practice and Public Health

The primary care office is a bad place for a primary care physician to do public health. The proper tools are not available, and physicians do not have the denominator data necessary to analyze the information (even if they were trained to do it). Primary care physicians need a public health entity that has the necessary resources and the willingness to collect information relevant to his/her practice and to communicate the information it has on a timely basis to support the primary care practitioner. At the same time the local health department is often not structured to meet the public health needs of the primary care physician. As noted earlier, this leads to lack of meaningful and/or timely communication between the two groups. We need to view the two groups as part of a single system and members of a collaborative team with common objectives—improving population and community health, sharing the same information systems, and serving the same patients and populations at the same time.

Primary Care, Public Health, and Mental Health

Many of the same comments stated above apply to the mental health system's support of primary care practice as well. It is estimated that as much as 30 to 40 percent of family relations are affected by some kind of mental health, behavioral, or substance abuse problem over time. Additionally, mental health and substance abuse problems are often dealt with in discrete, but uncoordinated systems of care (community mental health centers, employee assistance programs, worker's compensation, automobile insurance, and so forth). Rarely do these systems of care interact effectively with the primary care medical care system. Perhaps the local health department could play an integrating, standardizing, and coordinating role in these areas as well. The concept here is not dissimilar to the earlier discussion about managed care.

Public Health, Primary Care, and Organizational Issues

As noted earlier, public health departments must increasingly fulfill the role of ensuring population and community health. We also noted the reality of society's movement to a health care system and service environment increasingly characterized by managed care provided in a competitive market context. In fulfilling its responsibilities to ensure the health of populations, the public health department of the future will increasingly need to play a coordinating, standardizing, and monitoring role relative to the vast array of personal health and community-based social services. This will be necessary to ensure access to populations by increasing the efficiency and effectiveness of local markets for health care services.

To accomplish this critical and mission-related objective, public health departments (or some other appropriate community health agency) assuming responsibility for ensuring access and service must assure the appropriate function of the health care market as well. One of the most important functions to be accomplished in this regard will be to ensure the standardization and availability of information to health providers and managed care organizations and to consumers—individuals, employers, and government program sponsors. To accomplish this critical function it will be particularly important for public health departments or other designated community health agencies to establish strong operational relationships with managed care organizations and with emerging integrated delivery systems, many of which are combining hospitals and primary care physicians in the same organizational structures.

These operational relationships must be based on standardized information exchange and a strong emphasis on communications. Many of these emerging systems have broader resource bases than solo or small-group primary care practices, and it may therefore be easier in many cases to emphasize the development of primary care and public health communications relationships between the health department and the medical directors of these emerging organizations. In communities where there are significant medical and nursing training activities in the area of primary care, as well as training activities in public health, it may also be important to develop ongoing communications systems, as well as to standardize training program emphasis on primary care and preventive health services within the community.

By developing these roles and relationships it will also be easier and quicker to establish standards and to conduct health services research, to determine more efficient and effective information flows and organizational forms to improve population and community health.

Finally, significant opportunities exist for health departments, schools of public health, and schools of medicine to collaborate with each other and with these emerging systems of care—sharing in research and in training for the future. These partnerships, and those with managed care organizations and emerging integrated health delivery systems, will be critical to ensure the future health of populations and communities. Unless these relationships are properly developed and managed by health departments, on the basis of a realistic local assessment of local market conditions for health services and its future direction, major opportunities for improving population and community health will almost certainly be lost.

The above observations seem to have a single common denominator. All represent significant discontinuities at the critical interface between the traditional population- and community-based services of public health and the emerging personal care system required to provide the base of integrated clinical and preventive services—in a population and community context—essential to maintain and/or improve population and community health in this period of transition to a more market-oriented health economy. All seem to result from decades of separation of education, practice, research, professional culture, perspective, and accountability structures for the health professionals and organizations that must now increasingly work in partnership and in common organizational structures to succeed in achieving common objectives.

The implications of these observations are profound for both public health and medicine—education, practice, and research—as we approach the 21st century. In the next section, we will explore these implications and suggest a number of future directions for both public health and primary care.

Improving Community Health Through an Integrated Community Health System

We have concluded that there is a need to visualize a health care system that includes a number of elements acting as a regularly interacting or interdependent group of elements forming a unified whole, with the overall goal being to improve the long-term health of population(s). The health care system must accept significant (but not necessarily total) responsibility for this. If we accept the fact that our existing and compartmentalized independent systems of primary care and population health are not achieving this objective either efficiently or effectively, if at all, we must now begin to suggest an alternative model for the future.

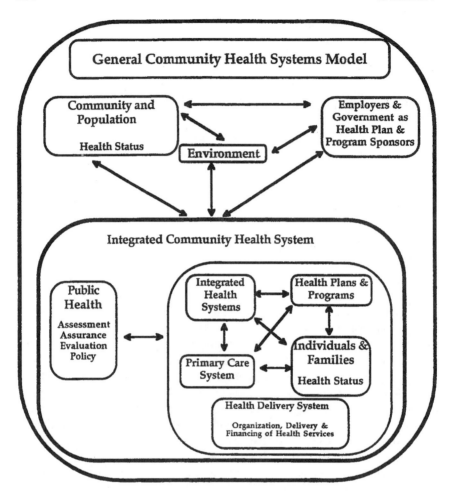

FIGURE F-3 General community health systems model.

Figure F-3 suggests the key elements, their conceptual interrelations, and their fundamental interactions within a general community health systems model.

Although Figure F-3 is somewhat complex, we believe it is generally accurate in portraying what is an inherently complex set of roles, responsibilities, relationships, interrelationships, and interactions. Perhaps this observation is important for policy makers, since it is clear that we, as a society, have not designed or accepted such a "system" to achieve our "clearly defined objectives" efficiently. This observation, of course, begs the significant policy question of: (1) whether we should *wish* to; (2) the economic question of whether we *must* (in order to continue to obtain reasonable services at affordable cost); and (3) the significant legal and political questions of whether we *can,* and under what circumstances and constraints. In any event, the development of a community health systems perspective may be the single most important conceptual reorientation necessary to ensure population and community health over time.

In evaluating such a systems concept and assuming the objective of "fulfilling society's interest in fulfilling conditions in which people can be healthy" (3, p. 7), it is important to define essential organizational requirements for optimal system performance. These may be summarized as follows:

1. Objectives must be clearly defined to achieve population health status targets.

2. System operating elements and critical relationships among elements must be clearly defined; responsibilities must be defined, agreed upon, and accepted; performance measurement systems defined (for the system as a whole and for each element of the system); and incentive systems must be designed to ensure that individual and system objectives are met.

3. Information systems, record-keeping systems, and information access policies must be designed and standardized to support the operation and outcomes evaluation of all elements of the system individually and to support the operation and outcomes evaluation of the system as a whole.

4. Population-based assessment, education, and resource services must be available as and when necessary to support the discharge of system element responsibilities. Assessment and resource services must be related to the populations for which individual practitioners and other operating elements of the system have direct responsibility.

5. Ongoing programs of quality assessment must be established, as must programs of continuing improvement, including continuing education of individuals, families, community organizations, school systems, employers, health plans, and providers.

6. To ensure that such a system operates effectively, it is essential to have appropriately trained personnel. Some of the training will occur within the system through the ongoing performance improvement process.

Ultimately, these integrated community health systems must depend on the educational establishment to train a broad range of health professionals (not only primary care physicians) appropriately to work in such a systems environment. In addition to any basic technical skills, educational programs must emphasize such elements as systems thinking and future orientation, how to achieve effectiveness through interdisciplinary teams, integration of diverse skills and information elements as a basis for critical analysis, organization and management skills (at varying levels of sophistication), and continuous evaluation and improvement skills.

Parenthetically, the adoption of these educational outcome objectives will mean significant change for educational institutions and programs, for those bodies that accredit them, and, finally, for the educators, themselves.

As an old Vermonter once said, "If you don't know where you're go'in, any road'll get you there." It's a tall order for change, but a necessary one to achieve the long-term results in population health maintenance and/or improvement that we all desire.

We submit that the key elements of an integrated model have already surfaced, in pieces. They simply have not been linked, integrated, or properly supported, however. Specifically, we refer to the functions of public health as outlined in Figure F-1 and the integrated system of primary and preventive care (P&PC) for clinical and preventive services outlined in Figure F-2. When the two are combined with each P&PC and the community health agency focuses on monitoring and supporting the health improvement of the same specific populations—in an information environment defined and supported through an integrated community health information network and in a context within which the health status impacts of improvements in environmental and occupational health policy and programs are understood and integrated (even if these policies and programs are not, as is most often the case, under the control of the health department)—a model for an integrated community health system emerges, as outlined in Figure F-4.

We note that such a system does not require a merged financial, business, or operating organization. It simply organizes and standardizes the market environment within which population-based providers will function. To this end it also standardizes technical, educational, marketing, and evaluative information flows within the market, thus leading to higher levels of public accountability and more efficient market function. Note that this model emphasizes accountability to the community for the overall functioning of the market for health insurance and for the results in terms of population health improvement, provider coordination, and consistency of public expectations.

With such a system in place and with proper attention paid to policy objectives and public accountability, its ultimate operation can only be positive relative to the dilemma presented by the "iron triangle" of cost containment, quality, and access noted by Kissick (Figure F-5).

Finally, the perspective of all systems elements is moved to the population(s) served within the community through its various health plans. Once the system is organized from the population perspective, health status expectations and accountabilities are established, the infrastructure providing universal provider access to standardized information on a real-time or other timely basis is in place, and the capitated reimbursement mechanisms and per capita performance measurements and operating systems are developed and aligned, the overall system should begin to work much more effectively than today's system does to improve the health of the community and its populations.

Although it is important to begin our overall recommendations with a gen-

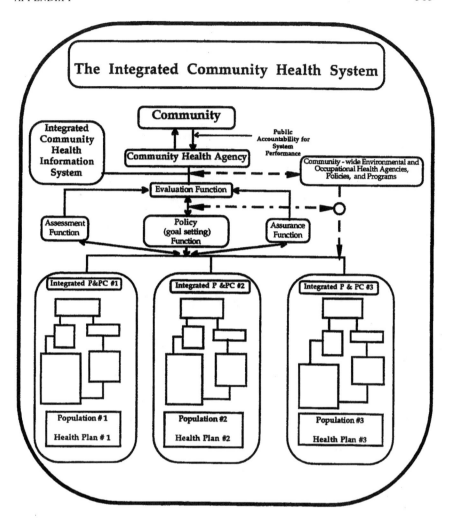

FIGURE F-4 The integrated community health system.

eral model, we are under no illusions regarding the difficulty of realigning the system to produce this result. We would simply note that if society as a whole and our political and commercial systems, specifically, want the nation's (public and population) health system to produce the results that can be achieved through a simultaneous and synergistic reorganization of the public health and primary care systems—operating in a capitated and competitive market context—we will need to move in this direction.

As public and purchaser dissatisfaction with increasing health costs and the

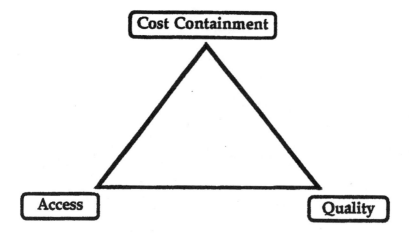

". . . in which cost containment, quality, and access have equal angles, representing equal priorities, and an expansion of any one angle compromises one or both of the other two."

Kissick (1994, pp. 2–3)

FIGURE F-5 Cost containment, access, and quality.

diminishing value per dollar spent on health care or on taxes required to support publicly sponsored health care programs increase, changes of this kind are more likely to occur. This will be exacerbated by an increasing public recognition and understanding of the importance of environmental and occupational health programs on personal, family, and community health status. These feelings are likely to occur and intensify over time, because an increasingly unstable combination of popular dissatisfaction, political pressure, and increasing purchaser concern will create an environment forcing more and more dramatic systemic change.

FUTURE DIRECTIONS AND ISSUES FOR CONSIDERATION FOR HEALTH POLICY, PUBLIC HEALTH, AND PRIMARY CARE: MOVING TO TOMORROW'S INTEGRATED COMMUNITY HEALTH SYSTEMS

Although it is important to create a vision for the future, it is also important to offer suggestions for the present. Many of these suggestions, of course, come directly from observations presented earlier.

1. Legislators (federal, state, and local) and health departments (local and

state) should move from a categorical focus to a population focus. This simple move would do more to reorient the entire health system than many other steps that could be taken.

2. Health departments and affiliated community-accountable not-for-profit entities should assume leadership roles in the development of community health information networks (CHINs). They should also assume responsibility for the standardization of data transfers and automated record information required for entry into the CHIN.

3. Health departments should develop a service perspective and mentality to serve the primary care system, integrated health provider networks, and emerging managed care organizations. Specifically, many of the difficulties noted earlier had to do with the lack of communication, the difficulty of communicating, and the categorical nature of health department responsibility assignment versus population- or community-focused responsibility assignment.

With personnel assigned to serve populations, the providers (hospitals and medical providers) and the health plans serving those same populations and focusing on the same populations and communities, there is a much higher likelihood of improved health outcomes for little or no additional expenditure of funds.

4. Health departments working collaboratively with providers and health plans should make greater efforts to coordinate community services affecting community health status (e.g., health aspects of social and educational services) and to offer this as a service to primary care providers within the community and to managed care plans. The net effect of this action would be to support the community and population service responsibilities of providers and health plans and to support the community served by the health department.

5. Although health departments should take the lead in ensuring the development of publicly accountable CHINs, it will be important to develop the networks in such a way as to facilitate and encourage the functioning of the competitive market for health insurance and competition on the basis of cost, quality (including service), and access among competing health plans and providers. From a public policy standpoint, this should have the effect of improving quality and reducing cost over the long run. This strategy will also support cultural values of entrepreneurism, pluralism, and independence on the one hand, while it will provide necessary public accountability and market facilitation services on the other.

6. Just as federal and state legislators and state and local health departments can move to a population and community perspective on their own volition, such a move would be facilitated by coordinated decisions of federal agencies responsible for assessment programs (Centers for Disease Control and Prevention [CDC] the Environmental Protection Agency, etc.) and for program organization and reimbursement (Health Care Financing Administration, CHAMPUS, etc.) to change their views to a population and community perspective, building the capabilities of the state and local health department infrastructure and policy

apparatus to assume the population-based management and information network management responsibilities suggested above. It should be noted that a relatively "simple and coordinated" federal policy decision of this sort will accelerate reorientation of the entire public health and primary care systems.

7. A simpler step to assist health departments to reorient their perspective would be for CDC to require state and local health departments to report statistics by population segments aligned by logical primary care markets and service areas. Aligning the statistical perspective of markets and service areas, disease prevention and control, and primary care will ultimately realign the perspectives and ongoing communications patterns of population health and primary care professionals. Noted, at this point, is the fact that multiple health plans and primary care systems will likely serve each primary care market area. In spite of this fact, however, the alignment of health statistics will be of greater assistance to all involved in problem identification, solution implementation, and ongoing assurance activities.

8. Health departments should build collaborative service relationships with managed care plans and integrated health delivery networks to provide population- and community-focused continuing education programs in the areas of prevention to primary care providers within their networks. This action taken in concert with several of the actions noted above should build positive relationships and improve primary care system communications.

9. In defining the "primary care system" we must be certain to include a broad base of community-based practitioners, all of whom provide some aspects of "primary care" to a community's residents. These will include dentists, physical therapists, nurse practitioners and midwives, pharmacists, sports medicine physicians, visiting nurses and other home care professionals, and psychologists, among others. Of course, some of these practitioners practice in association with primary care physicians; others do not. In any event, community- and population-based primary care information systems and coordination systems must ultimately capture the activities of these practitioners if the picture of our "community primary care system" is to be complete.

10. Most of the primary care physicians consulted complained of the significant amount of time "wasted" in processing paperwork. On the other hand, the public health system requires high-quality, timely, and complete information to discharge its community assessment, evaluation, assurance, and policy roles appropriately. With proper attention to the development of standards for record-keeping and for electronic information transfers and with the role of facilitating the development of such systems, it is likely that the efficiency and effectiveness of the primary care system would be improved significantly. The assessment, evaluation, policy, and assurance functions of the health departments would be improved substantially as well.

11. As populations throughout the nation diversify in terms of language and culture, primary care practitioners need assistance in serving those populations.

This is particularly true from a community health education perspective and from a cultural sensitivity perspective. With public health and primary care practitioners aligning their perspectives on the same populations, it is more likely that these important issues will be addressed more effectively.

12. Health departments and primary care providers cannot align their perspectives on populations and ignore issues of mental health, behavioral issues, and substance abuse issues. Although the mental health system often functions independently of both, it must be effectively integrated with the primary care system if the health of populations is to improve.

13. Health departments should develop a service focus by placing high-quality, population-related, and timely surveillance and environmental data on electronic data systems easily available to primary care providers. By providing them with more and more relevant services, long-term communications and relationships should be enhanced.

14. The federal and state governments, health departments, schools of public health, schools of medicine, managed care plans, and integrated provider networks should place a greater emphasis on organizational research, health services research, information systems research, and health policy research to improve the population health system. Without such a commitment to improving the organization and financing of the delivery system, we will not be able to move as swiftly to improve primary care system functionality.

15. Governing authorities involved with the accreditation of primary care residency training programs (specifically, family medicine, internal medicine, and pediatrics), working in partnership with interested private foundations and with public health leaders, should develop recommendations for a standardized model for training primary care physicians (including training in population health concepts and skills) and for encouraging schools of public health to train population health professionals in the skills and methods previously outlined to support the community practices of primary care physicians. Both should be trained in team settings to work collaboratively and longitudinally to improve the health of the populations commonly served.

Additionally, arrangements must be made to train and/or retrain existing primary care providers in the elements of population-based and preventive medicine. Overall, the training and retraining needs of health professionals will be significant, and they will be critical to the ultimate success of the program, as ultimately defined. The importance of adopting such principles by the Council on Graduate Medical Education and other accrediting bodies for graduate and continuing education of primary health professionals cannot be overemphasized.

16. A significant practical and policy question involves the mechanisms which must be contemplated to move to the type of model suggested herein, particularly considering the extremely powerful market forces involved and the extraordinarily powerful local and state political positions of large health plans. It seems to us that change of this magnitude must be facilitated nationally, per-

haps by setting national data transfer standards, assignment of certain monitoring and assessment responsibilities under federal health care programs (Medicare, Medicaid, Federal Employee Health Benefits Program, and CHAMPUS) to state and local health departments or specially chartered community benefit organizations, etc. In short, the federal government can use its market power to define the structure of the future system and its accountability mechanisms. If the federal programs define the need for these changes in a clear, coordinated, and consistent way across all markets, the markets and their supporting structures will change, and will do so in a relatively short period of time.

Most of the suggestions presented above call for fundamental change at the individual program or health department level. This arises from the dramatic changes in the markets for health services and in the significant restructuring, already under way, of our primary care provider, health plan and integrated community health delivery systems. Transformation of their structure, perspective, and financing affects public health by creating an even greater imperative for a conceptual reorientation in that area. Both public health and primary care providers must therefore seek and move together to a new paradigm in which both are collaborators and teammates, developing and operating from the common perspective of the population(s) that the two of them jointly serve. In this light they also must serve each other, if the health of their population(s) is to improve.

One overarching and additional important observation must be made at this juncture, however. The preceding suggestions tend to assume that all citizens have required access to the necessary clinical and preventive services through organized plans of care. Unfortunately, this is not the case, and the situation appears to be worsening as the nation's employer-based health insurance system encounters the stresses and strains of international competition. One is led to an unavoidable conclusion. If we accept the premises inherent in this paper, we must also move to ensure appropriate access to clinical and preventive services for all. This conclusion begs the question of the responsibility for financing such access, which could occur at each, or a combination thereof, of the federal, state, county, city, and community levels of jurisdiction on either a publicly funded or voluntarily funded (or a combination of both) basis.

Although it may seem that a number of new roles are being suggested for government and it may, in fact, be the case, many feel that government is the only entity that can rationalize the market and the rules of the game. In short the roles suggested are for rulemaker, honest broker, standardizer, market facilitator, and community quality ensurer. All of these roles are essential if public health and primary care are to improve the health of populations. Government in some form (or affiliated, publicly accountable entities) may be the necessary vehicle to ensure population health. It is important to note above all that this paper conceptualizes a clear separation between the appropriate role of government in the foregoing facilitation capacities and the appropriate role of government as a payer and, if necessary, as a provider.

If the changes suggested herein are adopted or largely adopted in communities, we will have effectively moved to COPC. We have concluded that the COPC model requires the following elements to ensure widespread adoption and success:

- Access to and support of local and state health policy structures and mechanisms, with broad support of national health policy.
- Broad bases of organizational support to provide and fund necessary staff support, including more highly organized forms of medical practice (e.g., comprehensive primary care group or multispecialty group practice forms of organization).
- Capitated revenue flows to align incentives and to support development of clinical and preventive service structures.
- Access to comprehensive, automated information flows and structures, integrating to the maximum extent information regarding community health issues, risk factors and risk behaviors, and longitudinal clinical information.
- Greater integration of primary care training supporting the COPC model or at the minimum the integrated clinical and preventive services model.

The importance of the availability of good information to support population (county) based primary care was noted by Lashof, above, and additionally by Barbara Starfield:

> The development of technology for collecting and processing information will certainly facilitate achievement of the initial steps in COPC. Improved medical technology will expand the definition of health needs; as existing problems are solved, new challenges at another level of need will emerge. Community-oriented care may not be achieved everywhere, or to the same degree in all places. But the concept is now appropriate for consideration as the challenges of the twenty-first century approach. (16, pp. 194–195).

The changes suggested herein are simple and complex at the same time. Mutual changes to a population perspective, service orientation, organizational structure, communications skills and patterns, and rapid movement to a modern information technology base to support population health improvement will lead us where we need to go. Several of these issues were addressed by Joyce Lashof in her 1991 Plenary Address to the AHCPR Conference on Primary Care Research:

> spectrum of community health problems is more difficult initially but in the long run far simpler than developing separate programs for each risk factor and disease. . . . We must experiment with new models that break out of the categorical mode, and we must develop the methodologies for evaluating the impact of programs on the health of populations . . . the development of a true partnership

between public health and primary care remains an unrealized goal. Yet such a partnership is essential if we are to achieve the goals of Healthy People in the Year 2000 (8) to mount a county-wide effort to integrate medical care and public health across the

The question is, of course, familiar—will we have the leadership vision and fortitude, the management skills, and political will to move there and in time?

FINDING OUR WAY: THE LEADERSHIP CHALLENGE

Throughout this paper we have suggested the need for a paradigm shift to improve the health of populations by restructuring the relationship between public health and primary care, as the nation's health care system itself is in the process of restructuring. In fact, we have suggested ways in which the population health system (the public health and primary care team) can work together to assist communities (society) in fulfilling their interest in ensuring conditions in which people can be healthy. This is, of course, the mission suggested by IOM in 1988 (3). Having said this, however, we must acknowledge both the degree and completeness of the change required for state and local public health departments to support our evolving market-oriented structure, particularly in the case of those populations categorically supported for the past 50 years and for those populations for which public health has been the "provider of last resort."

Ultimately such a vision and the required reorientation of existing large bureaucratic structures, a task analogous to turning a huge, lumbering oil tanker in a very short distance, is unachievable without four vital resources: political vision combined with appropriate amounts of courage, and willing and appropriately trained personnel and committed leadership supported by adequate resources. To this end the challenges for the nation's schools of public health, medicine, nursing, and allied health professions have never been greater. Just as it is necessary for public health and primary care practitioners to form a population health team, it will be necessary for these professional schools to form their own educational teams to teach population health and to reorient their perspectives and those of their colleagues within the university. The task is daunting, but essential.

Although critically important, the subject of resources may be easily addressed, in the relative and conceptual senses. If the suggestions outlined earlier relative to using existing federal program resources to define system requirements in the areas suggested herein are used, many, if not most, of the required resources to support the reorientation can be provided efficiently through that method. It will take a change of this sort and magnitude, however, to accomplish the task.

The subject of leadership deserves special attention, however, and may turn out to be the most significant question of all. We were particularly taken with a recent report from the Milbank Memorial Fund "Leadership in Public Health"

(17). In that report Molly Coye, William Foege, and William Roper each discuss different aspects of public health leadership and conclude that public health leadership must, in many ways, reinvent itself. Perspectives must be changed to become more global and to measure effectiveness over longer periods of time and to develop new systems and strategic thinking skills, as well as organizational and political skills, team management, and motivational skills (18). This is a tall order for any profession.

We share their concerns, yet we would submit that leadership development to support population health improvement paradigms is critical for primary care and public health professionals alike if our nation's ambitious, long-term goals are to be achieved and its substantial long-term challenges are to be met. In this regard, it will be most important to create a common vision of a system such as we have proposed and a clear understanding of their individual roles and of their shared and collaborative roles within such a system required to achieve its single objective improving the health of populations.

THE INTEGRATED COMMUNITY HEALTH SYSTEM: CLINICAL AND PREVENTIVE PERSONAL HEALTH SERVICES PROVIDED IN A COMMUNITY CONTEXT FROM AN INTEGRATED PERSPECTIVE

The recommendations of this paper challenge all of us to adapt our thinking to the market-based and community health-oriented realities of the years ahead. Whether or not any of us agree with such an evolution, the challenge for all will ultimately be how we will work collaboratively to make such a system work to improve the health of populations and communities. At the same time all will have to work collaboratively to ensure appropriate access to service.

The move to an integrated system of care such as that suggested in this paper is not without significant risks and difficulties. We suspect that the perspectives of population health professionals and personal health professionals will continue to exhibit tensions vis á vis priorities and resource allocation. To a large degree this is healthy. It is healthiest, however, when these perspectives operate within the same organizational and accountability structure—whatever that may be. It is also healthiest when these tensions are acknowledged as being appropriate to reach the best result for the populations and communities served—and when those populations and communities have a significant voice in guiding the decision processes of the organizational structures within which these critical decisions are made.

Increasingly, we will see the tensions evolving between the publicly accountable and voluntary components of our community health systems and the investor-owned (and non-community-oriented) elements serving our community health needs. We believe that these tensions can be appropriately managed to produce a positive health result for the community. We also believe, however, that we may have to seek or develop new organizational methods and public-private political structures to balance the competing requirements of community and shareholder accountability. It is entirely possible that the growing complexity of our communities, combined with the increasing recognition of the need to develop new ways to bridge the public-private chasm will lead us in the directions of exploring Schauffler's Community Based Health Promotion and Disease Prevention (CBHPDP) partnership concept, referenced earlier (6).

In any event, Schauffler recognizes the complexity of organizing the complete spectrum of community-accountable population-based and personal services required to create an environment within which health can be assured. Thus, a community, in the context of CBHPDP, is defined by its people, institutions organization, and locality.

Many of our communities are experiencing growing economic, cultural, and ethnic diversity; significant inequities in health status have accompanied this diversity. As a result, it is imperative that we recognize the important role communities must play if we are to improve and maintain the health status of our population. Two choices are available: (1) we can continue down the current path and support models that fragment care and focus only on the individual as the unit of prevention interventions, thereby risking an increase in the health status gaps that exist between the most advantaged and disadvantaged subgroups of our population; or (2) we can build a model for the twenty-first century that recognizes the diversity of our communities by developing a multidisciplinary, intersectoral approach that encourages and supports the significant role communities can and must play in promoting health and preventing disease (6, p. 9).

The difficulty of achieving this result and of reconciling the tensions described above between the community-accountable and non-community-accountable components of our integrated health system must not be underestimated. Ultimately, this is a problem that must be solved through our political system—local, regional, state, and national.

As we survey the path suggested in this paper, we ask, will it be risky to move in the direction(s) suggested? Ultimately, we also ask, will it be even more risky to make no movement at all?

REFERENCES

1. IOM. *Community Oriented Primary Care: A Practical Assessment, Vol. 1.* The Committee Report. Washington, D.C.: National Academy Press, 1984.

2. IOM. *Defining Primary Care: An Interim Report.* Washington, D.C.: National Academy Press, 1994.

3. IOM. *The Future of Public Health.* Washington, D.C.: National Academy Press, 1988.

4. Partnership for Prevention. Prevention Is Basic to Health Reform: A Position Paper from an Expert Panel. Washington, D.C.: Partnership for Prevention, March 1993.

5. Lashof, J. Public Health and Prevention. Presented at Public Health Agencies and Managed Care: Partnerships for Health Conference, Atlanta, Ga.,1994.

6. Schauffler, H. H. Health Promotion and Disease Prevention in Health Care Reform. *American Journal of Preventive Medicine* 10(5)(Suppl.), 1994.

7. USPHS. *For A Healthy Nation: Returns on Investment in Public Health.* M. Gold and S. Teutsch, project co-directors. Washington, D.C.: U.S. Government Printing Office, 1994.

8. Lashof, J. Public Health and Primary Care. Pp. 323–330 in AHCPR Conference Proceedings: *Primary Care Research: Theory and Methods*, M. Grady, ed., Publication No. (PHS) 91-0011. Rockville, Md.: U.S. Department of Health and Human Services, 1991.

9. Rundall, T.G. The Integration of Public Health and Medicine. *Frontiers of Health Services Management* 10:3–24, 1994.

10. McGinnis, J.M. and Foege, W.H., "Actual Causes of Death in the United States." *Journal of the American Medical Association* 270:2207–2212, 1993.

11. Kissick, W. L. *Medicine's Dilemmas: Infinite Needs Versus Finite Resources.* New Haven, Ct.: Yale University Press, 1994.

12. Lee, P.R. Re-Inventing Public Health, Shattuck Lecture, Massachusetts Medical Society, 1994 Annual Meeting. Boston, Mass., May 21, 1994.

13. Thompson, R.S., Taplin, S.H., McAfee, T.A., Mandelson, M.T., and Smith, A.E. "Primary and Secondary Prevention Services in Clinical Practice: Twenty Years' Experience in Development, Implementation, and Evaluation. *Journal of the American Medical Association* 273:1130–1135, 1995.

14. Waitzkin, H. And Hubbell, F.A. Truth's Search for Power in Health Policy: Critical Applications to Community Oriented Primary Care and Small Area Analysis. *Medical Care Review* 49:161–189, 1992.

15. Kukulka, G., Christianson, J.B., Moscovice, I.S., and DeVries, R. Community Oriented Primary Care: Implementation of a National Rural Demonstration. *Archives of Family Medicine* 3:495–501, 1994.

16. Starfield, B. *Primary Care: Concept, Evaluation, and Policy.* New York, N.Y.: Oxford University Press, 1992.

17. Coye, M.J., Foege, W.H., and Roper, W.L. *Leadership in Public Health.* New York, N.Y.: Milbank Memorial Fund, 1994.

G

Committee Biographies

NEAL A. VANSELOW, M.D., is a Professor of Medicine at Tulane University School of Medicine. He served as Chancellor of Tulane University Medical Center from 1989–1994 and as a Scholar-in-Residence at the Institute of Medicine during the 1994–1995 academic year. He has served as Chairman of the Department of Postgraduate Medicine and Health Professions Education at the University of Michigan, Dean of the University of Arizona College of Medicine, Chancellor of the University of Nebraska Medical Center, and Vice President for Health Sciences at the University of Minnesota. He is an allergist who received his training in internal medicine and allergy-immunology at the University of Michigan.

Dr. Vanselow was chairperson of the Council on Graduate Medical Education (U.S. Department of Health and Human Services), chairperson of the Board of Directors, Association of Academic Health Centers, and a member of the Pew Health Professions Commission. He has been a member of the Institute of Medicine since 1989 and has served as chair of the IOM Committee on the Future of Primary Care and co-chairperson of the IOM Committee on the U.S. Physician Supply. His areas of particular interest include the health care workforce and graduate medical education.

JOEL J. ALPERT, M.D., Professor of Pediatrics and Public Health at Boston University School of Medicine, graduated from Yale College and Harvard Medical School. Following completion of pediatric training at Children's Hospital in Boston, Massachusetts, St. Mary's Hospital Medical School in London, and military service in the U.S. Army at Fort Leavenworth, Kansas, he returned to

Children's Hospital as a fellow in Child Health and Chief Resident. He has served as Associate Professor of Pediatrics at Harvard Medical School, Medical Director of The Harvard Family Health Care Program, Chairman of the Department of Pediatrics at Boston University School of Medicine, and Director of Pediatrics at Boston City Hospital.

He has authored 132 papers, 65 abstracts, and two books. His major work has been in primary care education, delivery, and health care for disadvantaged children. He co-authored *Education of Physicians for Primary Care* in 1973 with Evan Charney. He is a member of AOA at Boston University, a member of the Society for Pediatric Research, and the American Pediatric Society. He received the Job Lewis Award for Community Pediatrics in 1991 from the American Academy of Pediatrics and the George Armstrong Medal in 1988 from the Ambulatory Pediatric Association of which he was president in 1969. He is a member of the Institute of Medicine and was on the governing council from 1992 to 1995. He has most recently been a member of the Institute of Medicine Board on Children and Families.

CHERYL Y. BOYKINS is the Program Director of The Center For Black Women's Wellness (CBWW), a community-based self-help organization committed to improving the quality of life for women and their families through empowerment.

A graduate of the University of Florida, Gainesville, she earned a B.A. degree in criminal justice. While completing undergraduate studies, she coordinated a continuing education program, job training and other support services as a correctional counselor in an innovative halfway house program designed to insure the smooth re-entry of incarcerated women into the community. In 1981, she began working as a health advocate at the Gainesville Women's Health Center.

Ms. Boykins attended the first National Conference on Black Women's Health Issues in 1983 at Spelman College, and in 1985 attended the United Nations (UN) End of the Decade Conference for women held in Nairobi, Kenya. Realizing the possibility of working with other women who understood the dual oppression of race and gender, she returned to Atlanta to accept a position coordinating self-help groups in public housing. She has continued to implement programs that develop self-help groups among women while building relationships with other local health and social service agencies. She has combined her knowledge and experience of criminal justice systems and health care for women to develop a grassroots model program into a reality that supports women individually and collectively in their overall health care needs.

Ms. Boykins and CBWW have been the recipient of many awards. She is currently a member of the Public Health Children's Initiative Task Force, Vice President of Parks and Recreation Advisory Council, Vice President for the Advisory Council of Summech Lane Trust and member of The Council of Elders for a Safe Place.

cAROLYN V. BROWN, M.D., MPH, is board certified in both obstetrics-gynecology and preventive medicine. Her career is deeply rooted in the direct provision of primary care, rural and outreach health care, psychosocial issues of health, access of populations to health care, and teaching.

Dr. Brown practiced in Alaska for 23 years at the private practice, institutional, academic, and public health levels of health care. She developed the first teaching curriculum for Alaska Native Health Aides. Her local and statewide work there involved women's primary health care issues, obstetric-gynecologic reproductive health care, and issues of psychosocial health care.

Dr. Brown was assistant professor of obstetrics and gynecology at the University of Vermont College of Medicine from 1988 to 1994. In this work, she continued a commitment to teaching primary care for obstetric-gynecology residents and students. In addition, she developed and taught the College of Medicine class in ethics for five years. Outreach health care was developed and implemented within the Department of Obstetrics-Gynecology. She authored the Vermont State Guidelines for Sexual Assault Examinations as well as the Vermont Health Department Guidelines for Evaluation of Family (Domestic) Violence for hospitals, emergency departments, and other health care facilities in Vermont.

She served on the American College of Obstetricians and Gynecologists (ACOG) committee in the development of *The Obstetrician-Gynecologist and Primary-Preventive Health Care*. She serves as chair of the ACOG District I Primary Care Committee.

In 1995 Dr. Brown returned to private practice in Burlington, Vermont, and continues her work in direct patient care, teaching, writing, outreach health care, and local-state-national health arenas.

PETE TONY DUARTE is Chief Executive Officer of Thomason Hospital in El Paso, Texas. Until 1992 he was Executive Director of Centro de Salud Familiar La Fe, Inc., El Paso, Texas, where he was responsible for administration and management of the largest community health center along the U.S./Mexico border.

He has also directed the programs of Project Upward Bound for the University of Texas at El Paso and was Assistant Professor, Department of Sociology. He has been a management consultant to the U.S. government and local governments and has directed the implementation and evaluation of health services and community development projects.

From 1965 to 1967 he was a Peace Corps Volunteer in the Dominican Republic. In 1964 he graduated from California State College, Hayward, with a

B.A. in Social Sciences. He received an M.A. in Sociology from the University of Texas at El Paso.

He has served on national committees and received many awards, including the Hispanic Magazine "Science Award," The National Conference of Christians and Jews "Extra Miler Award" in 1994, and the L.U.L.A.C. and District IV "Humanitarian Award" in 1995. He served as Board Member of COSSMHO in 1996.

PETER K. ELLSWORTH was elected President and Chief Executive Officer of Sharp HealthCare in March 1986. For 27 years prior to 1986 as an attorney in private practice, he represented Sharp on various matters. At the time of his appointment to Sharp as CEO, Mr. Ellsworth was president of the law firm of Ellsworth, Corbett, Seitman & McLeod, now known as Lindley, Lazar & Scales.

Mr. Ellsworth received his undergraduate and law degrees from Stanford University. Mr. Ellsworth is a member of the Executive Committee of the Greater San Diego Chamber of Commerce and is a member of the Executive Committee of the Chamber's CEO Roundtable. He served as President of Quality Net—a consortium of the largest not-for-profit hospitals in San Diego.

RAYMOND S. GARRISON, D.D.S., M.S., is associate professor and chairman of the Department of Dentistry at Bowman Gray School of Medicine in Winston-Salem, North Carolina. Dr. Garrison has been a member of the Department of Dentistry since 1981 and has served as Chairman since 1992.

Dr. Garrison received his B.S. degree from Davidson College and his D.D.S. degree from the University of North Carolina School of Dentistry. After finishing his undergraduate dental education, Dr. Garrison completed a one-year rotating dental internship at Baltimore City Hospitals in Baltimore, Maryland. The internship was followed by a three-year anesthesia residency at Baltimore City Hospitals and the University of Maryland. During his anesthesia training, Dr. Garrison completed a master's degree in pharmacology at the University of Maryland.

Dr. Garrison became a full-time faculty member of the University of Maryland Schools of Dentistry and Pharmacy in Baltimore in 1974. In 1978 Dr. Garrison joined the full-time faculty at East Carolina University School of Medicine in Greenville, North Carolina. At East Carolina Dr. Garrison started a general practice residency program within the Department of Family Medicine. In 1981 Dr. Garrison joined the full-time faculty at the Bowman Gray School of Medicine in the Department of Dentistry.

Dr. Garrison is active in many national organizations and committees. He is a fellow of the American Dental Society of Anesthesiology, the Academy of General Dentistry, the American Association of Hospital Dentists, and the American College of Dentists. He has a particular interest in accreditation, financing, and general practice residency educational programming in the hospital environment as well as in issues at the interface of medicine and dentistry. These include managed dental care reimbursement plans, access and treatment outcomes research, and integrated medical information systems. Other research areas include the teaching and use of conscious sedation in dentistry and complex restorative and esthetic dentistry.

LARRY A. GREEN, M.D., is Professor and Woodward-Chisholm Chairman of Family Practice at the University of Colorado. He is a graduate of Baylor College of Medicine in Houston. Dr. Green completed his residency in Family Medicine at the University of Rochester and Highland Hospital in 1976. Among the honors he has received are the American Board of Family Practice, Diplomate, 1976; recertified 1982 and 1989. Dr. Green's memberships include the Institute of Medicine; the American Academy of Family Physicians, North American Primary Care Research Group; Society of Teachers of Family Medicine; International Primary Care Network; Association of Departments of Family Medicine; Ambulatory Sentinel Practice Network. Dr. Green's major research interest is practice-based research. He has co-authored numerous publications relating to family practice medicine.

PAUL F. GRINER, M.D., is Vice President and Director of the Center for the Assessment and Management of Change in Academic Medicine (CAMCAM), Association of American Medical Colleges. This Center was formed in 1995 to analyze the impact of the changing health care environment on the academic programs of the nation's medical schools and teaching hospitals and to assist these institutions in managing the changes necessary to ensure the preservation of their academic and social missions. A graduate of Harvard College, Dr. Griner received his M.D. degree, with honor, at the University of Rochester School of Medicine and Dentistry in 1959. He completed an internship and residency in Medicine at the Massachusetts General Hospital and served as medical chief resident and fellow in hematology at Strong Memorial Hospital in Rochester. He remained on the faculty at Rochester, rising to the rank of Professor and held the Samuel E. Durand Chair in Medicine. From 1984 until 1995, he was General Director and Chief Executive Officer of Strong Memorial Hospital, the 720-bed teaching hospital of the University of Rochester.

As a nationally recognized authority on medical decisionmaking and the delivery of health services, Dr. Griner has published and lectured extensively on improving the efficiency and effectiveness of diagnosis and management, the assessment of medical technology, and directions in health policy. He has been a leader in the development of hospital programs designed to improve the quality and efficiency of patient care and chaired the efforts of a consortium of 12 university teaching hospitals to build the clinical information infrastructure needed to achieve these goals.

Dr. Griner participates in many professional organizations, most notably the

American College of Physicians, an association of approximately 85,000 internists, the largest medical specialty organization in the world. He served as both Chair of the Board and President of this organization, completing his term in 1995. Dr. Griner is also active in the Institute of Medicine and the Academic Medical Center Consortium (founding Chairman of the Board). He was a member of the New York State Governor's Health Care Advisory Board from 1990 to 1995 and served on the Mayoral Commission on the Health and Hospitals Corporation of the City of New York.

JEAN JOHNSON, RN-C, Ph.D., currently serves as Associate Dean of the Health Sciences Programs at The George Washington University School of Medicine and Health Sciences. She has been extensively involved in and provided national leadership in nurse practitioner education through her work with program development and as a commissioner on the Pew Health Professions Commission. She has also been an active participant in legislative and regulatory policy formulation to enhance the role of nurse practitioners through decreasing barriers to practice.

Dr. Johnson has also been a long-time advocate for improved care of the elderly, particularly those in nursing homes. She has worked to establish national standards for nurse assistant training and developed a nationally recognized educational program for this training. She currently maintains a clinical practice at a community clinic in Washington, D.C.

Dr. Johnson serves as a member of the Pew Health Professions Commission and Fetzer Foundation's Work Force to develop psychosocial curriculum for health professions. She is also the National Project Director for the Robert Wood Johnson Foundation's Partnership in Training Initiative.

P. EUGENE JONES, Ph.D., PA-C, is Associate Professor and Physician Assistant Program Director at The University of Texas Southwestern Medical Center at Dallas. He was a U.S. Navy hospital corpsman during the Vietnam era and completed physician assistant training in 1975. He has 15 years' experience as a physician assistant educator. He earned a B.S. in physician assistant studies from the University of Nebraska College of Medicine, an M.A. in health services management from Webster College in St. Louis, Missouri, and M.A. and Ph.D. degrees in education from the Clarement Graduate School in Claremont, California. His research interests include physician assistant practice in primary care and medically underserved communities.

HENK LAMBERTS, M.D., Ph.D., attended the University of Utrecht Medical School and the Medical School of Rotterdam (1958–1965) and received his Ph.D. from Leiden University in 1968. He founded the Ommoord Health Center in Rotterdam. He has been Professor of Family Medicine (University of Amsterdam, The Netherlands) since 1984. His main areas of interest are the development of the International Classification of Primary Care (ICPC) and its application in episode-oriented epidemiology in international family practice. This is now reflected in an epidemiological program (Trans) based on the data from the Transition Project—a large routine morbidity database in the Netherlands—and the introduction of an expert system-driven computer-based patient record (Transhis) for family practice that is in use in several countries.

Together with Maurice Wood (Virginia, U.S.) and Inge Hofmans-Okkes (Amsterdam, Netherlands) he is editor of *ICPC in the European Community With a Multilanguage Layer*. He is also the author of a Dutch textbook on Family Medicine.

Dr. Lamberts has been a Foreign Associate Member of the IOM since 1993.

PAUL W. NANNIS is Senior Program Officer at The Robert Wood Johnson Foundation. During the IOM Study on the Future of Primary Care he was Commissioner of Health, City of Milwaukee, Wisconsin. He was Executive Director of the 16th Street Community Health Center from 1976 to 1979.

He received a B.A. degree from Marietta College in Ohio and an M.S.W. from the University of Wisconsin. He is a member of many professional organizations and has served on boards and blue ribbon committees, including the Medical College of Wisconsin's Health Policy Institute, the Advisory Board of the School of Social Welfare at the University of Wisconsin and the National Health Service Corps Advisory Council for the U.S. Department of Health and Human Services.

R. HEATHER PALMER, M.B., B.Ch., S.M., is Director of the Center for Quality of Care Research and Education (QCRE) in the Department of Health Policy and Management at the Harvard School of Public Health. A pediatrician by training, Dr. Palmer turned early in her career to health services research and became a faculty member in the Department of Health Policy and Management at HSPH. Her prior research focused on evaluation of quality in ambulatory health care. Dr. Palmer is currently leading a research project funded by the Agency for Health Care Policy and Research called Understanding and Choosing Clinical Performance Measures for Quality Improvement: Development of a Typology as Principal Investigator and subcontractor to Mikalix & Co. She is also an investigator in collaboration with colleagues at the Beth Israel Hospital, on a study to validate the complications screening program.

Dr. Palmer also writes, speaks, and teaches about the theory and practice of quality of care measurement. Her book, *Ambulatory Health Care Evaluation: Principles and Practice*, has become a classic in the field. Her paper on defining and measuring quality for the IOM's Committee on "Medicare: A Strategy for Quality Assurance" is included in *Striving for Quality in Health Care: An Inquiry into Policy and Practice*. She also contributed the chapter on "Quality Management in Ambulatory Care" to *Health Care Quality Management for the*

21st Century, and a chapter on "Quality Improvement/Quality Assurance Taxonomy: A Framework for the Conference" in *Putting Research to Work in Quality Improvement*.

Dr. Palmer has contributed to policymaking about measurement of performance in health care through consultation to organizations in the public and private sector. She is on the Board of the Center for Clinical Quality Evaluation (CCQE) and on the Board of the Massachusetts Peer Review Organization. She serves on the National Performance Measurement Council of the Joint Commission on Accreditation of Healthcare Organizations (JCAHO), and on the American Medical Association (AMA) Expert Consultant Panel for Physician Performance Assessment, and for the National Academy of Sciences/National Research Council (NAS/NRC) on a Study on Performance Measures and Data for Public Health Performance Partnership Grants. She is also the Editor-in-Chief of the *Journal of the International Society for Quality in Health Care.*

Dr. Palmer earned her baccalaureate degree from Cambridge University, her M.B. and B.Ch. degrees (equivalent to the United States M.D. degree) from Cambridge University and the London Hospital Medical College, and a Master of Science degree in Health Services Administration from the Harvard School of Public Health.

BARBARA ROSS-LEE, D.O., is Dean of the Ohio University College of Osteopathic Medicine. In 1990, she became the first osteopathic physician to participate in the prestigious Robert Wood Johnson Health Policy Fellowship, where she served as Legislative Assistant for Health to Senator Bill Bradley. In August 1993, she was named Dean of the Ohio University College of Osteopathic Medicine—the first African-American woman to head a U.S. medical school. Ross-Lee has a strong background in health policy issues and serves as an adviser on primary care, medical education, and health care reform issues on the federal and state levels.

After receiving her Doctor of Osteopathy degree from the Michigan State University College of Osteopathic Medicine in 1973, she ran a busy family practice in inner-city Detroit for 10 years. She has worked throughout her career to address the health care needs of vulnerable populations—in particular, women, children, and minorities. This commitment mirrors the overriding mission of the Ohio University College of Osteopathic Medicine: to provide primary care physicians for the underserved areas of Ohio.

In June 1994, Ross-Lee was appointed to a four-year term with the 18-member National Advisory Committee on Rural Health for the U.S. Department of Health and Human Services. Ross-Lee is a Fellow of the American College of Osteopathic Family Physicians, Director of the American Osteopathic Association Certificate Program in Health Policy, and a member of the Executive Committee of the American Association of Colleges of Osteopathic Medicine.

In addition to other awards, Ross-Lee received the Women's Health Award from Blackboard African-American National Bestsellers for her contributions to women's health and the "Magnificent 7" award presented by Business and Professional Women/USA. The latter award honors seven women in America who have made exceptional contributions to business and workplace equity.

SHEILA A. RYAN, Ph.D., R.N., F.A.A.N, came to the University of Rochester in September 1986 from Creighton University in Omaha, Nebraska, where she was Associate Professor and Dean from 1980 to 1986. During her tenure as Dean and Professor, School of Nursing and Director, Medical Center Nursing at the University of Rochester, she has been responsible for a reorganization of faculty governance, expansion of faculty tracks for promotion, the development of a strategic plan for the School of Nursing, the initiation of the Community Nursing Center, and program management and advancement of the Commonwealth Fund Executive Nursing Fellowship Program.

Dr. Ryan earned her B.S.N. from the University of Nebraska, her M.S.N. in Psychiatric Nursing from the University of California, San Francisco, and her Ph.D. in clinical nursing research from the University of Arizona. She received the Citation for Alumnus Achievement Award in 1989, and was elected as a Fellow of the American Academy of Nursing in 1987, and elected to the Institute of Medicine, 1992 and as treasurer of the National League for Nursing in 1993. She has received numerous awards for Outstanding University Teaching and Professional Advancement.

Locally, regionally, and nationally, Dr. Ryan lectures in the areas of health care reform, informatics, faculty practice, and financial models of managed care. Dr. Ryan is a past member of the Advisory Committee of the Pew Charitable Trust's Health Professions Commission, and currently serves on the Health of the Public National Advisory Committee. She serves as an adviser to several corporate organizations, numerous national foundations, is a board member for local health institutions and has served on many community commissions.

RICHARD M. SCHEFFLER, Ph.D., is Professor of Health Economics and Public Policy at the School of Public Health and the Graduate School of Public Policy, University of California at Berkeley. He is the director of the Robert Wood Johnson Scholars in Health Policy Research Program and the Chair of the doctoral program in Health Services and Policy Analysis. Dr. Scheffler was a Fulbright scholar in the Czech Republic in 1993 and the founding director of a National Institute of Mental Health Research Center on the Organization and Financing of Care for the Severely Mentally Ill. Before coming to Berkeley in 1981, he was on the staff of the IOM and was the study director of the 1978 IOM report, *A Manpower Policy for Primary Health Care*. Dr. Scheffler has taught classes in health economics and public policy, health services research, international health care economics and micro-economics. His published research includes studies of health care workforce policy, managed care, the economics of preventive health measures, and mental health care delivery systems.

WILLIAM L.WINTERS, JR., M.D., is board certified in cardiovascular diseases and internal medicine and is Professor of Medicine and Deputy Chief in the Department of Medicine at Baylor College of Medicine. He is also on the Senior Attending Staff at the Methodist Hospital and has been on the Board of Directors and President of the Medical Staff.

He received a B.S. degree from Northwestern University and an M.S. from Temple University. He received his M.D. from Northwestern University Medical School. Dr. Winters did an internship at Philadelphia General Hospital, a residency in internal medicine, and a fellowship in cardiology at Temple University Hospital. He was a Director of the Cardiovascular Clinical Research Center, the General Clinical Research Center, and the Cardiac Care Unit between 1961 and 1968 at Temple University School of Medicine.

Dr. Winters is a member of many professional societies. He was President of the American College of Cardiology from 1990 to 1991. He was also President of the American Heart Association, Houston Chapter, from 1975 to 1976. Dr. Winters has received awards from the American Heart Association and has served on the editorial boards of several cardiology journals.

Index

Index

A

Academic health centers, 188, 206, 207
  interdisciplinary team training, 11
  mission of, in primary care, 9, 24, 144, 257
  role in primary care delivery, 111-112, 143-144, 173
Accessibility of services, 44, 47, 65-66, 240, 329
  in primary care definition, 2, 31, 32, 33, 45-46
  and workforce supply, 9, 20, 168, 169
Accountability
  in clinician-patient partnership, 57-58
  for efficient use of resources, 33, 49
  for ethical behavior, 33, 49
  for patient satisfaction, 33, 48-49
  of patients, 49-50
  in primary care definition, 2, 31, 33, 46-50
  for quality of care, 33, 46-48, 242-243
  research, 242-243
Accreditation organizations, 141, 193
  and primary care curriculum, 10, 186, 194
Acute care, 40-41

Advanced care planning, 85
Advocacy skills, 192
African Americans, 157, 195
Agency for Health Care Policy and Research (AHCPR), 218, 220, 221, 223-224
All-payer system
  for graduate medical education, 11, 202, 259
  for primary care training, 6, 10, 201-202, 258-259
  for research funding, 233
Alternative medicine, 126
American Academy of Family Physicians (AAFP), 190, 199
American Academy of Pediatrics, 199
American Board of Family Practice (ABFP), 208
American College of Obstetricians and Gynecologists (ACOG), 123, 190
American Society of Internal Medicine (ASIM), 122, 183
Asian Americans, 157, 195
Association of American Medical Colleges (AAMC), 182, 184
Availability of services, 8, 112-113, 253

B

Behavioral sciences, 81-82
Biomedical sciences, 3, 81, 191
Bureau of Health Professions (BHP), 198,
    199, 220

C

CALPERS (California Public Employees
    Retirement System), 139
Capital markets, 22, 108
Capitation payments, 114-116
    and mental health services, 115, 300-
        302
    and withholding of services, 327
    and workforce composition, 315
Caregivers, 35, 60
Catastrophic health insurance, 117
Centers for Disease Control and
    Prevention (CDC), 221
Certification and licensure, 10, 47
    after physician retraining, 11, 210-211
    examinations, 185
    of nurse practitioners, 159-160, 316
Chronic care, 2, 18, 41, 67
Classification, see Diagnostic
    classification and coding
Clerkships, 182-184
Clinical decisionmaking, 3, 39, 83-84, 355
    importance of continuity of care, 57
    and mental disorders, 86-87, 288, 293-
        298, 299
    by nonphysician clinicians, 320
    patient participation, 85-86
    theoretical bases, 81-83
Clinical nurse specialist (CNS) programs,
    161-162
Clinical trials, 236-237
    for mental health treatment, 287
Clinicians, 5, 148-149
    communication skills, 47, 82
    core competencies, 9, 188-194, 258,
        314
    in primary care definition, 29, 33, 36,
        44-45, 148
    salaried, 115, 116

see also Education and training; Nurse
    practitioners; Partnership with
    patients; Physician assistants;
    Physicians; Specialists and
    specialty care; Workforce
Coding, see Diagnostic classification and
    coding
Collaborative care, 71-72
    in mental health, 9, 136-137, 304-305,
        307
    see also Primary care teams
Communication and interpersonal
    relations, 47, 82
    training in, 10, 191, 194-195, 258, 307
Communities
    coordination of services within, 36, 43,
        71-72, 127
    in primary care definition, 3, 31, 32,
        33, 35-36
    research on, 243
Community-Based Public Health
    Initiative, 196
Community health information networks
    (CHINs), 365
Community-oriented primary care
    (COPC), 28, 30, 71, 133, 351-352,
        357, 369
Comorbidity, 80, 237, 289
    with mental disorders, 292-293, 295
Competencies, see Core competencies
Comprehensive care, 28, 68-69
    and care outcomes, 68-69
    integrated services, 32, 38-41
Computer-based patient records, 44, 57,
    69-70, 88, 125, 126, 142
Computer networks, 38
Consolidated Omnibus Budget
    Reconciliation Act, 197
Consortia, see Primary care consortium
Consultation/liaison (C/L) psychiatry, 305
Continuing medical education (CME),
    142, 192, 207
Continuity of care, 28, 29, 44, 69, 117-118
    and clinician-patient partnership, 56-57
    and mental health care, 302
    research, 241
    and service integration, 32, 43-44

Coordination of services, 32, 41-43, 55-56, 69-70, 88, 126
  research, 240-241
  specialty referrals and other services, 41, 55, 109-110, 124-126, 130-139, 131-132, 356
Core competencies, 9, 188-194, 258, 314
  for nurse practitioners, 192-193
  training, 5, 10, 183-184, 186-187, 188-194, 258
Costs and cost control, 14, 21, 64, 347-348
  patient resistance, 23, 39
  specialty care, 13, 63-65
  and technological innovation, 24
Council on Graduate Medical Education (COGME), 14, 170-171 202, 367
Cultural sensitivity, 36, 85-86
  training in, 10, 191, 194-196, 258
Culture and social norms, 35, 85-86, 329
Curricula, *see* Core competencies; Education and training

D

Data sources, 222-229
  development of national data set, 11, 224-225, 228-229, 260
  episodes of care, 79-80, 101
  patient interviews and surveys, 48-49
  patient records as, 48, 57-58, 227
  population-based surveys, 218, 223-224, 229*n*
  on workforce issues, 10, 170-171, 172, 257
  see also Medical Outcomes Study; Medicare Current Beneficiary Survey; National Ambulatory Medical Care Survey; National Health and Nutrition Examination Survey; National Health Interview Survey; National Medical Expenditures Survey; Netherlands Transition Project
Data standards, 12, 233-234, 261, 355-356
Definitions, *see* Primary care definition

Delivery of primary care
  academic health centers' role in, 9, 24, 111-112, 143-144, 173, 257
  coordination with other services, 109-110, 124-126, 130-139, 356
  diversity within, 109, 296
  organizational arrangements, 4, 108, 118-119
  professional roles in, 110, 119-126
  specialists' role in, 12, 41, 44, 110, 122-124, 238-239, 261
  to underserved populations, 4, 8, 111, 126-130, 255
  see also Financing of primary care; Infrastructure development; Integrated delivery systems; Managed care
Demand for clinicials, 156, 165-166, 167-168
  monitoring of, 5, 10, 170-171, 257
  see also Geographic distribution; Underserved population; Workforce
Dentists and dentistry, 44, 109, 125, 165
Department of Defense (DOD), 196, 221
Department of Health and Human Services (DHHS), 11, 12, 218, 219, 220, 223
Department of Veterans Affairs (VA), 109, 196, 221
Depression, 295, 297, 298, 302
Diagnosis, *see* Clinical decisionmaking; Early detection
Diagnostic and Statistical Manual for Mental Disorders (DSM), 79, 294, 295-296
Diagnostic classification and coding, 12, 228, 233, 234, 235, 261
  international systems, 79, 90, 218, 294, 296
Diagnostic tests, 84
Disease prevention, *see* Preventive care

E

Early detection, 41, 58-59; *see also* Preventive care
Educational levels, 71

Education and training, 5-6, 19, 167-170, 179-180, 307-308
  in ambulatory care settings, 10, 202-203, 258
  community contexts, 191-192
  continuing medical education (CME), 142, 207
  in core competencies, 5, 10, 186-187, 188-194, 258
  funding of, 5-6, 157-158, 166, 179, 181, 196-203, 257
  interdisciplinary approaches, 6, 11, 203-206, 259-260
  minority participation, 157, 169-170
  of nurse practitioners, 20, 159, 160-162, 200, 206, 316
  of physician assistants, 157, 196-200
  of physicians, 150, 156-158, 180-187
  see also Graduate medical education; Retraining of physicians; Undergraduate medical education
Efficiency and productivity, 15, 61-62, 115
  accountability for, 33, 49
  of nonphysician clinicians, 317-319, 321, 332
Elderly persons, 2, 18, 20, 60, 137, 138
Emergency care, 45, 65-66, 67, 111
Epidemiological studies, 82-83
Episodes of care, 56, 225-226
  comparison of U.S. and Dutch data sets, 89-101
  as unit of assessment, 48, 79-80, 226-228
Ethics and ethical behavior, 82, 192
  accountability for, 33, 49
Evidence-based medicine, 82-83

F

Faculty reimbursement, 197-198
Family members and relationships, 81, 191
  care givers, 35, 60
  in primary care definition, 3, 31, 32, 33, 35
  research on, 243

Family practice, 19, 63, 64, 77, 192
  residencies, 186-187, 199
Federated Council of Internal Medicine Curriculum Task Force (FCIMCTF), 189-190
Fee-for-service (FFS), 8, 114, 115, 116, 254, 314
  HMO payments to clinicians, 315n
  and mental health services, 300
Financing of primary care, 113-118
  impact on quality of care, 327-332, 355
  payment methods and mechanisms, 8, 115-118, 254
  universal coverage, 113-114, 253-254
  see also All-payer system; Capitation payments; Fee-for-service
First-contact care, 27, 28, 29, 38-39
  by non-medical professionals, 124-126, 165
For-profit ownership, 22, 108

G

Gatekeepers, 20, 39, 125
  in mental health services, 302
General practitioners, 19, 41n, 63, 64, 68, 190
Geographic distribution
  of managed care programs, 106-107
  of physicians, 64, 67, 158
  of primary care workforce, 10, 171-173, 257
Global capitation, 114-116
Graduate medical education (GME), 157, 185-187
  financing, 196-203
  Medicare support, 196, 197-198, 202-203, 259
  as a public good, 200-201

H

Health Care Financing Administration (HCFA), 128, 197, 221, 223, 224, 254

Health care reform, 7, 21, 113
Health care services, in primary care
  definition, 2, 31, 32-33, 37-38
Health Maintenance Organization Act, 20
Health maintenance organizations
  (HMOs), 20, 22, 63, 106, 107, 351
  payments to clinicians, 115
  staffing patterns, 322-327
Health promotion, 2, 3, 18, 58, 87-88,
  132, 134
Health services research, 236
HEDIS (Health Plan Employer Data and
  Information Set), 139
Hispanic Americans, 157
Hospital-based care, 13
  excess capacity, 21
  preventable, 66, 67
Households, *see* Family members and
  relationships
Humanities, 81

I

ICD, *see* International Classification of
  Diseases
Inappropriate care, 47
Income levels, 71
Information management, 3, 88, 142, 192
  and accessibility of services, 46
  in community contexts, 36, 44, 355-
    356, 361
  networks, 38, 365
  patient records, 43-44, 57-58, 69-70
Informed consent, 85
Infrastructure development, 141-143
  for research, 11, 218-219, 235
Insurance, 116
  mental health care coverage, 87, 297,
    299
  primary care disincentives, 116, 117,
    136, 137
  see also Universal coverage
Integrated delivery systems, 2, 18, 32-33,
  35, 38, 143
  accessibility, 45-46
  and clinician training, 206-207
  organization of, 22, 31, 107-108

Integrated services
  in community context, 352-372
  comprehensiveness, 32, 38-41
  continuity in, 32, 43-44
  coordination in, 32, 41-43, 126
  for mental health care, 303, 304-305,
    357-358
  in primary care definition, 2, 29, 31,
    32, 33, 38-44, 314
  research, 240-241
Interdisciplinary teams, *see* Primary care
  teams
Internal medicine and internists, 19, 20,
  77, 122, 156
  training, 186-187, 192, 194, 199-200, 209
International Classification of Primary
  Care (ICPC), 80, 90, 218
International Classification of Diseases
  (ICD), 79, 90
  and mental disorders, 294, 296
International medical graduates (IMGs),
  149

J

Judgment, *see* Clinical decisionmaking

K

Kaiser Permanente, 107, 320-321
Kellogg, W. K., Foundation, 134, 179,
  196, 222, 352
Korean Americans, 86

L

Latino populations, 195
Life-cycle curriculum, 191
Long-term care, 9, 60, 109, 114, 137-139,
  256

M

Managed care, 2, 18, 21-22, 64, 105-107,
  312, 356
  consolidation in, 22, 108

geographic distribution, 106-107
and information management, 355
and mental health services, 300-301, 302
and public health, 132-133, 134-135, 355
and underserved populations, 111, 118, 119, 127-128, 172-173, 327-328
workforce impacts, 106, 313-327
Market shares, 107, 108
Medicaid, 20, 22, 130, 167-168, 196
cost-of-care studies, 64
managed care arrangements, 22, 106, 127-128, 132
Medical Outcomes Study (MOS), 63, 68
Medical savings accounts (MSAs), 117
Medicare, 20, 22, 64, 116
graduate medical education support, 196, 197-198, 202-203, 259
managed care arrangements, 22, 106, 128
nursing education support, 200
Medicare Current Beneficiary Survey (MCBS), 224
Mental health
comorbidity, 292-293, 295
and insurance reimbursement, 87, 297, 299
prevalence of disorders, 289
relation to physical health, 3, 86-87, 237, 286-288, 299
research, 237, 306
Mental health "carve-outs," 109, 135, 136, 302-303
Mental health services, 9, 109, 135-137, 255-256, 285-308
collaborative care models, 9, 136-137, 304-305, 307
financing of, 87, 135-136, 300-304
parallel systems, 135, 304
research, 306-307
Mexican Americans, 86, 157
Minority groups, 85-86
medical education and training, 157, 169-170
see also Cultural sensitivity; Culture and social norms
Misuse of health services, 47
Mixed practices, 122

N

National Ambulatory Medical Care Survey (NAMCS), 77, 91-92, 97-101, 223
National Board of Medical Examiners (NBME), 185
National Center for Health Statistics (NCHS), 218, 223, 228-229
National Committee for Quality Assurance (NCQA), 139
National Health and Nutrition Examination Survey (NHANES), 223
National Health Interview Survey (NHIS), 91-92, 97-101, 223
National Health Service Corps, 171-172
National Hospital Ambulatory Medical Care (NHAMC) survey, 223
National Institute for Mental Health, 305-306
National Institutes of Health, 126, 221
National Medical Expenditures Survey (NMES), 223-224, 226-227, 228
National Organization of Nurse Practitioner Faculties (NONPF), 192
Native Americans, 157
Navajo, 85
Netherlands Transition Project, 80, 89, 90-91, 93-97
Nonphysician clinicians, *see* Nurse practitioners; Physician assistants
Nurse practitioners (NPs)
certification, 159-160, 316
core competencies, 192-193
education and training, 20, 159, 160-162, 200, 206, 316
in managed care settings, 320-321, 322-323
as physician substitutes, 315, 317-319, 322-323, 332
quality of care, 319-320, 333-334
responsibilities, 110, 162, 316
scope of practice, 10, 173-175, 258, 314-315, 332-333
supply, 160-162, 171, 316
work settings, 162, 316

O

Obstetrics and gynecology, 77, 110, 122, 123, 154, 209
Omnibus Budget Reconciliation Act, 197
Optometry and vision services, 109, 125
Orthopedists, 77
Outcomes of care, 67-70

P

Partnership with patients, 2, 3, 18, 44, 49-50, 53, 56-58, 61-62, 84-86, 329
  in primary care definition, 3, 31-32, 33, 36-37
  research, 241-242
  theoretical bases for, 81-82
Patient education materials, 142
Patient records
  in accountability systems, 48, 57-58
  as research data sources, 48, 57-58, 227
Patient satisfaction, 33, 44, 48-49
  with nonphysician clinicians, 319
Patients, in primary care definition, 31, 33, 34
Pediatrics and pediatricians, 19, 20, 77, 156, 192
  training, 186-187, 199-200
Performance monitoring, 114, 139-141, 256
  measurement, 9, 24, 47-48, 140, 141
Personal health care needs, 18, 53-54
  diagnostic clusters, 53-54, 77-78
  in primary care definition, 3, 31, 33, 37, 40
  research, 239-240
Pew Charitable Trusts, 134, 179, 221
Pew Health Professions Commission, 202, 204, 209
Pharmacy services, 109, 125-126
Physician assistants (PAs), 110, 162-163
  education and training, 20, 163-164, 198, 206, 316
  in managed care settings, 320-321, 322-323
  as physician substitutes, 315, 317-319, 322-323, 332

quality of care, 319-320, 333-334
  scope of practice, 10, 173-175, 258, 314-315, 332-333
  supply, 163-165, 171, 316
  work settings, 164, 316
Physicians
  demand and supply issues, 110, 149-153, 313, 315, 322-323
  education and training, 150, 156-158, 180-187
  geographic distribution, 64, 67, 158
  primary care supply and shortages, 19, 20, 154-158
  principal providers, 28, 41, 42, 123-124
  and public health professionals, 353-354
  retraining, 6, 11, 208-211, 260
  substitution with nonphysicians, 241, 315, 317-319, 322-323, 332, 334
  see also Specialists and specialty care
Pike Street Clinic Project, 303
Practice-based research networks, 12, 230-233, 260
Preferred provider organizations (PPOs), 106
Preventive care, 2, 3, 18, 41, 58-59, 70, 87-88, 132, 134, 192, 345
  actual practice of, 298
  in community context, 35-36, 71, 348-352
Primary care consortium, 7, 12, 141, 250-252, 261
Primary care definition, 1, 2-3, 8, 31-34, 104, 119-120, 252-253, 313
  development of, 29-31
  early definitions, 19, 27-29
Primary care teams, 2, 8, 42, 110, 120-121, 254-255, 313n
  as care coordinators, 55-56, 138
  in managed care, 327-332, 334-335
  training, 11, 203-206, 259-260
Principal physicians, 28, 41n, 42, 123-124
  specialists as, 41, 123-124
Productivity, *see* Efficiency and productivity
Professional societies, 193. *See also under names of individual societies*

Providers, *see* Clinicians
Psychiatry, 305
Public health, 29-30
  linkage to primary care, 9, 30, 60-61,
    88, 109, 131-135, 243-244, 255,
    342-372
  research on, 243-244
Public health nurses, 19
Public Health Service Act
  Title VII funds, 157, 196, 198-200
  Title VIII funds, 200
Puerto Ricans, 157

Q

Quality assessment, 47-48, 242
Quality of care, 3, 66-70
  improvement programs, 107-108, 256
  and nonphysician clinicians, 319-320,
    321-322
  performance measurement, 9, 24, 47-
    48, 140, 141

R

Randomized clinical trials (RCTs), 236-
    237
Referrals, 39, 70
  coordination of, 41, 55, 131-132
  incentives against, 115
  to mental health professionals, 86, 135,
    287, 302-303
Registered nurses (RNs), 158-159, 160
Relationships, *see* Collaborative care;
    Partnership with patients; Primary
    care teams
Requirements for clinicians, *see* Demand
    for clinicians
Research, 6, 216-217
  and clinical trials, 236-237
  on core concepts, 239-244
  data sources, 222-229
  data standards, 12, 233-234, 261, 355-
    356
  lead agency for, 11, 219-222, 260
  on mental health, 237

  on specialty care, 238-239
  see also Practice-based research
    networks
Residency, 5, 11, 186-187, 197
Residency review committees, 186
Resource-Based Relative Value Scale
    (RBVRS), 116, 254
Retraining of physicians, 6, 11, 208-211, 260
Robert Wood Johnson Foundation, 20,
    134, 179, 199, 221
Rural settings, 20, 111, 171-172
  demands on practice in, 129, 298
  managed care in, 106, 111, 127, 129-
    130, 172-173

S

Satisfaction, *see* Patient satisfaction
School outreach, 59-60
Scope of care, 40-41
Scope of practice, 5, 10, 23, 173-175, 258,
    314-315, 332-333
Screening programs, 87, 125
Self-care, 76, 86
Self-declaration, 208, 209
Self-efficacy, 81
Self-referral, 39, 70
Social functioning, 37-38
Social sciences, 3, 81-82
Society, *see* Communities; Culture and
    social norms
Society of Teachers of Family Medicine
    (STFM), 190
Socioeconomic conditions, 71
Southeast Asians, 195
Specialists and specialty care, 12, 13-14,
    24, 68, 106, 123, 153
  accessibility of, 13, 65-66
  clinical decision-making, 83-84
  cost issues, 13, 63-65
  imbalance in supply, 19, 20, 23, 122,
    155-156, 169
  quality issues, 66-70
  research on, 238-239
  role in primary care, 12, 41, 44, 110,
    122-124, 238-239, 261

Special-needs populations, 128-129, 255
State scope of practice laws, 5, 10, 23,
      174-175, 258
Stroke, 295
Substance abuse services, 109, 135
Substitution for physicians, 241, 315, 317-
      319, 322-323, 332, 334
Supply of professionals, *see* Workforce
Surveys, *see under* Data sources

T

Team care, *see* Primary care teams
Technical quality, 47
Technological innovations, 24
Telecommunication, 46, 88
Title VII funds, 157, 196, 198-200
Title VIII funds, 200
Traditional healers, 36, 126
Triage functions, 28, 118

U

Undergraduate medical education, 180-185
      competencies, 183-184
      curricular reforms, 182-183
      examinations, 185
      faculty, 185
      training in primary care settings, 5,
            181-184
Underserved populations, 171-172*n*
      and managed care programs, 111, 118,
            119, 127-128, 172-173, 327-328
      primary care delivery, 4, 8, 111, 126-
            130, 255
Underuse of care, 47, 49
Undifferentiated problems, 40*n*
Uninsured population, 22-23, 65, 66, 104,
      113
      in managed care markets, 107, 128

United States Medical Licensing
      Examination, 185
Universal coverage, 8, 21, 368
      financing, 113-114, 253-254
Unnecessary care, 47
Urban poor, 20, 111, 130, 171-173

V

Value of primary care, 2, 3, 14, 18, 52
      accessibility of services, 65-66
      for clinician-patient partnership, 53,
            56-58
      cost impacts, 63-65
      as guide through health system, 53, 54-
            56
      links with community and family, 53,
            59-61
      for preventive care and health
            promotion, 53, 58-59
      quality issues, 3, 66-70
      as route to appropriate care, 53-54
Vertical integration, 107

W

Workforce, 4-5, 9-10
      and care accessibility, 9, 20, 168, 169
      estimation methods, 165-167
      geographic maldistribution, 10, 171-
            173, 257
      imbalances in supply, 5, 169
      monitoring and data collection, 10,
            170-171, 172, 257
      nonphysician clinicians, 160-162, 171,
            316
      primary care physicians, 19, 20, 154-158
      specialists, 19, 20, 23, 122, 155-156, 169
      see also Education and training

DATE DUE

GAYLORD			PRINTED IN U.S.A.